Pathology Practice Management

Lewis A. Hassell • Michael L. Talbert • Jane Pine Wood
Editors

Pathology Practice Management

A Case-Based Guide

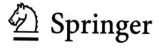 Springer

Editors
Lewis A. Hassell
Department of Pathology
University of Oklahoma Health
Sciences Center
Oklahoma City
Oklahoma
USA

Jane Pine Wood
McDonald Hopkins LLC
Dennis
Massachusetts
USA

Michael L. Talbert
Department of Pathology
University of Oklahoma Health
Sciences Center
Oklahoma City
Oklahoma
USA

ISBN 978-3-319-79439-6   ISBN 978-3-319-22954-6 (eBook)
DOI 10.1007/978-3-319-22954-6

Springer Cham Heidelberg New York Dordrecht London
© Springer International Publishing Switzerland 2016
Softcover re-print of the Hardcover 1st edition 2016

Printed on acid-free paper

Springer International Publishing AG Switzerland is part of Springer Science+Business Media (www.springer.com)

Preface

Most pathologists know almost nothing about practice management when they take their first regular positions. Despite many years of training, they risk financial stability, practice harmony, and professional satisfaction through trusting what may be categorized as a "gut feeling" about a practice opportunity. While some pathologists then learn through the "School of Hard Knocks," others gradually learn practice management through their early years in practice and progressively take control of their professional lives.

Practice management is a broad topic encompassing such diverse areas as billing and contracting, strategic planning, personnel and human resource issues, decision-making, and productivity. There are basic factual components, but the application of the principles of management is situation specific and best honed by experience. To increase the challenges, these factual aspects change as the health-care system changes and as the practice of pathology evolves.

Though highly trained specialist physicians, pathologists typically receive limited useful instruction and experience in practice management during residency and fellowship. Also, for most pathologists, the initial lure of medicine and pathology in particular was not arcane billing rules, the finer points of contracting, or a desire to address personnel issues. However, practice management issues are critical to day-to-day pathology practice, impacting quality, practice success, and professional satisfaction.

This book will provide relatively short didactic overviews of topics and concepts complemented by cases drawn from the experiences of the various authors. The cases are intended to illustrate approaches to common problems, provide a basis for discussion in a training environment or, for the more experienced leader, to stimulate thinking when faced with a particular practice management issue. We learned a lot from each other while assembling the didactics and cases for this book. We hope your experience is the same.

The authors have had a range of experiences as practicing pathologists, attorneys, practice managers, and consultants. We have also taught courses for the College of American Pathologists, United States and Canadian Academy of Pathology, American Society for Clinical Pathology, and American Pathology Foundation, along with other organizations, and feel blessed to have had the opportunities. But our best experiences have come from those with whom we have worked and networked. Our friends and colleagues have been the best teachers and sounding boards. Our thanks to you all.

This publication is designed to provide general background information to readers regarding a wide range of business, legal, financial, and billing topics. The publication provides general information rather than specific business, legal, financial, or billing advice. Because it is necessary to apply business, legal, and accounting and billing rules and principles to specific facts, always consult your professional advisor before using the information in this publication as a basis for a specific action.

M. L. Talbert et al.

Contents

Part III   Contracting

Part IV   Human Resources

Part V   Pathology Group Issues

Part VI   Better Practice Management

Part VII   Managing Risks and Opportunities

Contributors

Dale W. Bratzler Health Administration and Policy, College of Public Health, University of Oklahoma Health Sciences Center, Oklahoma City, OK, USA

Krista Crews ProPath, Dallas, TX, USA

Kimball Fisher The Fisher Group, Portland, OR, USA

Lewis A. Hassell Department of Pathology, University of Oklahoma Health Sciences Center, Oklahoma City, OK, USA

Amelia B. Larsen McDonald Hopkins, LLC, Cleveland, OH, USA

Linda McLean Department of Pathology, University of Oklahoma Health Sciences Center, Oklahoma City, OK, USA

Dennis L. Padget APF Consulting Services, Inc., Laguna Beach, CA, USA
The Villages, FL, USA

Karim E. Sirgi LambdaX3 International, Denver, CO, USA

Michael L. Talbert Department of Pathology, University of Oklahoma Health Sciences Center, Oklahoma City, OK, USA

Jane Pine Wood McDonald Hopkins LLC, Dennis, MA, USA

Part I
Money and the Practice of Pathology

Chapter 1
Health-Care Finance and the Pathology Practice

Michael L. Talbert

Overview

Case: Evaluating an Employment Opportunity

Nine years of training. Four years of medical school, 4 years of anatomic pathology/clinical pathology (AP/CP) residency, and a year of fellowship. US$175,000 of debt. A husband and two young children. You will be the primary breadwinner, and it is time to select the private practice job you have dreamed about for the past several years. You have interviewed with two groups, and both are interested in hiring you. By coincidence, both groups have six pathologists covering two hospitals in midsized cities in the Southeast near your parents. What do you need to know about the groups before a decision? How could such similar practice situations vary? Since you plan to buy a house and put down roots, how do you assess which situation is the most stable? What questions should you ask?

Understanding the fundamentals of practice management can help you understand the merits and potential risks of a practice situation. We will return to a discussion of the above scenario in Chap. 24 at the end of this book.

Many pathologists are drawn to medicine and hopefully pathology by the wonderful complexity of the human body, its range of maladies, and the variety of responses to disease. The pathology practice environment is similarly complex in that no two practice settings are identical, and no two practice environments present the same range of opportunities, threats, and financial milieu. When just looking from the outside of a practice opportunity (such as when evaluating a potential new job), one cannot immediately determine how successful a particular practice might be nor what the future trajectory of that group might be. But with an understanding of the environment, the internal structure and culture of the organization, and the skills and resources of the individuals within the organization, one might be able to reasonably forecast the future in that setting.

M. L. Talbert (✉)
Department of Pathology, University of Oklahoma Health Sciences Center, 940 Stanton L. Young Blvd., BMSB 451, Oklahoma City, OK 73104, USA
e-mail: michael-talbert@ouhsc.edu

© Springer International Publishing Switzerland 2016
L. A. Hassell et al. (eds.), *Pathology Practice Management*,
DOI 10.1007/978-3-319-22954-6_1

Practice Structures

Case: Can I Be a Partner in This Practice?

Dr. Carol Smith, now a fellow in surgical pathology, waited while her call was put through to Dr. Al Wright, her former residency program director. After exchanging greetings, Dr. Smith cut to the chase: "I am looking at joining a local community practice, but they said they don't have partners. I'd like to someday own part of my practice; am I being offered a poor deal?"

Discussion: Opportunities for partnership depend on the structure of a practice. If a practice opportunity involves a freestanding legal entity, such as a professional corporation (independent private practice) or a freestanding laboratory, it is possible to own stock and be a partner. How one obtains such stock may be through a buy-in which can occur at a particular time or be structured over a period of time during which a non-partner works for reduced compensation, or through a combination of the above. For partnership in a practice, the time frame for consideration should be specified in the initial employment agreement with that practice. The advantages of being a partner are potentially threefold: (1) Particularly on matters of great importance, a partner has more say (shares can be voted) than a non-partner; (2) partners typically divide and distribute excess revenues over expenses as bonuses or dividends (depends on legal/tax structure) to avoid having the practice pay taxes on profits; (3) should the practice or laboratory be sold, a partner would be entitled to a portion of the proceeds reflecting his/her share ownership in the entity. As such, partnership opportunity and status can be of great importance.

A partnership opportunity is not available in the typical academic practice since the pathologist is usually an employee of the state, university, or practice plan. Similarly, no partnership opportunity would exist if a pathologist were directly employed by a hospital or large laboratory. Finally, non-partnership tracks exist within some independent private practices. In these cases, the pathologist may have a different workload or schedule, a different pay package, and certainly would not enjoy the advantages of an ownership share of the practice. Non-partnership tracks are often used for part-time pathologists or for pathologists who are not expected to have an extended period of employment.

To simplify things, it can be useful to think about practice structures as being one of four types but with endless variations: academic, independent private practice, employed private practice, and commercial laboratory. Characteristics of an academic practice include the combined missions of clinical service, teaching, and research with the classic example being a university-medical-school-based practice with the majority of faculty physicians operating within some form of practice plan. The faculty could be wrapped into a common organization with the hospital or could be distinct. In the academic scenario, the pathology department may be virtually indistinguishable from the larger organization(s) or may function as an independent business unit with its own income statement and reserves. Most pathology departments operate somewhere between these extremes.

Legal Aspects of Practice Structures

There are many different types of legal entities in which pathologists can practice, all of which are established and governed by state law. Most pathologists in private practice have professional corporations or professional associations, which are corporations that can be owned only by licensed professionals.

Some pathologists practice through general business corporations in states where the use of a professional corporation or association is not mandatory. These corporate entities select either C corporation status or S corporation status from a tax-reporting standpoint, with the distinction between the C and S status being how the entity is taxed. This selection is typically made in consultation with the corporation's accountant.

Increasingly, pathologists in private practice use limited liability companies (or professional limited liability companies, depending upon the state) because these entities provide greater flexibility from a governance and tax standpoint. Occasionally, pathologists have limited liability partnerships, but these are not common. The importance of a corporation, limited liability company, or limited liability partnership is the protection afforded the owners from a liability standpoint. Although a pathologist always retains liability for his or her own actions, an appropriately formed and maintained corporation, limited liability company, or limited liability partnership can shield the pathologist from liabilities of the practice entity as well as the acts or omissions of the other pathologists in the practice. In contrast, partners in a general partnership share liability on a personal level for all acts or omissions of the practice and its pathologists.

The independent private practice represents the classic example of a private practice. The pathologists band together typically in a professional corporation (but there are other structures such as partnerships and limited liability companies), and, among the owners, decision-making is based on an equal-shareholder/partner/member concept or percentage ownership of the various owners. Practices can vary in size and have varying numbers of nonowners on a track to ownership, and possibly even pathologists on a nonownership track. Shareholder/partner/member status is typically done through a buy-in, which may range from token to substantial and which also can take the form of reduced total compensation during a variable number of pre-ownership years. In the independent private practice model, pathology groups typically contract for medical director services with the hospitals or laboratories they serve.

In the employed private practice model, pathologists are employed by a larger entity, typically a hospital or multispecialty group, with a direct reporting relationship up the leadership chain of the larger organization. While this lacks the independence and ownership aspects of an independent practice and is usually a bit less lucrative, being employed by a larger entity can be more stable with a degree of insulation from the significant business risks inherent in independent private practice.

Commercial laboratories range from privately held freestanding laboratories to nationwide behemoths that handle massive numbers of specimens and trade on the New York Stock Exchange. Commercial laboratories may serve the full range of AP/CP testing or may limit themselves to one or a few specialty areas. In these settings, the pathologist may be a salaried employee with productivity targets and limited say or responsibility in the business of the practice, may be independently contracted by the laboratory, or may be part of a group that is contracted by the laboratory.

Practice sizes may vary as well from solo practitioners to groups or departments of 50 or more pathologists. With increasing practice size typically comes greater specialization of pathologists and enhanced ability to capitalize (invest in) improvements in the practice. Larger practices usually can afford and often require more sophisticated management with a nonphysician practice administrator and more sophisticated human resources (HR) and legal support.

Thus, practice environments can be as variable as the practices themselves.

> Key Concept
> Pathology practice models and pathology practices differ in:
> Mission
> Size and scope
> Funding model and incentives
> Security offered
> Culture
> All should be considered in employment decisions.

Overall Financial Considerations

Case: How Do I Get Paid and for What?

Shortly after Dr. Carol Smith took a position with Good Health Hospital, the chief of pathology met with all five pathologists and told them, "Administration says we are operating in the red. If we can't raise revenues or cut expenses, they will need to take action like freezing hiring, denying raises or even cutting salaries by a small amount. What can we do to cut expenses?" By this time, Dr. Smith is having a hard time listening as her head spins with the thought of reduced income in the face of large school loans and a new mortgage. Need to raise revenues? Salary cuts? How can this happen in a country that spends the most per capita on health care?

Discussion: Understanding how pathologists are paid is absolutely key in this time of great change in health care. The following description will detail the various ways that pathologists are paid. Importantly, there are many things pathologists do that are not directly compensated or that may not be compensated at all. These include committee work, tumor boards, waiting for a frozen section, research support, and education. Each of these activities, though, are important for visibility, interaction with other members of the health-care team, and, ultimately, for maintaining a job or the contract to provide services. As health care slowly transitions towards payment for value and outcomes and away from fee-for-service where more services performed = more money, pathologists will increasingly need to show how they are adding value. For example, what value do pathologists add at tumor board? Do they change diagnoses previously made at other institutions? How often do they change or accelerate a patient's treatment based on their interactions at tumor board? Can this be quantitated? Other examples: (1) Can one quantitate the impact of a pathologist-initiated blood utilization program on decreasing immunosuppression, volume overload, and, perhaps most easily, total cost? (2) Can deploying a molecular viral identification test more quickly rule in or rule out viral meningitis and save hospital bed days? (3) Can pathologist-driven personalized medicine testing in colon cancer specimens lead to faster assignment to therapy, less testing when not needed, and better identification of those patients who may benefit from this workup? Can this effect be quantified? These are just a few examples of how pathologists can and do add value and how we will need to clearly demonstrate the value added in the future.

The US health-care system is not a system in the true sense of the word. It is a complicated, sometimes overlapping collection of various providers and payment schemes. Some areas, like the Veterans Administration, are better organized while others, such as individual practitioners and the uninsured population, are less so. Furthermore, as of this writing, there are truly monumental forces at work, some related to the Patient Protection and Affordable Care Act (aka Obamacare) and some driven by other forces.

The scope of the US health system is also debatable. Do we include public health and preventive care? What about health-related products such as Botox? A helpful way to understand how things work relative to practice management issues is to consider, in general, how money comes into a pathology practice. We can then consider changes that are occurring, with their attendant challenges and opportunities.

As we examine where money comes from in the health-care system, we can split pathologists' services into two general categories: (1) diagnostic work for individual patients such as surgical pathology and cytopathology and (2) medical direction such as quality assurance, designing protocols, hospital committee work, and laboratory direction. Diagnostic services for specific individual patients are described and billed using Current Procedural Terminology (CPT, see side bar, page 23) codes, a descriptive system maintained by the American Medical Association. For pathologists' purposes, CPT codes describe AP services and some CP services. For example, CPT code 88305 describes a diagnostic biopsy such as a typical gastrointestinal (GI) biopsy while 88342 describes an immunohistochemical stain. Payment is based on the CPT code submitted for a service and many pathology cases have multiple CPT codes reflecting multiple parts and additional studies such as histochemical or immunohistochemical stains. This is classic fee-for-service where payment is made for a specific service. A practice leader should have a strong working knowledge of the CPT-coding system. If not, there are seminars and online courses on coding in addition to any coding "experts" currently present in your practice.

Payment for Diagnostic Work for Individual Patients

Case: How Much Will I Be Paid for This Diagnosis?

Dr. Mike Taylor put the slide on the stage and quickly confirmed that the tissue was a section of gallbladder with a cross section of the cystic duct. He patiently examined the slide, confirming the typical changes of a chronic obstructive process while carefully excluding dysplasia or carcinoma. Seeing no other unusual features, he depressed the pedal of his digital dictation system and carefully said, "Diagnosis—Gallbladder: Chronic cholecystitis with cholelithiasis." He added billing codes and indicated there were no quality issues. Dr. Taylor then leaned back in his chair and thought aloud, "Wow, I just signed out my first case." Pausing a moment, he next thought, "I wonder how much money we'll collect?"

Discussion: How much a pathologist collects for a particular service varies depending on the service performed and for whom it is performed. In this section, we will discuss how a service is coded for billing purposes, which in turn determines the charge that is assigned; the actual payment is determined by the type or lack of health insurance coverage a patient has. If a patient has typical indemnity insurance, payment will usually be on a contractual basis and reflect a fee schedule set between the insurance company and the pathologist/practice. For patients with Medicaid, Medicare, Tricare, or Champus, the so-called federal payors, the rates are determined and not negotiable (but may vary between programs and geographic location). Patients with no coverage (so-called self-pay) may pay nothing, may pay the full charge, or may pay something in between, sometimes following a brief negotiation with the pathologist's billing office. Practically, most pathologists provide services without knowledge of a patient's health insurance coverage and accept that payments will vary. This is often the most practical approach given that a submitting healthcare provider will typically submit specimens reflecting a range of patient coverages.

For diagnostic work, there are four major payor categories: Medicare, Medicaid, insurance/managed care and other contracts, and the uninsured or self-pay. Medicare merits the greatest discussion because its payment scheme and rates often serve as a model for other payment sources.

Medicare is a federal government program overseen by the Centers for Medicare and Medicaid Services (CMS), which is part of the Department of Health and Human Services. Medicare covers persons 65 and older, persons under 65 with certain disabilities, and those of any age with end-stage renal disease or amyotrophic lateral sclerosis. Medicare has four parts: Part A, which covers hospital inpatients, skilled nursing, home health, and hospice; Part B, which covers physicians' services, outpatient hospital services, and medical equipment; Part C, Medicare Advantage or Medicare Managed Care; and Part D, Medicare prescription benefit. Much of Part A hospital inpatient payments are done using a prospective payment system where a single payment is made to the hospital based on the patient's underlying illness and comorbid conditions, the diagnostic-related group (DRG) payment. For Medicare Part B billing, which covers physician services for specific patients, payment is based on relative value units (RVUs) or the relative resources required to provide a particular service. The original RVU system values were derived from the Harvard Resource-Based Relative Value Scale study, but RVUs can change with time through the addition of new procedures or revaluing of existing RVUs. Once one knows the RVUs or resources assigned to a particular service, such as processing and diagnosis of a skin biopsy, then the payment from Medicare can be calculated by multiplying the RVUs by the current Medicare conversion factor (CF). The Medicare CF is typically set annually based on statute and congressional action. In concept, the payment system is fairly simple (RVU $\times$ CF = payment), but at any time, some aspects are under review or subject to political wrangling. Also, one can probably grasp that most all physicians would be impacted by changes in the CF, while predominately pathologists would be impacted by say, revaluing of RVUs for a frozen section.

Medicare Part B payment has additional complexities of importance to the pathologist. For many AP services, slides and reports must be made, forming the technical component (TC), in addition to the professional diagnostic work performed by the pathologist, the professional component (PC). The two, TC and PC, can be combined into a "Global Fee":

$$\text{Global Fee} = \text{Professional Component} + \text{Technical Component}$$

TC and PC may also be paid separately using a modifier (TC for Technical Component and -26 for Professional Component) appended to the CPT code. In the clinical laboratory, some services have a defined PC, such as: 86077 Blood bank physician services; difficult cross match and/or evaluation of irregular antibody(s), interpretation, and written report.

RVUs are more complex than we have stated so far. In fact, the RVU for the PC is composed of three components: actual physician work, practice expense, and malpractice.

$$RVU (PC) = RVU (Physician\ Work) + RVU (PC\ Practice\ Expense) \\ + RVU (Malpractice)$$

Similarly, TC RVUs are calculated by summing RVU subcomponents for TC practice expense and malpractice:

$$RVU (TC) = RVU (TC\ Practice\ Expense) + RVU (Malpractice)$$

So how might one calculate an individual payment for a service using RVUs? The CMS website provides a fee schedule search function that also yields RVU values (http://cms.gov/apps/physician-fee-schedule/search/search-criteria.aspx).

The CF is also available on the CMS website and as of September 2015 is US $35.9335.

So we can calculate for the 2015 National Average Medicare Physician Fee Schedule:

- 88305 PC = [RVU (Work) + RVU (PC Practice Expense) + RVU (Malpractice)] $\times$ CF = $[0.75 + 0.33 + 0.01] \times$ US$35.9335 = US$39.1675 = $36.17
- 88305 TC = [RVU (TC Practice Expense) + RVU (Malpractice)] $\times$ CF = $[0.94 + 0.01] \times$ US$35.9335 = US$34.1368 = $34.14
- 88305 Global = US$39.1675 + US$34.1368 = US$73.3043 = US$73.30

There is yet another complexity before we actually collect a dime. Geographic Practice Cost Indices (GPCIs) are used to adjust individual RVU components to account for geographic variations in costs to provide services. For example, it is less expensive to run a practice in, say, Oklahoma City than many other places in the country. As such, PC RVUs in Oklahoma City are adjusted downward in 2015 for RVU (practice expense) and RVU (malpractice) by factors of 0.872 and 0.845, respectively.

For the PC

$$RVU (PC) = RVU (physician\ work) (GPCI) \\ + RVU (PC\ practice\ expenses) (GPCI) \\ + RVU (malpractice) (GPCI)$$

2015 Oklahoma Medicare Fee Schedule

$$88305\,PC = [(0.75 \times 1.000) + (0.33 \times 0.872) + (0.01 \times 0.845)] \times US\$35.9335$$
$$= US\$37.59$$

(National Average 88305 PC = US\$39.17)

So, if you provide Part B services, just submit the appropriate and complete CPT codes to Medicare with the proper documentation, and you can calculate the payment you can receive using data from the CMS.gov website.

Key Concept
CPT codes determine payment via linkage to RVUs for both technical and professional component work.

An additional point to be aware of is that Medicare adjusts payments to physicians through its Physician Quality Reporting System (PQRS) which entails specific reporting in select cases that, as a good lab, you are probably already doing coupled with specific codes to report that you did the right thing. We encourage you to look more closely at the PQRS process particularly if you have significant payments coming from Medicare. Initially, there were modest percentage increases in all of an individual's Medicare payments for correctly reporting an appropriate percentage and number of eligible cases. For 2014 and beyond, there are increasing penalties for nonparticipation/non-reporting. For 2015, there are eight measures for pathologists, the five original involving breast cancer resections, colorectal cancer resections, radical prostatectomy cases, biopsies with Barrett's esophagus, and cases with Her-2/Neu immunohistochemical stain reporting, and three new for 2015 measures involving lung cancer and melanoma reporting. Failure to report in 2014 resulted in a 2% penalty applied to *all* Medicare Part B payments to be made in 2016. Participation in 2015 PQRS will impact the 2017 PQRS adjustments and 2017 value-based modifier (CAP Today November 2014).

Medicaid is a joint federal and state program using basic federal benefits but with significant state-to-state variability. Individual state programs set their own payment rate structures that are CPT-code-based but which usually pay less than Medicare. Medicaid is subordinate to Medicare for patients who have both benefits.

Insurance and managed care cover a range of products and payors. Historically, indemnity insurance had limited or no utilization controls, less focus on preventative care, and higher patient premiums than for other types of insurance, corresponding to a higher degree of patient autonomy or choice, and hence utilization. The term managed care covers a range of products and payment systems but typically involves targeted contracting and utilization controls. Payments from insurance and managed care can range from a percentage of billed charges to a negotiated (or take-it-or-leave-it) fee schedule, often some percentage of Medicare payments, to some form of "capitation" in which providers receive a set sum per month for all services provided to a patient or group of patients ("per-member-per-month" agreements). For patients who do not have any insurance or who are self-pay, the individuals are billed, and collections are quite variable from individual to individual. Usually, collections from this subset of patients are relatively limited.

Recent Trends and Changes

More recently, we see a growing call to move away from fee-for-service coupled with a trend to link payment rates to process and outcome measures. There is often a downside possibility for providers as well as upside potential (shared savings). In an attempt to reduce health-care costs, both federal and private insurers are experimenting with bundled payments and accountable care organizations (ACOs). Bundled payments use a larger single payment for either a range of services or a range of providers in an effort to reduce total payments. Providers may thereby be encouraged to reduce services or negotiate among themselves to achieve the savings. ACOs are groups of providers, sometimes including hospitals, that organize to become "accountable" for managing care across a population or chronic disease to encourage providers to better coordinate care in return for potential shared savings. For these new and growing models, it is important for the pathologist to be aware of what is happening in their service area and be proactive where possible by improving care pathways, test utilization, information management, and overall care coordination.

In April 2015, physicians rightly cheered the repeal of the sustainable growth rate (SGR) formula which was designed to limit the growth in Medicare payments to the growth in gross domestic product. Enacted by legislation in 1997, the SGR would have led to dramatic reductions in payments for Medicare services, but the cuts were routinely blocked by Congress with a series of legislative actions that blocked full implementation of SGR such that the indicated cuts in Medicare payments to physicians would have exceeded 20%. In fact, at the time of SGR repeal, a scheduled decrease of 21.2% in physician payments for Medicare patients hung over physicians as a distinct threat. While it is always treacherous to speculate on political wranglings, the SGR "fix" was a challenge because, on the one hand, repeal of the SGR has significant costs in federal dollars over a 10 year period in a time of substantial federal deficits, while on the other hand, a one-time cut in Medicare payments of the magnitude indicated (greater than 20%) would probably have disrupted provision of Medicare services creating access issues for America's seniors and creating undue hardship for some medical practices.

However, while newspapers and the mainstream media reported the SGR repeal and lauded the bipartisan nature of the legislation (Medicare Access and CHIP Reauthorization Act of 2015), there are other aspects of the legislation that are very significant. Put simply, the legislation will attempt to use increasing incentive payments to drive the change away from fee-for-service. The current system of incentives will run as previously designed through 2018, with annual fee payment increases of 0.5% through 2019, and then no payment updates through 2025. Beginning in 2019, a new incentive program, the Merit-Based Incentive Payment System (MIPS), will consolidate the existing programs (PQRS, value-based modifier, and meaningful use of electronic records) into a new 100-point measure with increased payment modifications (positive and negative) based on performance. Alternatively, providers with significant participation in "alternative payment mechanisms" such as ACOs, bundled payment arrangements, and medical homes would see a 5% bonus through 2024 with payment rates increasing faster than traditional fee-for-service in 2026 and beyond.

While much will become clearer through rule-making and actual implementation, the legislation has created drivers of growing strength that will encourage, or pressure, depending on your viewpoint, physicians to pursue the alternative payment mechanisms. Once again, this is a challenge for pathologists and pathology practices to appropriately position themselves in their local environments. As the alternate payment delivery models grow and develop, how do pathologists position themselves to ensure their professional services are appropriately valued?

Payment for Medical Direction

Case: Payment for Medical Direction

Dr. Carol Smith, AP/CP-boarded and now doing a surgical pathology fellowship, was perusing her e-mails and read and then reread the following message: Hello, Dr. Smith. You've been recommended as a possible medical director for our Clinical Laboratory Improvement Amendments (CLIA)-certified toxicology lab. We pay generously and only require one afternoon visit per quarter. Please reply to this e-mail if you would like more details.

Discussion: A pathologist should be paid for medical direction. Medical director work requires expertise and entails risk, and therefore should be compensated. Ideally, compensation should be similar in magnitude to a similar effort invested in signing out AP. A number of ways to establish reasonable compensation will be explored in this book. In this case, a freestanding toxicology lab is looking for a medical director who would have their name on the CLIA certificate and hence be responsible by law for the medically related aspects of the lab. While the e-mail indicates a rather minimal time commitment, any potential medical director would want to be sure enough time was accounted for to fulfill his/her duties (duties are delineated in CMS publication Clinical Laboratory Improvement Amendments (CLIA) *Laboratory Director Responsibilities*, Brochure #7; http://www.cms.gov/Regulations-and-Guidance/Legislation/CLIA/Downloads/brochure7.pdf). As well, ensuring that a laboratory reports accurate test results is an ongoing challenge and depends on having competent, motivated personnel, proper testing platforms, and close adherence to established processes and procedures. Therefore, in evaluating an opportunity such as that described in the e-mail, you must be sure compensation is adequate for the full job while also establishing that a good job can be done in that particular situation.

The second major category of work performed by the pathologists is medical direction. A medical director (such as laboratory medical director or director of surgical pathology) regularly provides professional services and oversight in quality assurance, validation, designing protocols, reviewing procedures, personnel oversight, medical staff issues, and education of physicians. These services are needed for quality health care, are valuable, and should be compensated. Typically, such services are compensated through a negotiated contract with the hospital laboratory, and payment should reflect the effort involved at compensation levels appropriate for practicing pathologists. There are many available educational tools for negotiating a contract for laboratory direction and many approaches. Pathologist effort can be determined by percentage full-time equivalent or on an hourly basis. Payment rates can reflect national norms for pathologists or can be developed using an updated and adjusted reasonable compensation equivalent (RCE) payment amount as described in the Federal Register and periodically updated by CMS. It is critically important to develop ongoing relationships with people such as senior hospital administrators who ultimately would be negotiating this contract with you and educate them over time about how you and your fellow pathologists add value. For example, you might meet weekly with your hospital administration, updating your groups' progress and demonstrating your involvement while always asking for feedback and input on ways to improve your service. A good source of further information on this topic is the Practice Management Resource area of the CAP.org website.

The funds to pay for medical direction come to the hospital from two major sources. Within the Part A, DRG payment to the hospital is a portion that covers pathologist medical direction services, but the actual amount has never been specified for the federally related DRG payments. As such, the pathologist must directly negotiate for that payment and ideally would do so using time or value added as a basis for payment. For non-Medicare/non-Medicaid or Champus/Tricare (i.e., non-federally based payors), the pathologist may either assume the hospital is being paid by the insurance companies and negotiate for additional payments to cover these services or bill the so-named professional component of clinical pathology. For the PC of CP, the pathologist bills the patient/patient's insurance by the test. While some insurers resist paying these bills, the process is described by the American Medical Association and has withstood repeated legal challenges.

Key Concept
Major sources of pathology revenue under government payment system:
Medicare Part A = Medical direction services provided on behalf of Medicare patients generally
Medicare Part B = Services provided to individual, identifiable Medicare beneficiaries

Some practice settings may also have other contractual sources of revenue, such as revenue derived from governmental or industry contracts or grants (e.g., provision of forensic autopsy services, collection, or management of clinical trial samples or other research grants) or revenue related to non-patient care services they may provide, such as review of legal materials, collection of biospecimens, or similar activities. Since these are generally a minor component of pathologist income, they will not be further dealt with in this work.

Beyond this brief overview of money flows through the US health-care system of interest to a pathologist, we encourage you to continue learning about health-care finance, as change is sure to be a constant. In particular, the payment rules, mechanisms, and amounts are rapidly evolving with the implementation of the Patient Protection and Affordable Care Act and the growing tendency of insurance companies, states, and the federal government to evolve their systems in response to an inexorable rise in overall health-care expenditures. Good sources of information are knowledgeable individuals in your own practice or institution, the College of American Pathologists' (CAP) *Statline* publication, online educational programs by a number of providers, and programs at national meetings of organizations such as the American Pathology Foundation (APF), American Society for Clinical Pathology (ASCP), and CAP.

Case: The Stable Practice

Dr. Jack Paris is AP/CP-boarded and recently completed a surgical pathology fellowship. He is currently 2 months into a genitourinary pathology fellowship. Dr. Paris enjoys diagnosing surgical pathology specimens and teaching but believes he would be happy in almost any practice setting that allowed him to see interesting cases. Dr. Paris generally tuned out during management lectures throughout residency and lets his wife worry about bills and investments. Just thinking about these things raises his heart rate and blood pressure. While contemplating what type of practice positions to apply for, Dr. Paris thinks aloud, "What type of practice would be most stable so I wouldn't need to worry about money and business?"

Discussion: Each practice is on its own trajectory with some practices thriving, some just surviving, and others destined to fail or dissolve. Therefore, you must "kick the tires" of any employment opportunity under consideration (see case at the beginning of this chapter). That said, logic suggests that a position in a commercial laboratory, where changing workloads and quarterly business performance will be closely matched with professional staffing, may offer less stability than many other practice settings. Another potentially less stable setting would be an independent private practice that is not dominant in its market. Regional hospital affiliations and mergers will drive changes in pathology providers and create winners and losers. Hospital-employed pathologists are in a middle group for stability as hospitals continue to align, realign, merge, downsize, or simply close. Academic practices would, on average, tend to be the most stable due to their size and multiple missions. For example, it seems almost inconceivable (perhaps we will eat our words) that the only state-based medical school/academic medical center in a state would be allowed to close, although significant pressures and changes would not be unexpected. For the individual academic pathologist who is a low performer, though, the risk will remain high as academic centers continue to respond to resource pressures in their three missions of clinical service, teaching, and research.

Case: How Do I Pay for Myself?

Dr. Cindy George suddenly felt uneasy. The AP/CP-boarded and fellowship-trained medical microbiologist had felt that her first annual evaluation as a faculty member at State University was going well. Her chairman, Dr. Sparks, had been very complimentary about her ability to work with hospital personnel to introduce two major testing platforms in her first 8 months on the job. The residents were suddenly excited about microbiology, and two were even contemplating fellowships in medical microbiology. The chairman of medicine, an infectious disease physician, had commented several times to Dr. Sparks that Dr. George was a great hire. Everything about the evaluation had been going well until Dr. Sparks showed Dr. George the collected Part B PC revenue that had been attributed to her in her first 8 months on the job: US$612.00. "Six hundred and twelve dollars?" A sudden sense of panic seized Dr. George as she thought, "I'm about to get fired."

Discussion: Pathologists are paid in multiple ways for their professional services, and, in the academic setting, teaching and research are paid for (if they are paid for at all) through other mechanisms. For her professional services, Dr. George could be compensated through a medical directorship contract (most likely a component of a larger agreement) representing Part A monies from CMS with or without hospital monies for nonfederally covered patients. If her practice billed the PC of CP, collected money could be attributed to Dr. George's efforts. As well, certain specific Part B services, such as transfusion reaction investigations that Dr. George might perform on call, could provide additional revenue. Money for teaching can be from a variety of sources: state money, hospital money, or a pass-through of Medicare, graduate medical education (GME) money being the most common. Dr. George could also receive research-related money from a component of salary on grants or through contracted research, for example, from a contract with a pharmaceutical firm investigating a new antibiotic. Therefore, one would not expect Dr. George to have significant Part B collections. Her salary would more likely be covered by payments for medical direction, PC of CP billing, teaching, and research.

Case: In Vivo Microscopy

In vivo microscopy (IVM) is a relatively new technology with the potential for pathologist involvement that has matured the furthest as a tool to guide endoscopic identification and biopsy of Barrett's esophagus. One application of IVM allows for endoscopic evaluation of mucosa very much resembling histologic evaluation at low power (optical coherence tomography) and higher power (confocal laser microscopy). This allows for identification of the highest yield areas for biopsy of Barrett's esophagus with or without dysplasia. IVM can also help map lesions for endoscopic mucosal resection. IVM is performed by the endoscopist during upper endoscopy, but, arguably, the best person to interpret these "near-histology" studies would be the pathologist. There is a CPT code for this interpretation that would not be billed by the endoscopist (the procedural code cannot be billed with the IVM interpretive code by the same physician), so a pathologist could bill this code and not directly compete with the endoscopist's coding/billing.

Questions for discussion:

1. For late 2015, the average Medicare global fee for IVM interpretation (CPT 88375) is US$48.15. If this technology is indeed an analog of histology and will continue to find new approaches and the pathologist should be involved, how can you or your practice be involved?
2. Does it make sense for a pathologist to work side by side with the endoscopist during endoscopy for say 20 plus minutes for reporting of a global payment of US$48 and change? (Do you even know where the endoscopy suites that provide such studies are located?)
3. Is there a more efficient way for the pathologist to be involved, either through enhanced information technology or by nonconcurrent IVM interpretation that would occur separate from the endoscopy?
4. Should you think of participation in IVM by your group as a loss leader to gain experience and be a player in the future, or would it be better for your practice to take a "watchful waiting" approach to this technology with the attendant risk that the technology is embraced by other specialties such that pathology involvement at a later time is no longer practical?

Resources

1. *Pathology Service Coding Handbook*, American Pathology Foundation (updated and released to current subscribers each calendar quarter), see at www.apfconnect. org
2. www.cap.org →Practice Management Resources
3. "Your CPT Questions" in *CAP Today*
4. *Statline* available at CAP.org
5. CPT Manuals from AMA (www.amapress.org)
6. AMA CPT Codes and Resources link (www.ama-assn.org)

Chapter 2
Trends Towards Outcomes, Accountable Care, and Value-Based Purchasing

Dale W. Bratzler

Case: A Glimpse into the Future

Dr. Lucy Yu, chair of pathology at Mid-State University Medical Center, felt a sudden sense of fear as she stopped to consider the big picture. As chair of the faculty practice plan's finance committee, which oversaw contracts and finances for the nearly 600-strong group, she had been so focused on the execution of the meeting that she had not fully realized the discussion's potential impact on her department. The committee was meeting with the state's Medicaid Chief Medical Officer (CMO) to discuss a proposal to intensely manage congestive heart failure patients and diabetics with the goal of reducing hospitalizations and ultimately total care expenditures for these chronically ill patients. The CMO promised to fund several case managers and provide IT support with the potential additional gain to the practice of sharing half of any savings over projected expenditures for these patients.

Dr. Yu and the committee were excited at the potential savings but were even more interested in gaining experience with intensive case management for chronically ill patients. But as Dr. Yu reveled in the possibilities, it suddenly occurred to her: but what about pathology? How do we fit in this model?

Discussion: Two related trends are evident in this scenario: (1) the move to manage patients outside the hospital with the goal of keeping them healthy rather than waiting until acute care is needed, (2) delivering less acute care and reducing unnecessary care. Although, in some cases, more intense or frequent testing may facilitate managing patients outside the hospital, both trends otherwise run counter to how most pathologists have positioned their practices. Pathologists have thrived for years by doing testing, and more testing was generally better. While adapting to less testing is relatively straightforward, how to use our expertise to help manage patients at home and to improve the health of populations are areas in which few pathologists have had much experience. As the health-care system continues to move towards maintaining health in addition to mitigating sickness, pathologists must take on new roles. Will we bring our IT expertise to bear and provide seamless reporting across all environments? Can we design testing algorithms that focus on maintaining health? Or will we have a very limited role in the outpatient and even "pre-outpatient" (home) environments?

D. W. Bratzler (✉)
Health Administration and Policy, College of Public Health, University of Oklahoma Health Sciences Center, 801 N.E. 13th St., CHB 128B, Oklahoma City, OK 73104, USA
e-mail: dale-bratzler@ouhsc.edu

© Springer International Publishing Switzerland 2016
L. A. Hassell et al. (eds.), *Pathology Practice Management*,
DOI 10.1007/978-3-319-22954-6_2

Transformation of the US health-care system and payment models was inevitable. In 2013, US health-care spending reached \$2.9 trillion annually, approaching 18% of the gross domestic product. Prior to passage of the Affordable Care Act, it was widely acknowledged that the Medicare Trust fund would enter deficit spending by approximately 2017. At the same time, there was growing consumer recognition that the costs of health insurance and the amount of out-of-pocket co-pays and deductible payments were outpacing rates of wage growth. The ever-increasing expenditures on health care in the USA were not sustainable and reports from the Institute of Medicine (http://resources.iom.edu/widgets/vsrt/healthcare-waste.html) highlighted that up to 30% of health-care spending is wasted on things such as unnecessary clinical services, excessive administrative costs, inefficiently delivered services, prices that are too high, fraud, and missed prevention opportunities.

Besides the rising costs of health care, there was also broad recognition that there were widespread gaps in the quality of health care. Many studies demonstrated significant variations between providers of care on a host of quality metrics including process of care measures and outcome measures. Although the USA has the most expensive health-care system in the world, we rank last on indicators of efficiency, equity, and outcomes as compared to other industrialized nations (http://www.commonwealthfund.org/publications/fund-reports/2014/jun/mirror-mirror). While the USA has developed the best "sick care" system in the world with a focus on high-tech, complex, hospital- and specialty-based care that is very costly, our population is generally not healthy when compared to many other countries.

Another factor driving transformation of the health-care system is rising consumerism. Consumer groups have promoted policies of transparency particularly related to quality and costs of care. These efforts aim to expand choices for patients armed with better information about the quality, patient experience of care, and cost of care, resulting in informed treatment decisions and selection of providers and care systems.

With this background, a number of laws have been passed and implemented over the past decade that have promoted transparency related to health-care quality and have started shifting the way that health care is financed. In 2003, the Medicare Prescription Drug, Improvement, and Modernization Act created the first requirements for collection and public reporting of quality metrics for hospitals. Hospital quality transparency was enhanced in 2005 with implementation of the Deficit Reduction Act of 2005, which expanded the authority of the Secretary of the Department of Health and Human Services to add required public reporting of additional quality measures and increased the penalty for non-reporting. These efforts were not limited to hospitals. Congress authorized the Physician Quality Reporting System (PQRS) through the Tax Relief and Health Care Act of 2006, which provided incentives to physicians who report standardized quality metrics to the Centers for Medicare & Medicaid Services (CMS), and, as with the hospital reporting programs, penalties for failure to report. Similar efforts were implemented for other settings of care such as nursing homes, dialysis units, home health agencies, and cancer centers.

Passage of the Patient Protection and Affordable Care Act in 2010 accelerated transformation of the health-care system with many payment and quality provisions.

In addition to continued incentives for quality reporting and transparency, the act provided for a number of payment provisions to accelerate value-based payment for health-care services. For hospital systems, the law required modification of hospital payment based on quality of care through the Value-Based Purchasing (VBP) Program. For physicians, the act created the Value-Based Payment Modifier (VM) which mandated that by 2017 performance on measures of cost and quality of care is to be included for calculating payments to physicians. The act also provided incentives for physicians to join together to form "Accountable Care Organizations (ACOs)."

With the rapid trend to develop value-based contracting methods, a range of models has been developed to transform health-care payment to a system that rewards high-quality care and value. The models described below represent a progression that is characterized by increasing financial risk assumed by providers and greater need to coordinate across settings of care:

- *Payments for reporting*—widely implemented by CMS for many settings of care, there are incentive payments for reporting quality metrics for public release, and often penalties associated with failure to report the quality metrics. For example, there are hundreds of metrics that physicians can choose from, including measures developed by the College of American Pathologists, to report to CMS as a part of the PQRS program.
- *Incremental fee-for-service payments for value*—the hospital VBP Program and the physician VM exemplify this model. When physicians and hospitals can demonstrate higher quality of care and efficient delivery of service (high "value") through quality measures submitted to CMS or calculated through payment claims by CMS, there are small percentage adjustments to fee-for-service payments. For example, up to 2% of a physician's Medicare payment is at risk under the VM, but for physicians who demonstrate high-quality care at the lowest costs, there are incentive payments available above the typical Current Procedural Terminology (CPT)-based fee-for-service payments.
- *Bundled payments*—under this model, the health-care facility and providers enter into payment arrangements that include financial and performance accountability for episodes of care. Typically, these arrangements include a fixed payment for all services provided to the patient for the specific condition. An episode of care is the set of services required to manage a patient's specific medical condition over a defined period of time. These models typically result in improved coordination of care and reduce unnecessary care. While most of the initial bundled payment demonstrations have focused on discrete surgical procedures such as joint arthroplasty or cardiac surgery, there are multiple demonstrations ongoing for using bundled payments for chronic disease episodes.
- *Accountable Care*—ACOs are groups of doctors, hospitals, and other health-care providers who come together voluntarily to give coordinated high-quality care to their patients. The goal of these organizations is to provide coordinated care to ensure that patients, especially the chronically ill, get the right care at the right time, while avoiding unnecessary duplication of services and preventing

medical errors. There is considerable variation in the contracting models of accountable care that currently exist (Shortell SM, Health Affairs 2010). Tier 1 ACOs (such as the Medicare Shared Savings Program) involve providers receiving fee-for-service payment, but additionally, added incentives are possible, such as shared savings or bonuses, if per patient spending is below some agreed-upon target. Financial risks are increased in Tier 2 ACOs which typically include some mix of payment based on fee-for-service reimbursement, partial capitation, and bundled payments for some conditions. In these arrangements, the potential sharing of savings and bonuses is greater if overall spending for the patients is below the agreed-upon target; however, there is some risk to the ACO if spending is above the target. The greatest financial risk is found in Tier 3 ACOs. These organizations are often reimbursed through full or partial capitation based on the health of a population of patients, in addition to extensive bundled payments for a variety of conditions. There are greater potential rewards to the ACO, such as shared savings and bonuses, if overall spending is below some agreed-upon target; however, there is also increased risk if spending exceeds the target.

Key Concepts
Strategic choices for pathologists are -how to best use expertise when payments are based on value to the patients and organization rather than volumes of patients served, and-how to measurably impact newer measures of outcomes, rather than process.

Another major trend that has been implemented by CMS is the move away from process of care measures to a greater focus on outcomes of care. For hospitals, there has been a dramatic shift away from measures of care process to a variety of outcome measures such as 30-day mortality rates, hospital readmission rates, and infection rates. Not only are there fewer process of care measures that hospitals are required to report, the weighting of the scores for the VBP Program has shifted to emphasize other metrics including outcomes of care, costs of care, and patient experience. Similarly, in the early Medicare demonstrations for ACOs, a variety of outcome measures are used to assess quality performance and outcome measures (such as preventable admissions) are now routinely calculated for physician practices as part of the VM. CMS has increased the emphasis on outcome measures because they directly measure the end result of care, as experienced by the patient. By being more directly tied to results, they are also likely to be more relevant to, and more easily understood and embraced by, patients.

As providers become increasingly accountable for overall patient outcomes and costs of care, it is important for pathologists to understand these various payment arrangements. It is likely that they will impact both the volume of services provided and rates of reimbursement for those services. In January 2015, Secretary Burwell announced that CMS plans to have 90% of all Medicare fee-for-service payments tied to quality or value metrics by 2018 and plans to have 50% of all Medicare payments tied to alternative payment models—primarily ACOs and bundled payment arrangements—by the end of 2018. As noted in Chap. 1, with passage of the Medicare Access and CHIP Reauthorization Act of 2015 (MACRA), which resulted in the repeal of the sustainable growth rate (SGR) formula, beginning in 2019 physicians will either have to have a "substantial portion" of their revenues tied to approved alternate payment models or will be subject to the Merit-Based Incentive Payment System (MIPS), which will hold the practitioner accountable for quality and costs of care. This trend towards value-based contracting is not unique to CMS as an increasing number of private insurance companies are contracting with health systems and providers of care through various alternate payment models. Finally, as private insurers seek to develop value-based contracts, a growing trend is to organize "narrow networks." Narrow networks are health insurance plans that place limits on the doctors and hospitals available to their subscribers. The most restrictive plans will not pay for care received outside of the defined network. The other way for implementation is to charge higher co-payments when patients seek care from providers who are not part of the narrow network. With either implementation, the primary goal is to emphasize high-quality care at the lowest cost.

Case: The Push Toward Outcomes, Bundled Payments and Value-Based Purchasing

The fee-for-service environment in which payments are made on a per-service basis has been successful for pathology practices, other medical practices, and hospitals. The more services that were delivered, the more payments that would be received by the service providers. This was founded on the trust between a patient, society, and the professionals bound by oath to do no harm and deliver care in the best interest of the patient. With the growth of bundled payments, where payments are made for an episode of care and the growing focus of paying for value, where value is defined as better results for the resources invested or similar results for less resources (value = outcomes ÷ cost), health-care experts are predicting a significant transition away from fee-for-service payments. Some experts project a decline in fee-for-service to as low as 30% of payments by the end of the decade. One complication is that these changes will not occur evenly across the country, and some practices will be affected to a much greater extent than others.

1. What changes have you seen in your environment?
2. How have the changes affected your practice?
3. How will the further development of these trends affect your practice?
4. Are there advantageous steps your practice can proactively take?
5. Would it make sense to attempt to drive the changes in your environment perhaps through new models with major insurance companies or large local employers?

Resources
CAP.org website
   Statline available at CAP.org

Chapter 3
Coding and Billing

Dennis L. Padget, Lewis A. Hassell and Michael L. Talbert

CPT® Coding

Case: Simple CPT (Current Procedural Terminology) Coding

A right colectomy specimen consisting of 4 cm of terminal ileum, appendix, and 8 cm of colon with attached mesentery is received with a working diagnosis of colon cancer. The gallbladder is in a separate container. How would you CPT code this case?

Discussion: 88309 and 88304 would be used for the neoplastic colon and gallbladder, respectively. A separate code would not be assigned for the segment of terminal ileum or appendix.

CPT: Physicians' *Current Procedural Terminology* codebook published annually by the American Medical Association (AMA). Each 5-digit numeric code describes a unique physician medical service (e.g., frozen section diagnosis, consultation on referred slides) or laboratory test (e.g., glucose, Papanicolaou test (Pap test)). CPT codes (a.k.a. Healthcare Common Procedure Coding System (HCPCS) level I codes) must be used by physicians and laboratories

D. L. Padget (✉)
APF Consulting Services, Inc., 1540 South Coast Highway, Suite 204,
Laguna Beach, CA 92651, USA
e-mail: DennisPadget@embarqmail.com

L. A. Hassell · M. L. Talbert
Department of Pathology, University of Oklahoma Health Sciences Center, 940 Stanton L. Young Blvd., BMSB 451, Oklahoma City, OK 73104, USA
e-mail: lewis-hassell@ouhsc.edu

M. L. Talbert
e-mail: michael-talbert@ouhsc.edu

© Springer International Publishing Switzerland 2016
L. A. Hassell et al. (eds.), *Pathology Practice Management*,
DOI 10.1007/978-3-319-22954-6_3

when filing claims for payment by insurers and payers in accordance with the Health Insurance Portability and Accountability Act (HIPAA), and insurers and payers must use CPT codes when paying those claims.

CPT refers to (Physicians') *Current Procedural Terminology*. It is a system of 5-digit codes and descriptors used to describe or report medical services by physicians, laboratories, and other health-care professionals and providers (e.g., hospitals). For example, a colonic biopsy is an 88305 level IV surgical pathology gross and microscopic examination.

CPT codes are fundamental to our ability to be paid for our services, and pathologists are responsible for how their cases are coded even if they do not personally assign billing codes case by case. Therefore, all pathologists should have a working knowledge of CPT, and pathologists involved in the financial aspects of a practice should have an even greater knowledge of CPT.

Background

CPT is owned and maintained by the AMA. CPT is overseen by the CPT Editorial Panel, 11 of whom are nominated by the National Medical Specialty Societies, with the remaining members being nominated by the Blue Cross/Blue Shield Association, America's Health Insurance Plans, the Centers for Medicare and Medicaid Services (CMS), the American Hospital Association, and two members of the Health Care Professionals Advisory Committee. CPT was first published in 1966 and is now updated annually. CPT is mandated for reporting Medicare and Medicaid services as well as services to all other patients.

Now we use CPT coding for virtually all surgical pathology and cytopathology services and to describe services in the clinical laboratory. There are three different kinds of CPT codes: CPT I, a 5-digit code (such as 88305) used to report a service or procedure; CPT II, optional codes (composed of four digits followed by a letter) used to collect performance data such as documenting body mass index (BMI; e.g., 3008F BMI documented); and CPT III, a set of temporary codes composed of four digits and a letter used to track new technology and procedures such as 0066T, computed tomographic colonography (i.e., virtual colonoscopy). For the remainder of this discussion, we will use CPT to denote CPT I codes.

The AMA publishes several CPT publications. Every pathologist should have access to *CPT, Standard Edition: Current Procedural Terminology* which is a good resource for day-to-day coding questions. An advanced coding resource would be the American Pathology Foundation's *Pathology Service Coding Handbook,* initially authored and published in 2006 by a contributor to this textbook, Dennis Padget. Over time, you will learn the common codes, and for a pathologist involved in the financial management of a practice, you will have a sense of Medicare, Medicaid, and average insurance payments for the commonly used codes.

Within CPT, there are distinct groups of codes covering evaluation and management, anesthesiology, surgery, radiology (including nuclear medicine and diagnostic ultrasound), pathology and laboratory, and medicine (except anesthesiology).

Similarly, codes are grouped within the pathology and laboratory section of CPT into organ or disease panels, drug testing, therapeutic drug assays, evocative/suppression testing, clinical pathology, consultations, urinalysis, chemistry, molecular diagnostics, immunology, hematology, microbiology, infectious agent detection, anatomic pathology, cytopathology, cytogenetic studies, and surgical pathology.

The most common codes used by pathologists who assign codes (depends on how coding is set up in a practice) are cytopathology (88104–88199) and surgical pathology (88300–88399).

There are also modifiers that can add information or specificity to a code, for example, for 88305-TC, the modifier TC denotes technical component and describes the actual embedding, sectioning and staining of the tissue along with report construction, dissemination, and storage. The modifier -26 denotes the professional component for looking at the slide and rendering a diagnosis. The two components together form the global code such that

88305 (global) = 88305-TC + 88305-26.

The -26 and -TC modifiers are frequently used in pathology because the physician professional and the facility TCs are frequently performed and billed by different parties. For example, a hospital may perform and bill the facility TC for its inpatients and registered outpatients, while its independent contractor pathologists perform and bill the diagnostic (i.e., professional) component. Modifiers -26 and -TC assure that both parties can bill and be paid by government payers and private insurers for their respective contributions to individual patient cases, and at the same time payers and insurers have a way to confirm that they are not paying twice for the same overall diagnostic procedures. Of course, the fact that pathology CPT codes can also be billed as global services (i.e., no modifier -26 or -TC) provides a convenient way for independent laboratories to bill payers, insurers, and patients for specimens from private physician offices, ambulatory surgery centers, and other settings.

Other commonly used modifiers for pathologists are: GC for a service by a teaching physician when a resident actively participates; XS for a separate procedure based on different anatomic site, different specimen, etc.; and XU for a separate procedure based on nonoverlapping services (e.g., flow cytometry vs. immunohistochemistry, IHC). These modifiers are demanded by Medicare and often by private insurers as well. They are intended to add clarity regarding the circumstances in which services are rendered to assure payers that their coverage standards are properly followed. For example:

- It would be contrary to AMA guidance to report both a macroscopic intraoperative exam (CPT code 88329) and a microscopic intraoperative exam of frozen tissue (CPT code 88331) for the same specimen. By adding modifier XS (separate procedure/different specimen) to the 88329 code on the claim (i.e., 88329XS), the pathologist is able to confirm to the insurer that she is not "fragmenting" a single consultative service (i.e., a very serious compliance violation); rather, the addition of the XS modifier tells the insurer that one specimen was examined and reported macroscopically (88329XS) while an entirely separate specimen was examined and reported microscopically using frozen tissue (88331).

- A pathology consultant cannot bill for reexamining a special stain prepared by the referring laboratory and initially diagnosed by the other laboratory's independent contractor pathologist. However, if the pathology consultant deems it medically necessary to order an IHC stain from his lab to complete the consultation on the outside case (e.g., that stain was not part of the material received from the referring institution), he is entitled to separately bill for that additional work. Appending separate procedure/different encounter modifier XE to the 88342 code on the consultant's claim tells the insurer that the charge is separate and distinct, hence, separately payable from the slides prepared at the outside institution. The consultant in this instance would report 88323 for the examination of the material from the referring party, plus 88342XE for the in-house preparation and examination of the IHC stain, to receive proper payment for the entirety of the service.
- A resident microscopically examines a tissue biopsy and jots down her impression of the diagnosis. However, government payers and private insurers will not knowingly pay for the clinical work of residents. If a senior pathologist (i.e., the "teaching" physician) microscopically examines the relevant slides for the tissue biopsy and confirms or changes the tentative diagnosis of the resident prior to the release of the final report, the senior pathologist may then charge for the professional work. She tells the insurer that she personally performed the "critical portion" of the examination—hence, she is entitled to payment—by adding teaching physician modifier -GC to the 88305 CPT code on the claim.

The process for adding or changing a CPT code starts with the submission of a coding change request form which is available on the AMA Web site. This submission is usually done by a physician specialty society but may be made by the CMS. There is a separate coding change request form for pathology and laboratory which asks for information regarding methodology, recommended terminology, and a discussion of why current codes are inadequate. The request is reviewed by AMA staff which, assuming the request has not been evaluated before, forwards the request to the appropriate members of the CPT Advisory Committee which supports the CPT Editorial Panel and is composed predominantly of physicians representing the National Medical Specialty Societies that are present in the AMA House of Delegates. CPT Advisory Committee members comment on the request, and the request is referred to the CPT Editorial Panel. The CPT Editorial Panel meets three times a year and can either add or revise the relevant codes, table a decision, and perhaps request additional information or studies or just reject a request. At this point, successful new codes are referred to the AMA Specialty Relative Value Scale (RVS) Update Committee (known as "The RUC") to assign relative values to the new or modified code which leads us into how codes are linked to payment.

CPT codes are linked to payment through relative value units (RVUs). RVUs are like a common currency between services and specialties based on the resource-based relative value scale (RBRVS) that was designed as a logical payment system in that all services can be related or compared on the basis of units of service or RVUs. For instance, our colon biopsy has a total or global value of 2.04 RVUs. For our 88305 colon biopsy, the global RVU value is a total of the RVU for professional component, the pathologist's portion, and the TC which covers making the slides and reports. The professional component RVU is in turn a composite of RVUs for work, that is, the actual work done, practice expense such as the overhead costs to practice pathology, and malpractice. The TC RVU is likewise a combination of RVUs for direct costs and malpractice. For services to Medicare beneficiaries, payment is determined by multiplying the RVUs of the reported CPT code or codes by the conversion factor which is set by CMS. The conversion factor for the period beginning July 1, 2015 is \$35.9335. For example, the national allowance for CPT code 88305 (e.g., colon biopsy) is calculated as \$35.9335 times 2.04 RVU equals \$73.30 (global service).

Private insurers too are required to accept CPT codes from health-care providers under mandate of the HIPAA. However, at the present time, there are new practice and payment schema being tried, so we will probably, over time, see a diminution of the percentage of physician work compensated on the basis of CPT codes and RVUs (fee for service).

So how does one assign a code or codes to describe the services performed? We will start with surgical pathology and cytopathology since these are the areas in which pathologists will do the most coding and then get an overview of clinical laboratory coding.

First the basic rules: The unit of service is the specimen. Think of what is a separately identifiable surgical specimen. Each specimen will be assigned at least one code. If you have more than one specimen, such as two separately identified colon biopsies, say one from the sigmoid colon and one from the ascending colon, then you code two 88305 codes or, in shorthand parlance, 88305 times 2 or ×2. To further illuminate the separately identifiable concept, it is possible to have, for example, two skin excisions in one container that would be assigned two 88305 codes if there is a clear way to separately identify the excisions. For example, the requisition could state left back and right arm—suture on right arm to denote the two specimens and identify one as from the right arm and the other from the left back. For some complicated specimens, it is possible to code multiple codes. However, there are also specific scenarios where separately labeled specimens must be bundled together so that only one charge is allowed. An example of this is a mastectomy specimen with separately submitted axillary lymph nodes. It looks like two specimens but must be bundled or coded as one code because the 88309 code is used for a mastectomy with regional lymph nodes by definition (Table 3.1).

There are also codes for ancillary studies such as special stains and immunohistochemical stains that might be performed on a surgical pathology specimen which we will learn about later.

Table 3.1 Common specimens that must be coded singly even if received in separate containers (Source: Adapted from CPT-2015, American Medical Association)

	Bundled code	Exceptions
Uterus with fallopian tubes and ovaries	88309 (uterine tumor) or 88307 (nonneoplastic)	Ovary contains possible tumor
Mastectomy with regional lymph nodes	88309	Lymph node is designated as "sentinel" or otherwise indicated by surgeon to need separate attention
Larynx with regional nodes	88309	Surgeon requests evaluation of multiple lymph nodes by level

One of the most active areas of coding for a pathologist will be in surgical pathology. The basic codes range from 88300 gross-only code to the 88309 level VI gross and microscopic examination code which is used for the most complex specimens. We refer you to the CPT coding manuals for what each code covers because in surgical pathology we have a relatively limited number of codes to cover many different kinds of specimens. For instance, any gross-only specimen will be coded 88300. For code 88305, the AMA CPT coding manual provides a long list of covered specimens which is partially shown below. Similar lists exist for 88302, 88304, 88307, and 88309. The lists are fairly comprehensive, but if you cannot find a particular specimen type listed, the AMA instructs that you assign the code based on equivalent physician work; for example, an excisional Loop Electrocautery Excision Procedure (LEEP) cervical specimen with examination of surgical margins is commonly equated to other specimens in CPT category 88307.

For common code 88305:

- Abortion—spontaneous/missed
- Artery, biopsy
- Bone marrow, biopsy
- Bone exostosis
- Brain/meninges, other than for tumor resection
- Breast biopsy, not requiring microscopic evaluation of surgical margins
- Breast, reduction mammoplasty
- Bronchus, biopsy
- Cell block, any source
- Cervix, biopsy
- Colon, biopsy
- Duodenum, biopsy
- +54 others

Let us take a moment for a few examples: Billing for our 88305 colon biopsy example—if you had five separately labeled colon biopsies, you would code 88305×5. If you had three separately labeled colon biopsies, a stomach biopsy, and an esophageal biopsy, once again, the code would be 88305×5 to account for the five separately identified specimens.

Skin Specimens

For skin specimens, the codes are

88300   Surgical pathology, gross examination only
88302   Skin, plastic repair
88304   Skin, cyst/tag/debridement
88305   Skin, other than cyst/tag/debridement/plastic repair

Skin specimens have a limited number of codes. A gross-only skin specimen would be coded 88300, while skin from a plastic repair is 88302. A skin cyst, skin tag, or skin debridement is coded 88304 regardless of the size. All other skin specimens, including complex tissues such as excisions of melanoma and basal cell carcinoma with assessment of margins, fall under 88305, skin other than cyst, tag, debridement, or plastic repair. As such, a 4-mm punch biopsy of skin is an 88305 as would be an 8×4-cm skin excision for basal cell carcinoma with evaluation of the margins. When a portion of skin accompanies another specimen, such as the portion of skin surrounding a mastectomy or a bit of skin encompassing the biopsy tract from a soft tissue sarcoma resection, the skin portion is not usually coded in addition to the primary specimen unless there is some reason to do so. Such reasons may include additional pathology evident to the examining pathologist or specific instructions from the surgeon.

Breast

The codes for breast specimens are

88305   Breast, biopsy, not requiring microscopic evaluation of surgical margins
88305   Breast, reduction mammoplasty
88307   Breast, excision of lesion, requiring microscopic evaluation of surgical margins
88307   Breast, mastectomy—partial/simple
88309   Breast, mastectomy—with regional lymph nodes

We have already alluded to special cases with breast specimens. A reduction mammoplasty would be coded 88305. Of course, if you have separately identifiable bilateral reduction mammoplasties, you would have 88305×2. For a typical breast biopsy not requiring examination of the margins such as a needle biopsy or small incisional biopsy or an excisional discrete lesion such as fibroadenoma where the margin is not important, you would code 88305. For a biopsy where the margin is important, such as an excisional biopsy of an infiltrating carcinoma, 88307 is used since you need to evaluate and report the margins. A partial or simple mastectomy is also coded 88307, while a mastectomy with regional lymph nodes is 88309 even if you receive the axillary lymph nodes in a separate container from the breast tissue.

GYN Specimens

Gynecologic (GYN) specimens are coded using the following codes

88305	Endometrium, curettings/biopsy
88305	Polyp, cervical/endometrial
88305	Ovary, with/without tube, nonneoplastic
88305	Ovary, biopsy/wedge resection
88305	Uterus, with/without tubes and ovaries, for prolapse
88307	Cervix, conization
88307	Ovary, with/without tube, neoplastic
88307	Uterus, with/without tubes and ovaries, other than neoplastic/prolapse
88309	Uterus, with/without tubes and ovaries, neoplastic

For GYN specimens, 88305 is used to code endometrial curettings, biopsies, and polyps. A nonneoplastic ovary with or without its corresponding fallopian tube is also an 88305. For specimens representing a biopsy or wedge resection of an ovary, the code is 88305. A uterus for prolapse is an 88305, and because the description is with or without tubes and ovaries, use only a single 88305 code for a prolapsed uterus with tubes and ovaries. Even though this seems like a lot of tissue compared with an endometrial biopsy, codes are assigned based on average total work and closest match—in short, just follow the rules and code exactly as laid out in the CPT manual.

A cervical conization specimen is coded 88307 as is a neoplastic ovary with or without its corresponding fallopian tube. More work equals a higher code, generally speaking, but this is only true in an aggregate sense and does not apply to work expended on an individual case. Up-coding a particularly challenging nonneoplastic ovary is not allowed. There will be outliers on both ends of the coding spectrum. This is especially true for the 88305 code. If you have a nonneoplastic uterus with or without its adnexa that was not removed for prolapse (such as a specimen for endometriosis), it would be coded 88307. For a neoplastic uterus with or without tubes and ovaries, use the 88309. There is an exception to bundling together using the tubes and ovaries phrase for cases when the surgeon sends an ovary separately because of its own presumed pathology or if the gross findings indicate the ovary requires "separate and individual attention." For example, if the surgeon is doing a total abdominal hysterectomy with bilateral salpingo-oopherectomy (TAH-BSO) for endometrial adenocarcinoma (88309) but sees a 3-cm mass in the left ovary and sends it to you for a frozen section which reveals a hemorrhagic corpus luteum (a nonneoplastic ovary, 88305), one would code 88309 for the neoplastic uterus plus 88305 for the nonneoplastic ovary plus a code for frozen section (FS, 88331) as we will learn later (Fig. 3.1).

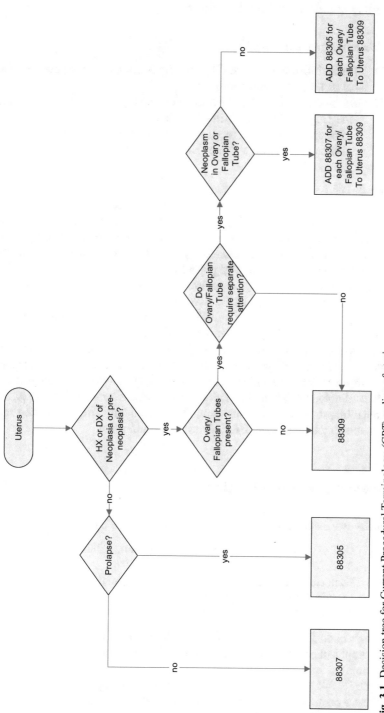

Fig. 3.1 Decision tree for Current Procedural Terminology (*CPT*) coding of uteri

Decalcification and Special Stains

For decalcification and special stains, the codes are

88311   Decalcification procedure (list separately in addition to code(s) for surgical pathology examination)
88312   Special stains including interpretation and report; Group I for microorganisms (e.g., acid fast, methenamine silver), each
88313   …Group II, all other (e.g., iron, trichrome), except stain for microorganisms, stains for enzyme constituents, or immunocytochemistry and immunohistochemistry

If you decalcify a specimen, you can code 88311 in addition to the specimen's other code or codes. It does not matter how many blocks or pieces you decalcify of a specimen; it is just one code. Also make sure you document in your report that you decalcified something. Ultimately, every code you report must be backed up by the surgical pathology report; otherwise, your charges are subject to prospective or retrospective denial by government payers and private insurers alike.

Special stains for microorganisms are coded 88312, while non-microorganism histochemical stains are coded 88313. You are permitted to bill one unit of special stain charge per different stain per different tissue block or preparation. For example, a periodic acid-Schiff (PAS) for fungi and acid fast bacilli (AFB) on two different blocks of a lung resection are reported as four units of 88312, with proper documentation in the pathology report. Medical justification for special stains should appear in your report: Why did you order the stain (i.e., what were you looking for), and what did you learn from it? With a few exceptions here and there (e.g., muscle and renal biopsies), special stains should be ordered only after the routine sections (e.g., hematoxylin and eosin; H&E slides) are examined.

Immunohistochemical Staining

Immunohistochemical staining utilizes the following CPT codes:

88342   IHC or immunocytochemistry, per specimen; initial single antibody stain procedure
88341   Each additional single antibody stain procedure (list separately in addition to code for primary procedure)
88344   Each multiplex antibody stain procedure

(Author's note: The fact that code 88341 follows 88342 in the preceding list is not a typographical error. The codes are out of numerical sequence in the official AMA codebook.)

Codes 88341 and 88342 apply when a pathologist reports an IHC stain using *qualitative* expression. A result is stated in qualitative terms if the report says simply that such and such a stain is positive or negative; for example, "the tissue stains negatively for cytokeratin" is a qualitative result.

Report one unit of 88342 for the initial qualitative single IHC antibody stain per different specimen. Report one unit of 88341 for each additional *unduplicated* single IHC stain (qualitative) documented for the same specimen. Note that, unlike special stain codes 88312 and 88313 discussed earlier in this chapter, the unit of service for IHC stains is the *specimen*, not the *block* or *preparation*. Furthermore, realize that if you are running a battery of several qualitative IHC stains on one specimen, it is totally arbitrary which one you think of as the "initial" stain for code 88342 reporting purposes.

Code 88344 comes into play when two or more separately interpretable antibodies can be simultaneously interrogated on one slide. You will encounter this situation mainly with an IHC multiplex stain such as prostatic intraepithelial neoplasia-4 (PIN-4, prostate) or the breast triple stain, which are single primary stains that come in one vial and require just one application, but they react to three unique antibodies by means of color and/or site (cell nucleus vs. cytoplasm) distinction. Typically, only one multiplex stain is performed per any given specimen.

Not every IHC multi-antibody, dual stain, or triple stain warrants reporting with code 88344. For code 88344 to be reported, the pathologist must be able to tell precisely which of two or three different antibodies is staining positive and which is not. Some IHC multi-antibody stains do not fulfill this requirement, such as AE1/AE3, which stains for two different antibodies, but the pathologist cannot tell whether it is the AE1, the AE3, or both that is/are positive in a given instance. The AMA instructs that an IHC "cocktail" stain be reported as a single-antibody stain (i.e., code 88342 or 88341).

Qualitative IHC is separate and distinct from quantitative/semiquantitative IHC: The former is not part of the latter from either a clinical or a billing perspective. Accordingly, it is never appropriate to report code 88341 or 88342 together with code 88360 or 88361 (see next paragraph) for the same IHC staining procedure on the same specimen. Furthermore, it would not be medically necessary to perform the same IHC stain by both qualitative and quantitative approach on the same specimen.

Two CPT codes are used for reporting quantitative and semiquantitative IHC or immunocytochemistry used to detect antigens in tissue.

88360 Morphometric analysis, tumor IHC (e.g., Her-2/neu, estrogen receptor (ER), progesterone receptor (PR)), quantitative or semiquantitative, per specimen, each single antibody stain procedure; manual
88361 Using computer-assisted technology

Codes 88360 and 88361 apply when a quantitative or semiquantitative result is determined and reported using the IHC staining technique. Quantitative/semiquantitative results are derived by counting the number of positive cells and expressing the outcome as a number, such as a "score" or the percentage of positive cells. A common method of "scoring" Her-2/neu IHC involves counting positive cells to a threshold number like 30%, combined with a subjective assessment of staining intensity:The 0–3+ score is deemed to be a semiquantitative result (*CAP Today*, February 2005). Report code 88361 for the IHC test if the counting is computer assisted, but for manual-counting method, report code 88360.

Pathologists frequently base their interpretation of a semiquantitative IHC stain on a visual approximation of the percentage of positive cells instead of actually counting cells. Practice guidance published by the College of American Pathologists confirms that, as regards the evaluation of IHC stains, the term "semiquantitative" covers a determination made by visual approximation as well as one made by literally counting positive cells (*Protocol for the Examination of Specimens from Patients with Invasive Carcinoma of the Breast,* CAP, October 2009).

The approved unit of service for codes 88360 and 88361 is each different single or multiplex antibody stain procedure per each different *specimen.* For example, a Her-2/neu, ER, PR, and Ki-67 by manual tumor morphometry on bilateral breast biopsies would be reported as 88360×8 (four different stains on each of two different specimens); however, the same four stains on two different blocks of the same specimen would yield just four units of 88360.

Intraoperative Consultation Codes

88329   Pathology consultation during surgery
88331   First tissue block, with frozen section(s), single specimen
88332   Each additional tissue block with frozen section(s)
88333   Cytologic preparation exam, first site, single specimen
88334   Cytologic preparation exam, each additional site, single specimen

For a gross-only type consultation, such as grossly evaluating a margin, the code is 88329. For frozen sections, the first tissue block frozen for any specimen is an 88331; any additional blocks from that specimen are coded 88332. For example, for a skin excision for which you freeze and interpret four blocks to determine the margins, you would code 88331×1 and 88332×3. If the four margins have been submitted separately and separately designated by the surgeon, they would represent four different specimens which would yield total codes of 88331×4. Once again, clear documentation of what was done is critical to ensure payment.

Intraoperative consultation by microscopic examination of a cytologic preparation (e.g., touch preparation or squash preparation) is reported with codes 88333 (first site per specimen) and 88334 (each additional site per specimen). If you examine four margins of a lumpectomy specimen using touch preparation (one slide per margin), you would report that as 88333 for the first margin and 88334 for each additional margin (e.g., 88334×3 for this example). It is completely arbitrary which margin you think of as the "first" margin from a CPT code perspective.

Some specimens, such as a lymph node, do not have margins per se, so two touch preparations examined intraoperatively for such a specimen warrant only one charge (i.e., 88333 alone). However, if two lymph nodes are presented to you as a single specimen for intraoperative examination, that would support an 88333 plus an 88334 coding scenario. Again, your report documentation is critical to correct CPT coding and third-party payer audit support.

You can report frozen section code 88331 and touch preparation code 88334 together for the same specimen in some instances. For example, you might examine the primary lesion in a lumpectomy specimen via frozen section and then separately examine three margins using touch preparation technique. With proper report documentation, you would report that as 88331 for the frozen section intraoperative diagnosis and 88334 × 3 for the cytologic preparation examination of three surgical margins. Never report codes 88331 and 88333 together for the same specimen.

Consultation on Referred Cases

88321   Consultation and report on referred slides prepared elsewhere
88323   Consultation and report on referred material requiring preparation of slides
88325   Consultation, comprehensive, with review of records and specimens, with report on referred material

When performing consultation on outside material, there are three codes to use. These codes do not apply if your physician associate in the group shows you a case. Rather, these codes are used when slides are referred from another institution for expert opinion, second opinion, or diagnosis confirmation (e.g., the patient is being transferred to your institution for advanced care or treatment).

Code 88321 is the most frequently billed code for consultation on outside slide cases received for second opinion or confirmatory review. One unit of charge is billed per each different outside case you receive for a given patient, but code 88321 is not chargeable for separate specimens within any given outside case. For example, if you receive slides for patient Jane Doe labeled by the outside institution as S14-1234 and additional slides for Jane Doe labeled S14-0329, you would report that as two units of 88321 (i.e., two different outside cases); but if S14-0329 had three separate specimens, those you would bundle under the single 88321 unit of service for that case. Code 88321 covers the examination of both routine sections and special stains, including IHC, that were prepared at the outside institution and initially diagnosed by the pathologist at that site; you cannot separately charge for ancillary services (e.g., 88313 or 88342) that were prepared at the outside institution.

You may determine that a special stain or IHC stain not performed at the outside institution is medically indicated to complete your consultation on a case that has been referred to you for expert opinion or second opinion. You order the stain from your lab using a block from the outside institution, and you report the interpretation in the consultation report. The primary consultation code is changed from 88321 to 88323 in this instance. (Code 88323 is substituted for 88321.) Furthermore, you are entitled to separately charge for the special stain or IHC stain that was performed in your lab, so you would add the appropriate CPT code to your claim with the necessary separate procedure modifier appended to it (e.g., 88313XE or 88342XE).

Comprehensive consultation code 88325 is reportable only if significant additional medical documentation is received with an outside case that is outside the norm. That might be a bone X-ray or an oncologist's clinical evaluation of the patient. Needless to say, comprehensive consultations are few and far between.

Your billing office must carefully attend to the patient account in relation to outside consultation charges once you have signed out the case. In particular, the billing people must determine the patient's financial class prior to releasing the claim, and the account may need to be adjusted to remain compliant. Medicare and Tricare limit consultation charges by pathologists to one per beneficiary per date of service, so the billing office may need to write off one or more 88321 units of service prior to releasing the claim to Medicare or Tricare. For example, if Jane Doe used by way of example earlier in this discussion were a Medicare beneficiary, the billing office would have to write off one of the two units of 88321 prior to sending the claim to the Medicare payment contractor.

Non-GYN Cytology

88104   Cytopathology, fluids, washings or brushings, except cervical or vaginal; smears with interpretation

88108   Cytopathology, concentration technique, smears, and interpretation (e.g., Saccomanno technique or cytospin)

88112   Cytopathology, selective cellular enhancement technique with interpretation (e.g., liquid-based slide preparation method), except cervical or vaginal

80305   Cell block, any source

For non-GYN cytology specimens for which direct smears are made and interpreted, 88104 is used. If smears are made after concentration (e.g., centrifugation or concentration technique such as cytospin), use 88108. 88112 is selective cellular enhancement technique with interpretation (e.g., liquid-based slide preparation method), except cervical or vaginal. This is the code used for non-GYN specimens in which a liquid medium such as ThinPrep medium is used. If you make and interpret a cell block, code 88305 is used. If you do additional special stains or immunohistochemical stains, add-on codes are used much like a surgical pathology specimen.

Note that it is not the specimen per se that drives the CPT code; rather, it is how the specimen is prepared that counts. A pleural fluid prepared as direct smears is reported as 88104, but one that is concentrated via cytospin is properly reported with 88108. It is critical to correct CPT coding and third-party payer audit support that your medical report contain unambiguous information about how each non-GYN cytology specimen is prepared: Use terms such as "direct smear," "cytospin," and "liquid based" to assure correct coding.

A cell block (code 88305) is separately chargeable with a cytologic preparation, provided it is adequately documented in both the gross description and the final diagnosis. However, it is never appropriate to report 88108 (concentration) and 88112 (cellular enrichment) together for the same specimen. Furthermore, stains applied to cytology specimens merely to achieve visualization of the cellular material and components on the slide (e.g., Pap stain, Giemsa stain, DiffQuik stain) are never separately chargeable, whether applied singly or in concert with one another.

For a non-GYN cytology specimen obtained using fine-needle aspiration (FNA) technique (see below), refer to CPT code 88173 regardless of how the specimen is prepared for microscopic evaluation. Realize that not all aspirations are "fine-needle" aspirations; for example, aspiration of a breast cyst primarily as a therapeutic measure commonly should not be coded as a "fine-needle" specimen.

Fine-Needle Aspiration

10021 FNA, without imaging guidance
10022 FNA, with imaging guidance
88172 Cytopathology, evaluation of fine-needle aspirate; immediate cytohistologic study to determine adequacy of specimen(s), initial evaluation episode per specimen
88173 Interpretation and report
88177 Additional assessment of specimen adequacy, each additional evaluation episode per specimen

For FNA, we have codes for both FNA performance and interpretation. CPT code 10021 is used for FNA without imaging guidance, while 10022 is used for FNA with imaging guidance. Codes 10021 and 10022 are in the surgery section of the official CPT codebook, but a cardinal rule of the AMA is that a physician may report any code in the codebook to accurately bill for the service he or she has rendered, regardless of where that code may be classified. In other words, the AMA says that the classification of codes by section (e.g., surgery vs. radiology vs. pathology) is merely for reader convenience but is in no way intended to limit a physician's ability to use codes in relation to services actually performed.

A pathologist who performs the FNA surgical procedure (10021 or 10022) is entitled to charge for the service in addition to the interpretation components of the case. The procedure must be appropriately documented in the patient's medical record and disclosed apart from the diagnostic work on the material generated by the procedure. The pathologist might document the surgical procedure in an "op note" separate from the cytopathology report, but that is not the recommended approach. Instead, it is best to include the procedure note as a separate section of the cytopathology report. Third-party payer auditors commonly do not think to look beyond the pathology report for evidence of the pathologist's work, so including the procedure note there will avoid possible challenge.

Immediate study (i.e., intraoperative) work to determine specimen adequacy for diagnosis is separately reportable using CPT codes 88172 and 88177. The unit of service is each different evaluation episode per each different specimen (i.e., anatomic site or lesion). Report code 88172 for the initial evaluation episode per specimen and add code 88177 for each additional evaluation episode for the same specimen.

An evaluation episode is not the same thing as a "pass," although they may be one and the same for a given episode. A new evaluation episode starts the moment the pathologist tells the clinician or radiologist that additional material is required, and the clinician or radiologist accordingly "sticks" the patient again. The pathologist's determination might have been made based on the examination of material from a single pass, or perhaps two or three passes were ready for examination by the pathologist when she entered the radiology suite.

It is imperative that cytopathologists properly and completely document their immediate study work to permit correct CPT code and units of service determination as well as third-party payer audit support for that work. Here is how it should be done.

Intraoperative Consultation

> Fine-needle aspirate, thyroid (lesion at one site):
> Evaluation episode #1:
> Pass #1: no epithelial cells identified
> Pass #2: no epithelial cells identified
> Evaluation episode #2:
> Pass #3: no epithelial cells identified
> Evaluation episode #3:
> Pass #4: no epithelial cells identified
>
> Pass #5: diagnostic material obtained
> The adequacy evaluation results were reported to Dr. Radiologist during the procedure at 1430 h (FNA episode #1), 1445 h (FNA episode #2), and 1500 h (FNA episode #3) on 1 May 2015.
> Immediate study performed by Jim Pathologist, MD.

The sample intraoperative consult report section above readily and unequivocally supports CPT code 88172 for the initial evaluation episode on the single-site thyroid lesion, plus two units of CPT code 88177 for additional evaluation episodes #2 and #3.

For FNA interpretation, there is code 88173 for the final interpretation and report. This covers all the various preparations that were made and interpreted, except for a cell block, which may be separately charged using CPT code 88305, with proper documentation in the report. Code 88173 is reportable per *specimen,* which basically covers all material from a single anatomic site or lesion. The material from three passes at a nodule in the upper pole of the patient's right thyroid is reportable as a single unit of 88173, but the material from separate nodules (e.g., upper and lower poles) in the patient's right thyroid would be reportable as 88173 × 2, assuming separate diagnosis lines appear in the final cytopathology report. The same caveats should be observed if a core biopsy is obtained in conjunction with the FNA procedure. The core may be billed separately (usually as an 88305 but for some organs as an 88307), and a cytologic touch preparation to determine adequacy may be done and billed. Proper attention to the documentation is critical, however, to being paid for these services.

Flow Cytometry

88184   Flow cytometry, cell surface, cytoplasmic, or nuclear marker, TC only; first marker
88185   Each additional marker (list separately in addition to code for first marker)

The CPT codebook provides separate codes for the facility technical and the physician professional components of flow cytometry immunophenotyping procedures. The codes shown above are only for the facility technical work. The hospital or lab reports code 88184 for the first marker in a panel plus as many units of 88185 as are needed to account for each additional *unduplicated* marker in the panel. Realize that which marker is deemed to be the "first" marker in a panel is totally arbitrary. Each marker must be identified in the laboratory report to support the charges.

One of three CPT codes is reported by the pathologist for the interpretation and report on a flow cytometry panel. Select from the following three codes, based on the number of total markers that were considered in the interpretation:

88187 if there are 2–8 markers
88188 for interpretation of cases with 9–15 markers
88189 for interpretation of cases with 16 or more markers

So, for example, working up a suspected lymphoma with ten markers would be coded 88184 for the first marker, TC, 88185 × 9 for the additional nine markers of the TC, and 88188 for the interpretation. Note that the professional codes are not added together for the same panel; for example, interpreting a panel of 24 markers is reported as one unit of 88189, not as one of 88189 plus one of 88187.

In Vivo Microscopy

The relatively new field of in vivo microscopy (IVM) has a small set of CPT codes.

For 2015, CPT code 88375 is used for interpretation reporting either real time or after the procedure for optical endomicroscopic imaging on a per procedure basis. Fortunately, since the gastroenterologist has specific codes for upper gastrointestinal (GI) procedures involving in vivo microscopy and the 88375 code cannot be reported by the same physician who codes for the endoscopy with endomicroscopy, the 88375 code is, for practical purposes, for the use of pathologists. There are also category III codes which would typically not be paid on a national basis for IVM performed on breast specimens, namely code 0351T for real-time interpretation of optical coherence tomography on excised breast or axillary lymph node tissue if performed real time and 0352T if performed non-real time. Use code 0353T for optical coherence tomography of a breast cavity intraoperatively and 0354T if performed in a non-intraoperative basis. It will be interesting to see how the IVM field develops and how pathologists will be involved in this new technology.

Clinical Pathology Services

Medicare and other government payers and private insurers recognize a limited number of clinical pathology interpretive and consultative services billed by pathologists for hospital patients as well as nonhospital patients (e.g., ambulatory surgery center). The services are divided into three broad classes, and each class is subject to its own coverage requirements.

Clinical lab test interpretation services are payable to pathologists in relation to a specific list of tests consisting mainly of hemoglobin electrophoresis (83020), protein electrophoresis (84165 and 84166), molecular diagnostics (G0452 for Medicare and Tricare), immunofixation (86334 and 86335), and crystal examination (89060). The patient's attending physician must request the interpretation of such a test by a pathologist, but the request may be accomplished via standing order of a hospital's medical staff. A concise interpretation by the pathologist must be posted to the patient's medical record for each test, and it must demonstrate the exercise of medical judgment and be signed and dated by the responsible pathologist. CPT professional component modifier -26 must be appended to the applicable CPT code on the claim filed on behalf of the pathologist.

Pathologist interpretation of abnormal peripheral blood smears and intervention for clinical input purposes related to certain physician blood bank services are also paid by Medicare and private insurers. A request by the patient's attending physician is usually not necessary to support the pathologist's professional charge. However, a concise interpretation must be posted to the patient's medical record by the pathologist, must be signed and dated, and generally must demonstrate some abnormality. The CPT codes associated with these services are 85060 (abnormal peripheral blood smear), 86077 (irregular antibodies), 86078 (transfusion reaction), and 86079 (authorization for deviation from standard blood banking procedure). These codes are *not* billed with professional component modifier -26 under normal circumstances.

The third category of clinical pathology services is clinical pathology consultations. CPT code 80500 applies to *limited* clinical pathology consultations, while code 80502 covers *comprehensive* clinical pathology consultations. (The latter code requires that the pathologist consider relevant patient history, other clinical findings, and material in the record beyond that available in the laboratory system alone.) The patient's attending physician must request the clinical consultation by the pathologist event by event; codes 80500 and 80502 cannot be supported by a standing order. An appropriate consultation report by the pathologist must be posted to the patient's medical record, it must be signed and dated by the pathologist, and it must demonstrate the exercise of medical judgment by the responsible pathologist. In general, the test result that is the focus of the pathologist's consultation must be abnormal. Medicare, other government payers, and private insurers generally view 80500 and 80502 charges by pathologists with a healthy degree of skepticism, but they nonetheless are payable if all the requisite conditions are fulfilled.

Clinical pathology consultative and interpretive services are subject to unique—and often illogical—coverage rules, depending on the particular payer. For example, Medicare permits billing abnormal peripheral blood smear interpretation code 85060 only if the patient was an inpatient of a hospital at the time the blood was drawn. It is best that you consult with your billing and compliance advisor before starting to charge for your clinical pathology services to ensure that all the prerequisites are fully in place.

> *ICD:* International Classification of Diseases, maintained and published by the World Health Organization (WHO). The clinical modification (CM) version of ICD is maintained by the Department of Health & Human Services (DHHS) Centers for Disease Control and the CMS. ICD CM codes describe unique medical conditions and ailments (e.g., basal cell carcinoma of the skin). The CM version of ICD must be used by physicians and laboratories when filing claims for payment by insurers and payers to comply with HIPAA, and insurers and payers must use ICD CM codes when paying those claims. The 10th edition of the ICD CM codebook (ICD-10-CM) was to be adopted by physicians, laboratories, payers, and insurers effective October 1, 2015.

ICD Coding

The *International Classification of Diseases* (commonly known by the acronym ICD) is maintained and published by the WHO. It is a taxonomy for use by researchers, public health officials, and others for uniformly describing, classifying, and tabulating data related to diseases, injuries, and causes of death. The 10th revision of ICD is currently in use around the world, with the 11th revision due for publication in mid-2017 per latest WHO projection.

The *Clinical Modification* version of ICD is what is used in the USA for purposes of claim filing by health-care providers and payment by government payers and private insurers. That version in the USA is maintained and published jointly by the Centers for Disease Control & Prevention and the CMS, both of which are part of the federal DHHS. The secretary of DHHS has directed that all health-care providers adopt ICD-10-CM for claim-filing purposes effective no later than October 1, 2015.

HCPCS: Healthcare Common Procedure Coding System, maintained and published by the DHHS CMS. HCPCS-I codes and CPT codes are one and the same. The 5-digit alphanumeric HCPCS-II (level II) codes describe pharmaceuticals, blood products, medical supplies and appliances, and other items not contained in the CPT codebook; they also describe some physician services in a way not compatible with the CPT codebook when necessary to fulfill Medicare policy. Physicians and laboratories must use HCPCS-II codes when filing claims for payment under Medicare Part B when mandated by program policy.

ICD is one of two national code sets that are mandated for use by health-care providers and payers (including private insurers) in the USA under authority of the HIPAA. The HCPCS, of which the AMA's *CPT* taxonomy is a major part, is mandated for use in describing individual medical services and procedures (e.g., frozen section, gross and microscopic tissue examination, IHC stain) via 5-digit codes. The ICD-10-CM taxonomy is mandated (effective October 1, 2015) for use in describing the clinical rationale for the medical services and procedures that were rendered on behalf of individual patients.

A pathologist's claim for a professional service rendered on behalf of an individual patient, whether it is billed with modifier -26 separate from the TC or as part of a global charge (combined professional and TC), must be supported by the applicable HCPCS/CPT procedure code as explained earlier in this chapter, plus at least one ICD diagnosis code that supports the medical necessity of the service. A claim missing one of those two codes—or a claim with an invalid HCPCS/CPT or ICD code—will be summarily rejected by the government payer or private insurer.

Federal law requires referring physicians to furnish the reason why a specimen is being sent to pathology for diagnostic examination. It also requires pathologists and laboratories to report the ICD code(s) on the claim for physician professional or global service that describes the outcome of the diagnostic examination. If a definitive pathologic diagnosis is available at the time your claim is filed, you are to report on your claim the ICD-10-CM code associated with that diagnosis as the reason for the examination. However, if a definitive pathologic diagnosis is not available (e.g., normal colonic mucosa), you are to report on your claim the ICD-10-CM code representing the reason the biopsy or polyp was sent to you for diagnostic evaluation, as that information was given to you by the referring physician.

The process for determining the principal diagnosis code associated with each patient case you work on is relatively straightforward, at least for many patients. Let us assume you receive a right middle lobe lobectomy diagnosed with adenocarcinoma and a separate brushing specimen from the left upper lobe diagnosed with "no malignancy seen." Start by looking in the ICD-10-CM Index under "Adenocarcinoma." The general reference says to "see also Neoplasm, malignant, by site," and you also notice listings for "alveolar" and "bronchiolar," both of which direct you to "see Neoplasm, lung, malignant."

Following the index instruction, you turn to the Neoplasm table and run your finger through the body site and organ listings until you reach "lung." You continue looking under "lung" until you reach "middle lobe," at which point you move your finger horizontally to the column headed "Malignant Primary." The code in that column is C34.2 which you jot down in preparation for the final step.

Now you go to the tabular list in the ICD-10-CM codebook. Flip through the pages until you find code C34.2. The descriptor for that code is "Malignant neoplasm of middle lobe, bronchus or lung," so you know you have got exactly the right code for the organ and diagnosis at hand. That is the code you post to the coding sheet to alert the billing office to enter that in the patient record for claim filing purposes.

(Out of curiosity, note that, had the specimen been the lower lobe, you would have had to select from C34.31 for right vs. C34.32 for left.)

What about the bronchial brushing for this patient? Your billing office will know to attribute the adenocarcinoma diagnosis (C34.2) to it (e.g., CPT code 88104) as well as the lobectomy (CPT code 88309) specimen on the claim. You diagnosed the patient with lung cancer, so it is not all that relevant that the patient went to the doctor complaining of a persistent cough. Looking up a code for the brushing specimen would be a waste of time, and it is not required in any event—our obligation is to report what is wrong with the *patient* (i.e., lung cancer), not what is going on with each individual specimen.

Assigning ICD codes to cases can be much more time consuming than determining HCPCS/CPT procedure codes, so the diagnosis coding function is frequently delegated to professional coders in the business office. Crib sheets can be very helpful from an efficiency standpoint, whether the actual coding function is performed by professional coders, the pathologists, or some combination of the two. Here is one sample crib sheet for cervical cases:

#carcinoma in situ [D06.x] (x=0 endocervix; 1 exocervix; 7 other parts; 9 unspecified)

#malignant neoplasms [C53.x] (x=0 endocervix; 1 exocervix; 8 overlapping; 9 unspecified)

Adenocarcinoma (C53.x @ #malignant neoplasms)

Adenomatous polyp (D28.7)

Cervical intraepithelial neoplasia [CIN] I (N87.0)

Cervical intraepithelial neoplasia [CIN] II (N87.1)

Cervical intraepithelial neoplasia [CIN] III (D06.x @ #carcinoma in situ)

Cervicitis, acute/chronic/unspecified (N72)
Cervicitis, follicular (N72)
Cyst (N88.8)
Dysplasia, mild (N87.0)
Dysplasia, moderate (N87.1)
Dysplasia, severe (D06.x @ #carcinoma in situ)
Endocervical polyp x/adenomatous (N84.1)
Endocervicitis, acute/chronic/unspecified (N72)
Exocervicitis, acute/chronic/unspecified (N72)
Hyperplasia, mild (N87.0)
Hyperplasia, moderate (N87.1)
Polyp x/adenomatous (N84.1)
Postmenopausal bleeding (N95.0)

Here is another sample crib sheet for skin specimens not diagnosed with a nevus or neoplasm:

Actinic keratosis (L57.0)
Cicatrix (L90.5)
Colloid milium (L57.8)
Cyst, skin, NOS (L72.9)
Dermatitis NOS (L30.9)
Epidermal cyst (L72.0)
Epidermal inclusion cyst (L72.0)
Epidermoid inclusion cyst (L72.0)
Fibrosis NOS (L90.5)
Follicular cyst (L72.8)
Hyperkeratosis (L85.8)
Irritated (inflamed) seborrheic keratosis (L82.0)
Juvenile lentigo (L81.4)
Keloid scar (L91.0)
Lentigo (L81.4)
Milium (L72.0)
Morphea (L94.0)
Pilar cyst (L72.11)
Rosacea NOS (L71.9)
Scar (except keloid; L90.5)
Scleroderma, localized (L94.0)
Sebaceous cyst (L72.3)
Seborrheic keratosis NOS (L82.1)

Obviously, ICD diagnosis coding requires diligence and care, just as does HCPCS/CPT procedure coding. The key for any given pathologist professional practice or laboratory is to determine the most cost-effective way to accomplish that ongoing task: (a) manual and/or crib sheet coding by professional coders, (b) crib sheet coding by the pathologists, (c) outside vendor automated coding, or (d) some combination. There is no "one size fits all" solution.

CPT Coding Exercises—Simple Cases

Case

A colonoscopy specimen consisting of five bottles labeled right colon, transverse colon, left, sigmoid, and rectum, each containing multiple tissue fragments.

  88305×5

Case

Cervical biopsies in four bottles labeled 3 o'clock, 6 o'clock, 9 o'clock, and 12 o'clock.

  88305×4

Case

Two skin biopsies in one container. One biopsy has a black suture. Requisition says right back and left arm; suture on left arm.

  88305×2

Case

A right thyroid lobectomy is received for frozen section. Frozen section reveals follicular variant of papillary carcinoma in the single frozen section block that is made. Later that day, the left thyroid is received in a jar labeled left thyroid.

  88307×2 and 88331 (for frozen section, FS)

Case (see Fig. 3.2)

A prostatocystectomy with unilateral 10-cm length of ureter for urothelial carcinoma, plus the bilateral pelvic lymph nodes. On microscopic exam prostatic adenocarcinoma is also identified.

  88309×2, 88307×3

Case

Your otorhinolaryngology (ORL) surgeon sends you six separate margins from a tongue surgery. You do frozen sections (six blocks) and report that while five margins are negative, #3 has at least high-grade dysplasia. Two additional pieces labeled 7 and 8 are received. You freeze these (single block each) and report that both are negative for carcinoma or significant dysplasia. The eight frozen blocks are forwarded to histology for permanent section processing. Three hours later you receive a hemiglossectomy specimen and a right radical neck dissection specimen consisting of adipose tissue from which you recover six lymph nodes.

  88331×8, 88305×8, 88309×1, 88307×1

Case

The orthopedic surgeon sends you a resection of a bulky intramuscular myxoid neoplasm with several margins marked. Additionally he sends two soft-tissue biopsies of additional lesions detected at the time of surgery. One is just synovitis, but the other appears to be a potential second neoplasm. (See Fig. 3.3).

  88307, 88305×2

Case

You receive the following specimens. No frozen section requested (see Figs. 3.4 and 3.5):

  Part 1: Larynx with lymph nodes
  Part 2: Right radical neck dissection
  Part 3: Anterior lymph nodes
  88307×2, 88309

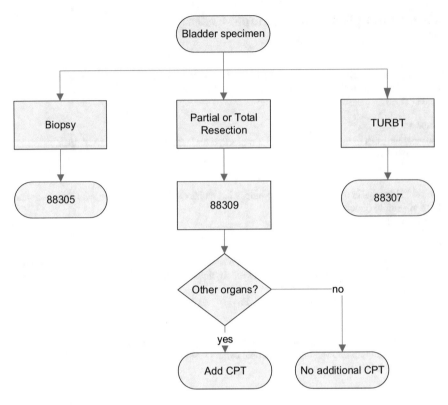

Fig. 3.2 Decision tree for handling bladder specimens. CPT Current Procedural Terminology, TURBT transurethral resection of bladder tumor

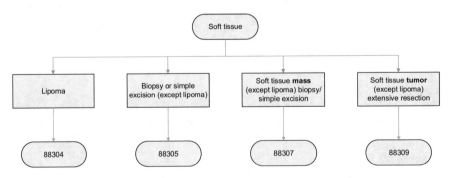

Fig. 3.3 Decision tree for soft tissue

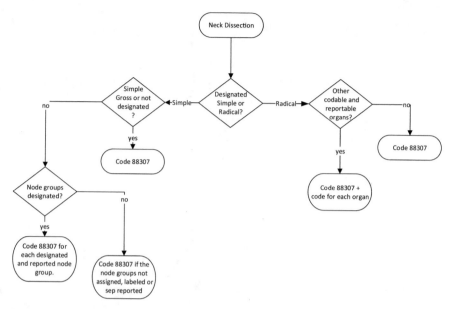

Fig. 3.4 Decision tree for neck dissection coding

Case

You receive the following:

Part 1: Left upper outer breast excisional biopsy; the diagnosis is fibroadenoma; the margins are negative.

Part 2: Left lower breast excisional biopsy; the diagnosis is infiltrating ductal carcinoma, the margins are negative.

88307, 88305

Case

You receive the three guided needle core biopsies of left breast. Each is separately designated as to location as left upper-outer (LUO), 9 o'clock, and 6 o'clock. LUO shows a complex sclerosing lesion with atypical features involving the entire specimen, and you suggest consideration of excision to further classify the abnormality. Nine o'clock shows fibrocystic change with focal calcification. Six o'clock shows ductal carcinoma in situ with extension to the margin of the biopsy.

88305 × 3 (three biopsies without the need to assess margins)

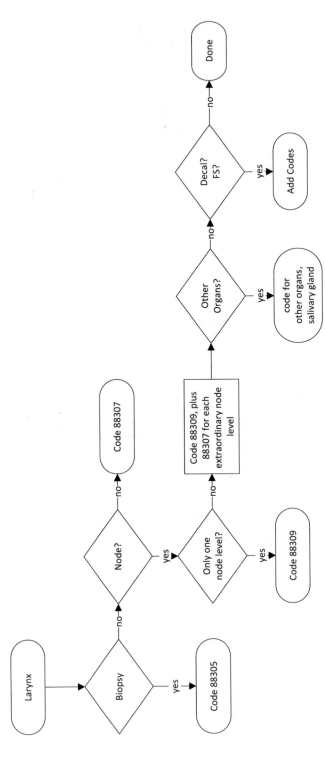

Fig. 3.5 Decision tree for laryngectomy

More Complex CPT Coding Cases

Case: FNA with IHC

You attend an interventional FNA on a deep mass in the retroperitoneal soft tissue. The radiologist performs two passes which the tech stains prior to your arrival. The first one is nondiagnostic, but the second one contains features that suggest a soft tissue neoplasm. You recognize it will need IHC, cytogenetic study, and possibly molecular analyses to nail down, so you suggest that a core biopsy sample would be very useful if possible. The radiologist complies with your suggestion and offers you two separately identified core biopsies. Touch preparations are performed on each one of these, and they are deemed to contain tumor suited for your IHC needs, etc. For sign-out, the following are reviewed: direct smears and a cell block from the FNA. Core biopsy sample H&E plus five IHC stains nonquantitative, plus a semiquantitative Ki-67 stain.

What CPT codes should be assigned to the pathology services associated with this case?

Case: Extensive Head and Neck Resection

You receive a composite Commando and oral resection that includes the left tongue, floor of mouth, mandible and portion of hard palate, maxilla, maxillary sinus and retromolar trigone, plus a left neck dissection including salivary gland, levels I–III lymph nodes, all separately designated. You take decalcified sections through the mandible and maxilla and separately report the tumor status for each of the three nodal groups. In addition, you receive four key margins for frozen section, each one block. The tumor ends up being a routine floor of mouth squamous cell, but it invades the bone of the mandible. In addition, there is a second tumor on the hard palate that does not involve the bone and areas of mucosal dysplasia elsewhere that do not involve the margins.

What CPT code or codes should be given this specimen?

Case: Whipple Procedure

You receive a Whipple procedure specimen which was performed for a tumor in the head of the pancreas. The specimen also includes common bile duct and a 10-cm segment of duodenum. The gallbladder is in a separate small container. You find 12 lymph nodes in the peripancreatic tissues. A frozen section of the pancreatic margin was requested at the time of surgery, which you did, but it required three blocks.

What CPT codes should be given this specimen (see Fig. 3.6)?

Case: Breast Lumpectomy

A breast lumpectomy specimen is received which has a close margin on gross intraoperative consult. The surgeon submits another specimen with oriented margins after your report. A sentinel lymph node is submitted for evaluation, but no frozen section is done. Three H and E levels on each of three blocks are done, with a pan-keratin IHC stain on each block as well.

What CPT codes should be given this specimen?

Case: Endoscopic Surgery

The gastroenterologist has provided you with several specimens during his endoscopic intervention on a 56-year-old with a history of esophageal dysplasia and a recently noted positron emission tomography (PET)-avid mass abutting the wall of the stomach. He biopsies two areas. He also does an endoscopic mucosal resection of an area of the esophagus with a nodule in the mucosa. He performs an ultrasound-guided needle aspiration of two different sites, one a mediastinal level 7 node, and you do an adequacy evaluation after the second pass which leads him to have you evaluate passes 3–4, which you indicate have an adequate lymphoid sample. He then turns to the perigastric mass and provides you with a needle aspirate for rapid assessment. You deem it nondiagnostic, and he gives you two more which are also acellular.

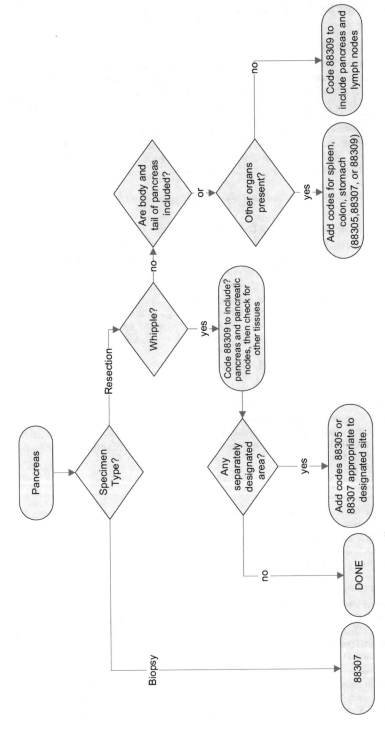

Fig. 3.6 Decision tree for pancreas coding

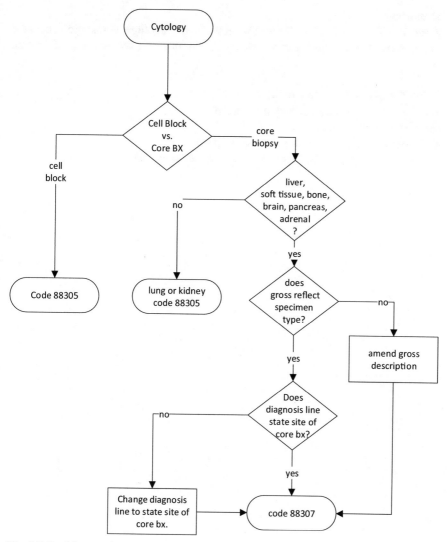

Fig. 3.7 Decision tree for cytology cell block and core biopsy (BX or bx) samples

He then opts to do a core needle biopsy of this and asks for a touch prep assessment which you do. You process these samples and provide him a comprehensive report of low-grade dysplasia in the two biopsies of esophagus and high-grade dysplasia not involving the margins in the mucosal resection sample. The perigastric soft tissue FNA smears are not diagnostic, but the core biopsy samples show a GI stromal tumor which you confirm using four immunohisto-chemical stains.

How should this scenario be coded (see Fig. 3.7)?

Resources

Pathology Service Coding Handbook, American Pathology Foundation (updated and released to current subscribers each calendar quarter), see at www.apfconnect.org.

"Your CPT Questions" in *CAP Today*
www.cap.org CPT Coding Resource Center
Statline available at CAP.org
CPT Manuals from AMA (www.amapress.org)
AMA CPT Codes and Resources link (www.ama-assn.org)

Chapter 4
Revenue Cycle Management

Dennis L. Padget

Overview

Revenue cycle management is the process by which health-care providers capture charges for services to individual patients, express those charges on insurance claims according to required procedure and diagnosis taxonomies (e.g., Physicians *Current Procedural Terminology* (CPT) and *International Classification of Diseases* (ICD)), submit claims, balance bill deductible and coinsurance amounts, and otherwise convert services rendered into cash in the bank. The goal of revenue cycle management is to turn services into cash as efficiently and effectively as possible.

As you might expect, revenue cycle management consists of numerous component functions that must be individually optimized for peak overall system efficiency. Furthermore, numerous decisions must be made initially when the system is first developed as well as ongoing as refinements and upgrades become available.

This chapter explores the key essentials of revenue cycle management for the pathology practice or independent laboratory. Decision variables are emphasized, with internal policy suggestions offered as appropriate.

D. L. Padget (✉)
APF Consulting Services, Inc., 1540 South Coast Highway, Suite 204,
Laguna Beach, CA 92651, USA
e-mail: DennisPadget@embarqmail.com

2347 Clearwater Run, The Villages, FL 32162-2308, USA

© Springer International Publishing Switzerland 2016
L. A. Hassell et al. (eds.), *Pathology Practice Management*,
DOI 10.1007/978-3-319-22954-6_4

Selecting a Billing Operation

Case: Selecting a Billing Operation

You and your colleagues have created a limited liability corporation, entered into a service contract with a community acute care hospital, and registered as participating physicians with Medicare and several large private insurers. Now it is time to think about generating a positive cash flow. Some trusted peers, over cocktails at a recent medical conference, told you the only way to go is an in-house billing operation, but others insisted you would be foolish not to contract with a commercial medical billing company. Which way should you go? Is there a rational process by which you can make this very important decision?

In-house versus contracted billing is a decision that all physicians and independent laboratories must make at least once in their life as a business. There is no "one size fits all" answer. Each approach has its advocates and detractors, and each has major as well as minor advantages and disadvantages. You will hear fabulous success stories as well as accounts of disaster with equal frequency and veracity for both in-house and contracted billing operations.

Table 4.1 summarizes the principal pros and cons associated with in-house and contracted medical billing operations. A narrative description of the pros and cons is also presented. Suggestions for weighing the advantages and disadvantages in your own decision-making process are also provided.

- *Front-End Capital*: Setting up an in-house billing operation requires substantial capital. A computer, software, office space, office equipment and furnishings, and numerous other items of major and minor equipment and supplies must be leased or purchased. Staff must be hired, and there will be at least a few weeks of downtime during which they finish setting up the office, develop operating policies and procedures, become thoroughly trained, and perform other tasks necessary before the first claim can be released. All of this must be funded via equity contribution of the physicians or owners, or through borrowed funds.

  Commercial medical billers are staffed and equipped to begin processing your charges and claims on "day one." There typically is no capital buy-in, security deposit, or other upfront cash required of new clients. Company representatives

Table 4.1 Key business considerations when choosing between in-house billing and a contracted service

Key business consideration	In-house operation	Contracted service
Significant front-end capital investment required	Yes	No
Substantial lead time before start-up required	Frequent	Infrequent
Upgrades and innovations readily implemented	Sometimes	Usually
Close involvement by physicians (owners) required	Usually	Seldom
Cost of operation correlated with volume of medical services	Seldom	Usually
Physicians (owners) have substantial control over operation	Yes	Somewhat
Attention to interests of physicians (owners)	Solely	Diverse
Financial and compliance risk is diverted	No	Somewhat

will meet with you and, if indicated, your clients (e.g., a hospital) to create the initial set of billing and collection policies, develop a fee schedule, establish data transfer links, and perform other tasks needed to get you going, all as part of its standard new client start-up service (i.e., no extra charge). There may be an additional fee charged by the commercial biller for an out-of-the-ordinary data link or other arrangement you want that is unusual or unique to your practice or laboratory.

- *Start-Up Lead Time*: As suggested in the immediately preceding point, it is unlikely that a "from scratch" in-house billing operation can be set up and "turned on" in fewer than perhaps 6 weeks. In contrast, an experienced commercial medical biller can probably have you up and running in 2 weeks or so, assuming there is nothing unusual about your medical operation. You must judge whether start-up time is an important consideration in your in-house versus contracted billing operation decision.

- *Upgrades and Innovations*: Claim-filing requirements change constantly, and some, such as the pending transition to International Classification of Diseases-10th Revision-Clinical Modification (ICD-10-CM) diagnosis coding (scheduled for October 1, 2015 at the time of this writing), have significant implications for the file structure, electronic claim field population, and related specifications for medical billing software. Furthermore, innovations in office equipment and electronics become available on a regular basis, and these may hold promise of staff productivity gains.

  Software and office equipment upgrades can be costly and time-consuming to research and implement. Depending on the size of your in-house billing operation and the technical savvy of the personnel, evaluating and implementing worthwhile innovations and upgrades can be challenging and may be quite expensive as well. Of course, a relatively small commercial medical biller will face the same challenges, whereas a larger contracted biller likely will be in a position to integrate upgrades and innovations with relative ease. The key takeaway from this discussion is that you need to take technology changes into account in your decision to go with an in-house versus a contracted billing operation.

- *Physician/Owner Attention*: Physicians and laboratory owners should always play an active role in the operation of their billing process, whether it is in-house or contracted. However, their role should in most instances be limited to setting and periodically validating operating and collection policies, participating in payer contract negotiations, approving capital and other major expenditures, monitoring performance, and other high-level matters. In general, it is not a wise use of valuable physician or owner time to become involved in the day-to-day operation of a billing and collection system.

  A knowledgeable, experienced, loyal, self-motivated manager is vital to the successful functioning of an in-house billing operation. With such a person on board, chances are the physicians or owners will have no need to involve themselves in anything other than performance-monitoring and high-level decision-making activities. Otherwise, it may be necessary for at least one physician member of the group to take a more active role in day-to-day operations.

A contracted billing operation, particularly when the company is well-managed, sufficiently capitalized, and has several pathology and laboratory clients, seldom requires more than high-level policy and performance-monitoring involvement by physician and laboratory clients. Due diligence during the proposal evaluation process is very important in these regards because a less-experienced or less well-managed commercial medical biller may require much more hand-holding or close scrutiny.

- *Fixed vs. Variable Cost*: In the short run at least, an in-house billing operation represents a fixed cost of the physician practice or laboratory. There is virtually no opportunity to reduce space, equipment, insurance, maintenance, and related costs if the volume of medical services rendered by the physicians falls due to seasonal or other factors. Similarly, labor costs typically cannot be quickly adjusted by more than a nominal amount to keep pace with changes in service volume; for example, if you practice in a tight labor market, it may be difficult to find a sufficient number of qualified people to handle a materially higher volume of medical service transactions. In general, it is best to assume that you cannot materially influence your in-house billing costs with less than 3 or 6 months' notice.

Commercial medical billers typically charge for their services based on a fixed percentage of collections. (Alternatively, a fixed fee per claim or transaction may be imposed.) Hence, the cost of billing automatically increases or decreases as the volume of medical services by the physicians or laboratory changes. (There will be a slight lag when compensation is based on a percentage of collections, because it typically takes an average of about 30–45 days to convert a medical service into a cash receipt.) This is an important advantage to physicians and laboratories that find themselves in a period of sustained growth or decline or whose volume of services tends to fluctuate due to seasonality or other reasons.

A common mistake made by physicians and laboratories when comparing commercial medical biller proposals is to focus on the percentage of collections or other rate of charge being offered. In particular, it is often assumed that the least costly proposal is the one with the lowest percent of collections quotation. What you should focus on is the *net* percent of collections; that is, percent of collections adjusted for the expected rate (percentage) of revenue converted to cash according to the experience of the commercial biller. A 4% of collections quotation as the biller's proposed charge to you may seem attractive compared to another biller's quotation of 5%, but that number suddenly becomes much less compelling when you factor in a finding that the first biller's average collection rate is 10 percentage points *less* than that of the second biller. "Save a dime, lose a dollar" is not a formula for financial success.

- *Physician/Owner Control*: Physicians and owners of laboratories will have greater or lesser need to control the billing operation depending mainly on personal preference. An in-house billing operation has the advantage of offering maximum control to physicians and laboratory owners. Of course, increased control may also mean increased time commitment, which may not be a wise use of valuable physician resources. On the other hand, contracting with a commercial medical biller does not—or at least should not—mean a complete loss of control.

Well-run commercial medical billers often go out of their way to ensure that client wishes, desires, and directives are integrated into the workflow for each client account. In short, contracted billing frequently permits pathologists to maintain satisfactory control of the overall operation, while avoiding getting caught up in workaday, mundane matters.

- *Focus on Your Practice/Lab*: There is no question that one possible advantage of an in-house billing operation is that the attentions of all its personnel are devoted 100% to your individual practice or laboratory. This dedication will be of greater or lesser importance depending on the personal philosophy of the physician members of a group or the owners of a laboratory. Of course, the value of a dedicated focus might be offset by factors such as a staff that is too small to readily keep up-to-date with the many external rule changes that regularly occur.

  A common advantage of a commercial medical biller is larger size due to service to multiple clients. The larger size accommodates economies of scale as well as intangibles such as expertise in the rules associated with particular physician specialties. Even though commercial billers have a fiduciary responsibility to multiple clients at any one time, most assign a client service representative to each individual account such that a close working relationship is established and maintained. In our experience, well-run commercial medical billers are able to give their individual clients personal attention to the extent that is satisfactory to most pathology practices and laboratories. Nonetheless, this is something you should include as part of your due diligence when evaluating a proposal from a commercial medical biller. Obviously, larger size does not guarantee better service—some of the most attentive commercial medical billers are relatively small.

- *Risk Diversion*: Little or no opportunity for diversion of financial or compliance risk exists when an in-house billing operation is conducted under the legal umbrella of the professional practice or laboratory. In that instance, the actions and omissions of billing and collection personnel flow directly to the employer, which is the same entity that employs the physician practitioners. Some financial risk may be diverted when the billing operation is set up under a separate service company, but you should confer with your legal counsel to determine if this is an alternative worth pursuing under your state statutes. Your general liability insurance agent will recommend coverage terms that take your in-house billing and collection operation into account.

  Under most circumstances, commercial medical billing companies are solely responsible for their own financial affairs and business risks; physician and laboratory clients typically do not share in the profits of these companies, nor are they liable for any losses that commercial billers might incur. Of course, you might suffer suboptimal collections via poor performance if the commercial biller you select is undercapitalized or falls on hard financial times. In addition, if a disaster such as a fire or lightning strike befalls your commercial biller and destroys its physical plant or computer system, all of your account receivable and related records could be lost if the biller does not have a robust disaster recovery plan in effect. You can protect yourself to a large extent by conducting necessary due diligence steps in advance of signing a contract with a commercial biller.

Furthermore, your insurance agent will advise you regarding business interruption and related coverage that will protect your company in case something untoward happens to your commercial biller, including misadventure of its employees, such as defalcation involving monies collected on your behalf.

A common misconception holds that physicians can transfer Medicare and other payer compliance risk to another party, such as an employer or commercial medical biller. Although there are technical nuances that come into play any time an allegation of compliance violation is lodged, you are best advised to disregard that advice. The truth is that, in most situations, physicians, group practices, and laboratories are liable for the accuracy and compliance of claims filed in their name, regardless of whether the claims are prepared and submitted via an in-house operation or a contracted billing agent. This is why it is recommended that physicians, group practices, and laboratories conduct periodic (e.g., every 6 months, but no less frequently than annually) internal audits of the claims and patient accounts that are managed by their in-house or commercial billers. (An independent expert might be retained to conduct the periodic audits to assure their thoroughness and impartiality.) Such internal audits will permit immediate correction of any identified issues and inappropriate claim preparation protocols and will help mitigate the compliance liability to which the provider will be held in case of challenge by a regulator or private insurer.

Key Concept
Using an external vendor for billing does little to reduce compliance risk.

The preceding discussion has been intentionally simplified by assuming that there are only two types of billing operations: completely in-house versus completely contracted. In reality, there are hybrid arrangements to take into account. A common hybrid arrangement uses in-house billing personnel who are employed by the physician group or laboratory, but the billing and accounts receivable management computer, software, and associated support are leased from a commercial medical biller. (Variations on this basic theme are found here and there.) A hybrid arrangement can mitigate the more significant disadvantages of both "pure" types of operations. For example, the initial capital investment can be reduced by a material amount, and upgrades and innovations would be the responsibility of the commercial biller. As stated earlier, there is no "one size fits all" solution to the billing operation decision: Feel free to "think outside the box," and realize that working with an experienced pathology/laboratory financial consultant may be a wise investment to help guide you through this very important process.

Another fact to consider is that the billing operation decision you make today need not last forever. Not infrequently, groups and laboratories start out with a contracted biller and later migrate to an in-house operation (or a hybrid arrangement) when growth in medical service volume and greater business maturity support the wisdom of that change. Circumstances may direct that movement in the opposite direction—from in-house to contracted—is the sensible course of action. The decision factors enumerated above apply in these situations with equal emphasis depending on the practice or laboratory start-up circumstance.

We conclude this section by repeating an exceedingly important point made a bit earlier: No matter the style of billing operation you select (in-house, contracted, or hybrid), the level of trust you have in your billing manager or client service representative, or any other consideration, you must objectively, closely, and continuously monitor the performance of your billing operation on an ongoing basis. Monitoring includes careful evaluation of the monthly collections and receivables reports as well as periodic audit of claims, remittances, and patient accounts. Monitoring is necessary to provide early detection of problems, mistakes, and persistent deviation from established policy. Failure to conduct appropriate monitoring activities on a regular basis can lead to suboptimal practice or laboratory financial performance at a minimum, or worst-case scenarios wherein federal or state regulators are poring through your records in preparation for compliance sanctions against you and your physician associates.

Key Concept
Built or bought, you still need to monitor and audit your billing system regularly.

Getting the Data for a "Clean Claim"

Case: Getting the Data for a "Clean Claim"

Your spanking-new state-of-the-art billing operation is all set up and ready to go! But wait a minute...how do we get the patient demographic and insurance information from the hospital to our biller? Where will the CPT procedure and ICD diagnosis codes for our cases come from? What about other "clean claim" information like referring physician, performing physician, Clinical Laboratory Improvement Amendments (CLIA) number, national provider identification numbers, etc.? Your head is about to explode!

Discussion: Relax...take six deep breaths...then calmly consult the following analysis of key billing data you need to collect and manage to file "clean claims" on a regular basis. In medical insurance parlance, a "clean claim" is one that is complete and accurate in all respects, such that it sails through the insurer's payment processing system without tripping an integrity edit—the claim is promptly and correctly paid the first time through. The prime objective of your in-house or contracted billing operation is to maintain as high a "clean claim" performance level as possible.

Four general categories of information are necessary to prepare a "clean claim". They pertain to the patient and his/her insurance coverage, the health-care setting and physician participants in the care of the patient, the medical services provided to the patient, and idiosyncratic data such as procedure code modifiers. The specific information that falls under each of the four categories is explained below.

1. *Patient Demographic and Insurance Information*: Commonsense information about the patient and his/her insurance coverage is critical to the preparation of a "clean claim." The patient's name (including middle initial), address, birthdate, sex, and telephone number are required. The insured person's name (including middle initial), address, birthdate, sex, and telephone number are required as well, if the patient and insured person are not one and the same. (The relationship of the insured person to the patient, including "self," must be disclosed.)

The name and address of the primary insurer are needed, as well as the group/plan number and the individual member identification number. The same information is required for any secondary insurer. A secondary insurer may be a plan such as a Medicare supplement that steps in to pay any deductible and/or coinsurance for which the patient/insured would otherwise be personally responsible. If the condition for which the patient received medical care is employment- or accident-related (e.g., auto), that information must be captured and reported too. Workers compensation or subrogation of liability may be implicated by an employment- or accident-related event.

Pathologists and laboratories are "downstream" health-care providers, meaning that they seldom have face-to-face contact with patients; instead, they receive medical orders from physicians or other providers with primary responsibility for the diagnosis, care, and treatment of individual patients. Having no convenient way to interview patients, photocopy insurance cards, and the like, pathology practice and laboratory business office personnel rely almost exclusively on other care providers (e.g., referring physicians, hospitals) to gather the requisite patient demographic and insurance information, validate the information as necessary, and pass it along to the practice or laboratory.

The vast majority of hospitals readily agree to pass along patient demographic and insurance data to ancillary service providers such as pathologists, reference laboratories, radiologists, and anesthesiologists. (It is in a hospital's best interests to ensure that ancillary service providers do not badger patients for the same information over and over again and that they can receive payment from insurers with little or no hassle.) Ideally, the subject information will be transferred to your billing office in electronic format by hospitals with which you have a service agreement. This will save your people significant time by not having to reenter the data into your billing system as well as eliminating the possibility of data entry error on your end.

Thinking about nonhospital referral sources, the current expansion of electronic medical record systems in this country may permit you to receive the requisite patient demographic and insurance information from at least some physician offices, ambulatory surgery centers, and other noninstitutional health-care providers in electronic format. However, experience indicates you will have to rely on a paper requisition—a form that you create, pay for, and distribute to referral sources—to gather this information in numerous instances. The requisition naturally will capture patient history, ordered procedures, and other relevant information beyond that simply in the realm of demographics and insurance.

Your billing office or agent will need to verify patient insurance coverage (and perhaps other information, such as insured person or even correct patient name and/or address) to a greater or lesser extent. Your office/agent may find that the information coming from hospitals and/or other referral sources is highly reliable, in which case their time spent on insurance verification will be nominal. On the other hand, your referral sources may not do a very good job of sending your office/agent accurate patient/insurance information, in which case the verification function may consume a significant amount of their time.

The official hardcopy Form-1500 (02-12) (Fig. 4.1; we will use Form-1500 as a framework for the next several items for discussion) used by physicians and laboratories when filing claims with Medicare Part B, other government payers, and private medical insurers provides space for signature by the patient/authorized agent (box 12) and the insured person/authorized agent (box 13). Under normal circumstances, it is not necessary for the patient/insured person to literally sign the claim form: Entering the phrase "signature on file" is sufficient, meaning that

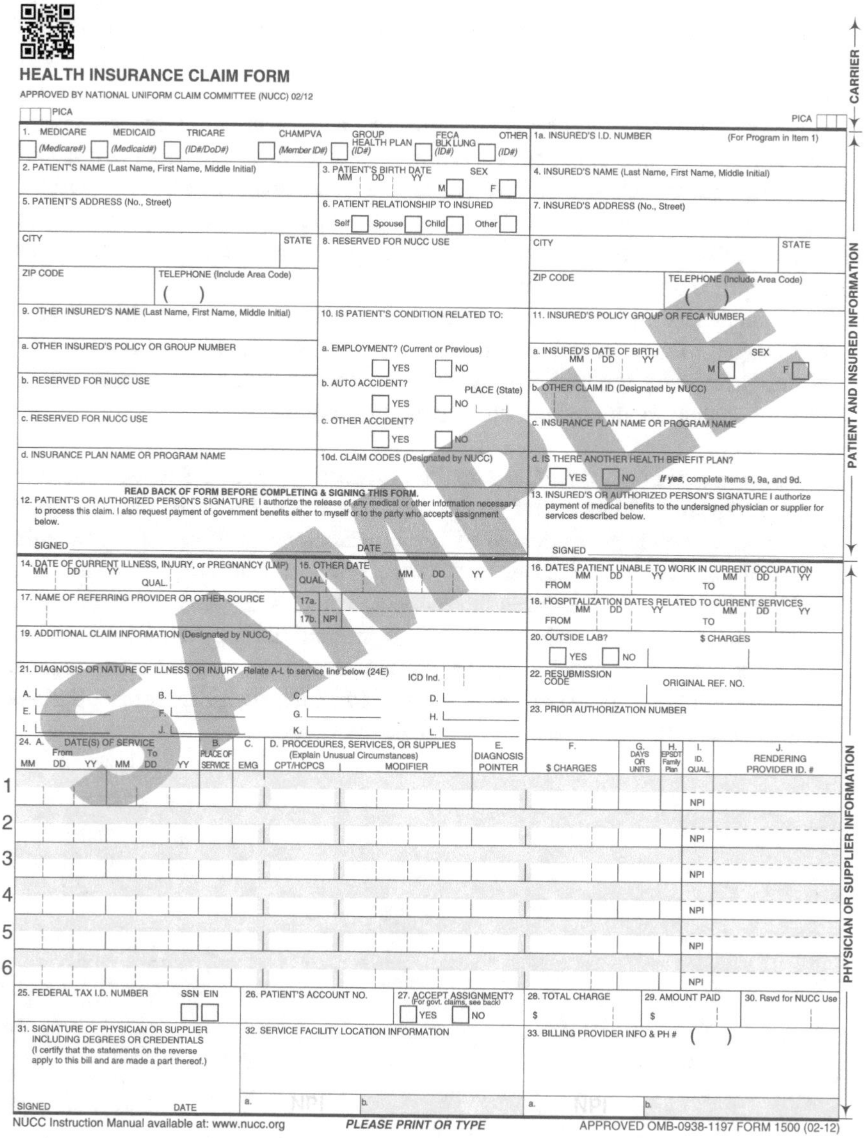
HEALTH INSURANCE CLAIM FORM
APPROVED BY NATIONAL UNIFORM CLAIM COMMITTEE (NUCC) 02/12
PICA PICA
CARRIER
1. MEDICARE (Medicare#) MEDICAID (Medicaid#) TRICARE (ID#/DoD#) CHAMPVA (Member ID#) GROUP HEALTH PLAN (ID#) FECA BLK LUNG (ID#) OTHER (ID#)
1a. INSURED'S I.D. NUMBER (For Program in Item 1)
2. PATIENT'S NAME (Last Name, First Name, Middle Initial)
3. PATIENT'S BIRTH DATE MM DD YY SEX M F
4. INSURED'S NAME (Last Name, First Name, Middle Initial)
5. PATIENT'S ADDRESS (No., Street)
6. PATIENT RELATIONSHIP TO INSURED Self Spouse Child Other
7. INSURED'S ADDRESS (No., Street)
CITY STATE
8. RESERVED FOR NUCC USE
CITY STATE
ZIP CODE TELEPHONE (Include Area Code) ( )
ZIP CODE TELEPHONE (Include Area Code) ( )
9. OTHER INSURED'S NAME (Last Name, First Name, Middle Initial)
10. IS PATIENT'S CONDITION RELATED TO:
11. INSURED'S POLICY GROUP OR FECA NUMBER
a. OTHER INSURED'S POLICY OR GROUP NUMBER
a. EMPLOYMENT? (Current or Previous) YES NO
a. INSURED'S DATE OF BIRTH MM DD YY SEX M F
b. RESERVED FOR NUCC USE
b. AUTO ACCIDENT? YES NO PLACE (State)
b. OTHER CLAIM ID (Designated by NUCC)
c. RESERVED FOR NUCC USE
c. OTHER ACCIDENT? YES NO
c. INSURANCE PLAN NAME OR PROGRAM NAME
d. INSURANCE PLAN NAME OR PROGRAM NAME
10d. CLAIM CODES (Designated by NUCC)
d. IS THERE ANOTHER HEALTH BENEFIT PLAN? YES NO If yes, complete items 9, 9a, and 9d.
READ BACK OF FORM BEFORE COMPLETING & SIGNING THIS FORM.
12. PATIENT'S OR AUTHORIZED PERSON'S SIGNATURE I authorize the release of any medical or other information necessary to process this claim. I also request payment of government benefits either to myself or to the party who accepts assignment below.
SIGNED DATE
13. INSURED'S OR AUTHORIZED PERSON'S SIGNATURE I authorize payment of medical benefits to the undersigned physician or supplier for services described below.
SIGNED
PATIENT AND INSURED INFORMATION
14. DATE OF CURRENT ILLNESS, INJURY, or PREGNANCY (LMP) MM DD YY QUAL.
15. OTHER DATE QUAL. MM DD YY
16. DATES PATIENT UNABLE TO WORK IN CURRENT OCCUPATION FROM MM DD YY TO MM DD YY
17. NAME OF REFERRING PROVIDER OR OTHER SOURCE 17a. 17b. NPI
18. HOSPITALIZATION DATES RELATED TO CURRENT SERVICES FROM MM DD YY TO MM DD YY
19. ADDITIONAL CLAIM INFORMATION (Designated by NUCC)
20. OUTSIDE LAB? YES NO $ CHARGES
21. DIAGNOSIS OR NATURE OF ILLNESS OR INJURY Relate A-L to service line below (24E) ICD Ind.
A. B. C. D. E. F. G. H. I. J. K. L.
22. RESUBMISSION CODE ORIGINAL REF. NO.
23. PRIOR AUTHORIZATION NUMBER
24. A. DATE(S) OF SERVICE From MM DD YY To MM DD YY B. PLACE OF SERVICE C. EMG D. PROCEDURES, SERVICES, OR SUPPLIES (Explain Unusual Circumstances) CPT/HCPCS MODIFIER E. DIAGNOSIS POINTER F. $ CHARGES G. DAYS OR UNITS H. EPSDT Family Plan I. ID. QUAL. J. RENDERING PROVIDER ID. #
1 NPI
2 NPI
3 NPI
4 NPI
5 NPI
6 NPI
PHYSICIAN OR SUPPLIER INFORMATION
25. FEDERAL TAX I.D. NUMBER SSN EIN
26. PATIENT'S ACCOUNT NO.
27. ACCEPT ASSIGNMENT? (For govt. claims, see back) YES NO
28. TOTAL CHARGE $
29. AMOUNT PAID $
30. Rsvd for NUCC Use
31. SIGNATURE OF PHYSICIAN OR SUPPLIER INCLUDING DEGREES OR CREDENTIALS (I certify that the statements on the reverse apply to this bill and are made a part thereof.)
SIGNED DATE
32. SERVICE FACILITY LOCATION INFORMATION a. NPI b.
33. BILLING PROVIDER INFO & PH # ( ) a. NPI b.
NUCC Instruction Manual available at: www.nucc.org PLEASE PRINT OR TYPE APPROVED OMB-0938-1197 FORM 1500 (02-12)
SAMPLE

Fig. 4.1 Form 1500 (02-12)

the patient gave you permission to file a claim against his/her medical benefits by signing an appropriate release in the possession of the primary health-care provider (e.g., hospital, referring physician office). Furthermore, the vast majority of the time your in-house or contracted biller will file claims electronically, which obviously does not support physical signatures.

As a "downstream" ancillary service provider, you have no choice but to rely on the primary health-care provider (e.g., hospital, referring physician) for three additional very important legal permissions from the patient: (a) release of medical information in your possession to the insurer as necessary to support your claim; (b) assignment of the insured's medical insurance benefits to you, which allows you to receive payment directly from the medical insurer; and (c) acceptance by the patient of responsibility to pay your claim if the medical insurer denies payment. Hospital registration forms that patients must execute prior to receiving other than emergency treatment commonly gather these permissions on behalf of provider-based physicians (e.g., pathologists and radiologists) in addition to the hospital itself. The requisition your laboratory or practice gives to noninstitutional referring providers (e.g., physician offices, ambulatory surgery centers) should accommodate capture of these permissions directly from the patient, unless an alternate arrangement is made with those entities. You are encouraged to work closely with your legal counsel or pathology consultant to ensure that these permissions from patients/insured persons are arranged with all referral sources, both institutional and noninstitutional.

2. *Health-Care Setting and Physician Participants in Care of Patient*: The standard physician and laboratory service claim record, whether hardcopy or electronic, accommodates disclosure of key information about the setting in which the services were rendered, the health-care provider who ordered the services, and the physician who rendered the services. The data elements and instructions discussed below are mandatory for Medicare and Tricare beneficiary claims; except as noted, they usually apply as well to private insurers and state Medicaid agencies, but you should confirm the extent to which any given insurer that you do business with may depart from these instructions.

NPI: Each physician and eligible healthcare entity (e.g., independent laboratory) that desires to serve and bill Medicare beneficiaries or the program must apply for and be assigned a National Provider Identifier. (Healthcare provider NPIs are mandated by HIPAA.) An NPI is unique to an individual physician or other healthcare provider in much the same way as social security numbers are unique to individual US citizens. In general, a claim for payment filed by a pathologist or independent laboratory must disclose the NPI of the ordering physician, the performing physician or laboratory, and the billing physician, group practice, or laboratory; a claim missing even one of those NPIs typically will be rejected by the Medicare contractor.

> *PECOS*: The Provider Enrollment, Chain and Ownership System is an Internet-based healthcare provider enrollment mechanism offered by the DHHS Centers for Medicare & Medicaid Services as a convenient alternative to hardcopy forms for that purpose. PECOS allows physicians, non-physician practitioners, suppliers (e.g., independent labs), and other healthcare providers to enroll in the Medicare program, make changes to their enrollment information, and confirm the information on file for their organization.

a. *Referring physician or other health-care professional*: The name and national provider identifier (NPI) of the physician or other health-care professional (e.g., physician assistant) who referred the pathology specimen to you or your lab must be reported in fields 17 and 17b (or the electronic equivalents) of the standard claim. The name entered must be that of an individual; it cannot be the name of a group or legal entity. Furthermore, the individual must be properly enrolled as a Medicare provider, must have a valid NPI, and must be registered in the Provider Enrollment, Chain, and Ownership System (PECOS). Refer to the official instructions for Form-1500 (02-12) for details on completing fields 17 and 17b.

   The referring physician whose name is reportable in field 17 may or may not be the same physician who admitted the patient to the hospital or who is otherwise designated as the patient's "primary" attending physician. The name disclosed in this field should be that of the physician or other health-care professional who actually extracted the pathology sample (e.g., biopsy, polyp, brushing) that you have received for diagnostic evaluation. Your billing office should always ensure that the name reported in field 17 of the claim corresponds to the name of the referring physician according to your pathology report.

   The NPI of the referring physicians and other health-care professionals who regularly refer pathology specimens to your practice or laboratory often do not appear on the hospital registration sheets or requisitions that come with specimens. Pathology and lab billing offices overcome this potential problem by building and periodically updating a table of referring physicians and the validated NPI for each. Hospitals typically are in a position to provide this information, or your biller can directly contact each referring professional's office.

b. *CLIA number*: The official label of field 23 of Form 1500 (02-12) is "prior authorization number," but Medicare and Tricare instruct pathologists and laboratories to report the CLIA number of the site where the pathology service was rendered in this space. Pathologists who perform all their work at a hospital are allowed to report the hospital's CLIA number in this field, provided the hospital gives its permission to the pathologist or group. (A pathology group or solo practitioner could apply for its own CLIA number for the hospital's histology and/or cytology laboratory, but that is not necessary under usual circumstances.) Many private insurers do not require pathologists or laboratories to report a CLIA number on their claims, but you should check with your state Medicaid agency and the major private insurers in your area to confirm their instructions in these regards.

A pathologist billing only the physician professional component or a laboratory billing the global charge (professional and technical components combined) reports the CLIA number of the site where the pathologist performed the microscopic examination, regardless of where the technical component was performed. On the other hand, a laboratory billing only the technical component of a pathology service should report the CLIA number associated with the site at which the technical component was conducted. The CLIA number in field 23 should correspond with the "service facility location information" reported in field 32 of the claim (see next).

c. *Service location*: The name and address (including zip code) of the facility at which the billed service(s) was performed must be disclosed in field 32 of Form-1500 (02-12), with the NPI entered in field 32a if applicable. The address reported in this field should correspond with the CLIA number you reported in field 23 (see immediately preceding topic). A pathologist billing just the professional component or a laboratory billing the global charge (professional and technical components combined) reports the name and address of the site where the pathologist performed the microscopic exam, regardless of where the technical component was performed. A laboratory billing just the technical component of a pathology service reports the name and address associated with the site at which the technical component was conducted.

A common misconception is that the name and address reported in field 32 must relate to the "place of service" code reported in field 24B. In point of fact, fields 32 and 24B are unrelated to one another—they need not correspond in any way. Information about field 24B is provided later in this section.

d. *Rendering provider NPI*: The NPI of the pathologist who personally performed each billed medical service must be disclosed in field 24J of Form-1500 (02-12). The NPI in 24J of each claim line is to correspond with the medical service that appears in CPT/Healthcare Common Procedure Coding System (HCPCS) code format on that claim line. For example, if Dr. Smith performs the frozen section consultation and Dr. Jones performs the permanent section examination, Dr. Smith's NPI is to appear in 24J of the 88331 claim line and Dr. Jones' NPI is to appear in 24J of the 88307 claim line. The performing physician associated with each medical procedure for a case must be validated by reference to the final pathology report.

The Department of Health and Human Services (DHHS) Centers for Medicare & Medicaid Services (CMS) national office and individual Medicare administrative contractors (MACs) differ at times in their guidance regarding field 24J of claims by independent laboratory providers for anatomic pathology services. Some MACs indicate that field 24J of claims by independent labs should either be blank or should be filled in with the NPI of the billing laboratory. Other MACs and the CMS national office advise that the NPI of the actual performing pathologist is to be entered in field 24J, the same as with claims by hospital-based pathologists. We generally recommend that the CMS national office guidance be adopted, but if you have written instructions from your local MAC to the contrary, you should be protected from compliance challenge if you follow your MAC's contrary instructions.

> *MAC*: A Medicare administrative contractor administers Medicare program policy and pays healthcare provider claims under contract with the DHHS Centers for Medicare & Medicaid Services. A MAC may administer only claims from Part B providers (e.g., physicians, laboratories), from Part A providers (e.g., hospitals, skilled nursing facilities), or both. The US is divided into ten payment jurisdictions, with eight MACs currently contracted with CMS to administer the federal Medicare program in the ten jurisdictions.

   e. *Billing provider*: Field 33 of Form-1500 (02-12) is to be populated with the name and address of the billing provider (e.g., pathology group practice or independent lab), which is the entity that is entitled to receive payment on behalf of the performing physician(s). The NPI of the billing provider is to appear in field 33a, and its federal employer tax identification number (FEIN) goes in field 25. Each physician employed by or contracted with the billing entity—either a physician professional organization or an independent laboratory—should formally reassign his/her right to bill for his/her personal services to individual patients to the billing entity. Form 855-R accommodates reassignment from the individual physician to his/her employer or principal.
   f. *Signature of physician or supplier*: Form-1500 (02-12) field 31 accommodates the name ("signature") of the performing physician or other provider representative who is certifying to the accuracy and veracity of the information in the claim as filed. Inserting the name of the performing physician in this field can be problematic, especially when more than one physician is involved in a particular patient's case. The recommended policy is to simply insert "signature on file" in field 31, which is permitted by CMS guidance. Alternatively, the name of the practice or laboratory administrator might appear in that space, signing as an authorized representative of the pathology practice or laboratory.

3. *Medical Services Provided to Patient*: Two fields, #21 and #24, of the standard Form-1500 (02-12) accommodate detailed reporting of pertinent diagnosis and medical service information relevant to each patient. The diagnosis information is used by insurers to verify the medical necessity of the care rendered by the pathologist as well as coverage within the terms of the patient's medical policy with the insurer. The procedures performed field (#24) is where you report detailed information, expressed in five-digit CPT/HCPCS code format, about the medical services conducted by the pathologist to diagnose the patient's ailment or condition. The data in the two fields—that is, ICD diagnosis codes and CPT/HCPCS procedure codes—are mandatory in relation to all government and privately insured patients. The primary source of the diagnosis and procedure information that goes in fields 21 and 24 is the final pathology report, as more fully discussed below.

a. *Diagnosis information*: Federal law requires referring physicians to provide relevant clinical diagnosis and medical history information on patients when ordering diagnostic tests and procedures such as pathology examinations and radiology studies. It also requires pathologists, radiologists, independent laboratories, and other "downstream" health-care providers to report relevant diagnosis information on their claims for services to Medicare, Tricare, and state Medicaid beneficiaries. Private insurers also require relevant diagnosis information on claims by pathologists, independent laboratories, and other health-care providers.

Diagnosis information reported on Form-1500 (02-12) must be expressed using the clinical modification version of the ICD maintained and published by the World Health Organization. The taxonomy in use in the USA as of the date of this writing is the 9th edition (ICD-9-CM), but the 10th edition (ICD-10-CM) is to be adopted by all health-care providers, private insurers, and government payers on October 1, 2015 according to the mandate of the DHHS CMS. Narrative diagnoses are not accepted by payers and insurers: Diagnoses must be posted to field 21 using the approved numerical (ICD-9-CM) or alpha-numerical (ICD-10-CM) code taxonomy.

Referring physicians are not required to submit clinical diagnosis and/or medical history information to "downstream" health-care providers using the ICD-9-CM or ICD-10-CM code taxonomy. However, if they elect to provide narrative clinical diagnosis or medical history information, it must be at a sufficiently detailed level to enable the "downstream" health-care provider to convert it to the applicable diagnosis code(s) as necessary for that provider to file its claim to the government payer or private insurer.

Pathologists and laboratories commonly receive clinical diagnosis and/or medical history information from referring physicians on the test requisition (or order entry screen in the case of an automated system) or request for consultation. Independent laboratories are forbidden by Medicare policy from looking in their medical record databases for past clinical diagnoses for individual patients; the only approved source of that information is the referring physician. While pathologists should use various means of gathering information regarding a patient's medical condition when diagnosing a patient's specimen, pathologists are discouraged from researching hospital or clinic electronic health record databases for diagnosis information on individual patients for data that may end up being reported in item 21 of their insurance claims; for example, knowing the outcome of a recent radiologic imaging study may be helpful in establishing a differential diagnosis for a complex surgical pathology case, but "fishing" for clinical information to support a diagnosis of "benign colonic mucosa" might very well be viewed as a major compliance infraction by a pathologist. Pathologists should strenuously resist referring physician requests to "see electronic health record (EHR)" and should instead insist that they proactively provide relevant clinical information with each laboratory requisition or order as required by federal law.

A critical nuance to consider when setting up your ICD data capture system is the source of the diagnosis to report in relation to claims for clinical laboratory tests (e.g., Pap tests, molecular tests, common blood chemistry tests) versus anatomic pathology procedures that are paid via the Medicare physician fee schedule. Government payers and many private insurers insist that the laboratory's claim for a clinical test be supported by the referring physician's clinical diagnosis (i.e., the reason the test was ordered) as the first-listed (primary) diagnosis; any abnormality detected by the clinical lab test(s) may be added as a secondary diagnosis. The prescription for claims for anatomic pathology procedures is just the reverse: The definitive pathologic diagnosis is to be the first-listed (primary) diagnosis, assuming one is available at the time the claim is filed. Any relevant clinical diagnosis may be added as a secondary diagnosis on the anatomic pathology claim at the sole discretion of the billing provider, and that will be the source of the primary diagnosis as well if there is no definitive pathologic diagnosis available for the case. The best source of information on ICD diagnosis codes for anatomic pathology cases is the final pathology report file.

Diagnosis coding for pathology services has materially different rules compared to the much larger clinical specialties such as surgery, internal medicine, and family practice. Nonetheless, pathology professional coders tend to be trained in the larger specialties, so they inadvertently miscode or over-code pathology cases. For example, common misconceptions about pathology cases include: (a) each different *specimen* must be assigned a unique ICD code; and (b) as many clinical diagnoses should be reported on the claim as possible. The truth is that the official ICD guidance and instructions published by CMS confirm that pathology claims are to report the one or two diagnoses that reflect the patient's most significant *current* diagnosed condition (i.e., by the pathologist). Mistaken adherence to myths about ICD coding for pathology cases results in significant wasted time and risk of medical necessity denials.

The APF is an excellent source of correct information about the true and proper way to determine and assign ICD diagnosis codes to pathology cases. Education and guidance is provided via periodic conferences and webinars as well as detailed instructions in the APF's electronic text *Pathology Service Coding Handbook*.

b. *Procedure information*: Detailed information about each billable procedure furnished by the rendering pathologist is reported in field 24 of the Form-1500 (02/2012) claim. The source of the information depends on the datum: Some comes from the referring physician via the order entry screen or requisition, but the critical data in terms of money claimed and collected comes from the final pathology report. (Performing provider field 24J is certainly critical, but it was discussed earlier, so that information is not repeated in this section.) How you collect the data depends on the extent to which your order entry, medical reporting, and other information systems are computerized and integrated—never underestimate the power of a well-designed manual (i.e., hardcopy) information system.

- Date of Service (24A): The date of service for pathology technical component services and clinical lab tests is defined by Medicare as the date the specimen (e.g., biopsy, Pap fluid, blood, urine) was collected from the patient. This datum should appear on the order entry screen or the requisition from the referring physician, and it should be faithfully disclosed in the pathology or laboratory report as well.

  Medicare has not, as of the date of this writing, released a formal definition of the date of service for the professional component of physician diagnostic procedures such as radiology and pathology examinations. Some contractors and private insurers define the date of service for diagnostic physician procedures as the date the "service" was "performed"—whatever that may mean! (You do a frozen section tonight, the gross exam tomorrow morning, issue a preliminary report the next day, and release the final report the day after that once the fluorescent in situ hybridization (FISH) results are available—what is the "service"? What is the "date of service"?) Absent a specific instruction from a particular contractor or private insurer, most pathologists and laboratories define the date of service for the physician professional component as the date of specimen collection, the same as the technical component. (That policy minimizes patient and insurer confusion as regards pathologist and hospital claims and statements, and it is the only way an independent laboratory can bill global fees for pathology services to nonhospital patients.) Nonetheless, some pathologists report the accession date or the final report date as the date of service in item 24A of the Form-1500 (02/2012).

- Procedures or Services (24D): Post in this column the CPT or HCPCS-II code that accurately describes each billable procedure that you rendered to the patient during the encounter. The source of this data should be—or at least should be confirmed by—the final pathology report. More will be said in a moment about who should assign CPT or HCPCS-II codes to your cases, and an overview of the CPT/HCPCS-II taxonomy is provided in another chapter.

- Diagnosis Pointer (24E): The data in this column merely links each procedure code in item 24D to the ICD code in item 21 to which it relates. If ICD diagnosis codes are being properly determined, most claims will link all procedures to the same ICD code line (or two lines in a minor number of situations).

- Charges (24F): The usual and customary charges you bill to insurers and patients per CPT or HCPCS-II code are set in advance and are posted to each claim by your business office or billing agent. The amount reported per any given line of the claim is merely the product of the preset fee per the applicable procedure code times the number of service units rendered on that date to that patient.

- Units (24G): Pathology cases quite frequently involve multiples of the same type of service or procedure; for example, multiple biopsies (e.g., skin, prostate), multiple special stains (e.g., iron, reticulin), and/or multiple qualitative immunohistochemistry stains (e.g., CD20, S100, Vimentin). In general, multiples of the same CPT or HCPCS-II code for a case are reported on one line of the claim using the "units" column (24G). For example, three skin biopsies received for a patient on the same day will be displayed on the claim as "88305" in column 24D and "3" in column 24G.

4. *Idiosyncratic Data Required by Payers/Insurers*: Professional coders and billers will tell you that frequently there is little or no "rhyme or reason" to the claim specifications individual payers and insurers demand of providers to achieve "clean claim" status. As one example, private insurers often do not want the CLIA number reported on the claim, and instructions for procedure modifier usage (see topic below) usually differ from one insurer to the next. Very often the only way one can determine a particular insurer's "clean claim" requirements is trial and error, and then there is no guarantee that its requirements will not change in a month or two.

We could devote significant space herein to the arcane and idiosyncratic data requirements of payers and insurers, but the long-term value of that information would be doubtful. Therefore, we will focus instead on the two most significant topics of ongoing interest to pathology coders and billers: procedure code modifiers and "place of service" codes.

a. *Procedure code modifiers*: Modifiers are two-digit alpha, numeric, or alphanumeric codes that are appended to the regular CPT or HCPCS-II procedure code to clarify the scope, context, or circumstance regarding the procedure as it affects payment or coverage. By way of example, the most frequently-used procedure code modifier in pathology is "26": When modifier "26" is appended to a CPT code, it means the physician performed and is billing just the professional component of the service—another provider (e.g., hospital or independent lab) performed the technical component and is billing separately for it.

Proper use of procedure code modifiers is critical to the claim preparation process. Failure to append a modifier such as "26" (professional component only) or "TC" (technical component only) will result either in denial of the claim (e.g., the payer detected a mismatch of procedure code, without the expected "26" modifier, and place of service) or overpayment (e.g., payment at the global service rate instead of professional only). In another situation, failure to append the appropriate "separate procedure" modifier will lead to summary denial of at least one charge line due to suspicion by the payer that you have broken up one procedure into two or more component parts (a very serious compliance violation known as "fragmentation") or that some of the procedures were not truly medically necessary.

The procedure code modifiers used most frequently by pathologists and laboratories today are "26" (professional component only), "TC" (technical component only), and "59" (separate procedure). (Modifier 59 may be used with some private insurance claims inasmuch as Medicare substitutes four alpha modifiers to break down separate procedure reporting into more discrete circumstances: Different encounter (XE); different specimen, anatomic site or lesion (XS); different physician (XP); and nonoverlapping procedures (XU).) Teaching physicians must append modifier "GC" to their procedure codes to confirm that they—not a resident or fellow—personally performed the critical portion of the procedure.

As earlier intimated, the instructions for procedure code modifier usage quite frequently vary from one Medicare contractor or private insurer to another. This is particularly true in relation to "separate procedure" circumstances and situations where multiple units of the same CPT or HCPCS-II code are eligible for billing with the same date of service on a claim. Your billing office personnel or commercial billing agent must become thoroughly familiar with the rules for modifier use by the Medicare contractor, Medicaid agency, and private insurers in your service area to ensure maximum "clean claim" performance and payment turnaround.

b. *Place of service*: A "place of service" code must be reported in item 24B of the Form-1500 (02/2012) by physicians, laboratories, and other Part B healthcare providers. The place of service code-set consists of several two-digit items intended to denote where the service(s) being billed was rendered. The codes most commonly reported by pathologists and laboratories are 21 (hospital inpatient), 22 (registered hospital outpatient), 11 (physician office or clinic), 24 (ambulatory surgery center), and 81 (independent laboratory).

In some instances, the place of service code serves to judge whether the billing provider is entitled to payment for the global service (professional and technical components combined) or only the physician professional component. A pathologist or independent laboratory is eligible for payment only for the physician professional component from Medicare when the place of service is 21 or 22 (hospital inpatient or registered hospital outpatient respectively) inasmuch as only the hospital in which the patient was registered at the time of specimen collection may bill the program for the technical component. On the other hand, a pathologist or independent laboratory may claim payment for the global service if the specimen was extracted during a physician office or clinic visit (POS 11), at a free-standing ambulatory surgery center (POS 24), or at an independent laboratory (POS 81). (Under certain circumstances a pathologist may purchase the technical component of an anatomic service from an independent laboratory or a hospital and bill the global charge to Medicare.)

The majority conventional wisdom historically and today is that the place of service code for pathology and laboratory services should reflect the type of facility that was being visited by the patient when the specimen was extracted. For example, if a biopsy is taken during a physician office visit, the pathologist or independent laboratory should report POS 11 (office or clinic) on the claim for processing and examining the biopsy even if the professional and/or technical component is performed at an independent laboratory. On the other hand, some providers and advisors believe that the place of service code for pathology services should be based on where the technical processing of the specimen occurred. (In our opinion, the former viewpoint is the better supported and more appropriate interpretation.)

Medicare's guidance to pathologists and independent laboratories regarding proper place of service reporting is in a state of flux as of the date of this writing. One longstanding instruction from Medicare indicates that place of service for Medicare claim purposes is determined by the type of facility being visited by the patient when the specimen was obtained. However, nearly 2 years ago, Medicare told radiologists to base the place of service code on where the technical component was performed, unless the patient was registered at a hospital at the time the film or image was taken. We anticipate that when Medicare finally gets around to issuing the pathology and laboratory-specific guidance that it promised about 2 years ago, it will confirm the longstanding instruction.

Key Participants and Allocation of Responsibilities

Case: Who Does What?

Jones and Associates just want to practice medicine, pathology in particular. Whenever possible, they try to farm out the scut-work tasks so that they can do what they do best, run labs and make diagnoses. As a result, when a large medical billing company serving mostly surgical and radiology practices offered to do their billing for a mere 5% of collections, they were overjoyed and felt they had landed a bargain. In a clause in the contract, they noted that the company was also willing to assign CPT codes and ICD codes for an additional 0.5% of collections. They quickly signed the Business Associate agreement allowing access to the protected health information (PHI) contained in all their reports and let the billing and coding begin. Things seemed to be going well until they performed an audit 6 months into the agreement and discovered that a growing percentage of claims were being rejected, and therefore not collected, and moreover, that their audit sample of surgical pathology cases revealed over 10% of cases either under- or over-coded. What was going wrong?

Discussion: Resubmission of selected rejected cases after review of the codes and other data revealed that ICD code selection may have been in part responsible, while examination of the under- or over-coded cases seemed to indicate that the human-assisted computer algorithm being used to assign CPT codes was failing at the human review stage. In other instances, the data to justify some of the codes appeared to be missing from the report.

You have identified all the billing and clinical information needed to file complete and "clean" claims to government payers and private insurers, and you have planned out exactly where each datum will come from. But you are still not 100% certain how to allocate the various data gathering and transmittal responsibilities among your physician associates and the billing staff. Who is in the best position to undertake key activities such as CPT procedure and ICD diagnosis code determination? The information in this section will make important suggestions for key participants in the revenue cycle management process and allocation of responsibilities.

The pathology medical report is by far the most important document to consider when setting up a complete revenue cycle management system for a professional practice or laboratory. Under normal circumstances, government agents and private insurers view the pathology report as the exclusive document relied on for purposes of verifying billed charges (i.e., procedure codes) and medical necessity (i.e., diagnosis codes). Pathologists must, therefore, recognize when dictating their medical reports that they not only are communicating with the referring physician, but coders in their billing office and outside government and private insurance auditors as well.

Pathologists must, at a minimum, be familiar with the fundamental procedure and diagnosis coding principles, conventions, rules, and nuances in order to prepare complete and clear reports that will permit professional coders to accurately determine or confirm the billable charges and primary diagnosis for each case. They must learn and faithfully use in their reports the CPT-oriented key words that will assure uneventful third-party payer audits, and they must become familiar with the "red flag" words that will cast doubt on the medical necessity of ancillary services such as special stains. In short, pathologists are intimate and indispensable participants in the revenue cycle process, even though they may not literally take part in the determination of individual procedure or diagnosis codes.

The essential data elements that go into a valid claim for pathology or laboratory services were enumerated in the preceding section of this chapter. In this section, we discuss the role of various people who might participate in the process on behalf of the pathology group or the laboratory. The role of the individual pathologist may be limited to generating the medical report, or it may be enlarged into a couple of other necessary areas.

1. *Accessioning*: Accessioning personnel play a vital role in the revenue cycle as well as the medical reporting processes. They must, of course, verify that the specimens received correlate exactly with the requisition. But, additionally, they should ensure that all the essential patient demographic and insurance information has been provided as well as required information about the referring physician, patient history, and current clinical diagnosis. A mechanism should be in place whereby the referring physician is immediately contacted to resolve any discrepancy and acquire missing essential information. If available, the electronic health records system might be consulted to answer questions about the patient and referring physician, but recall that it is the responsibility of the referring physician to provide the clinical history and diagnosis.

A fairly common feature of many anatomic pathology medical reporting software systems is the ability to assign billing codes (e.g., CPT or HCPCS-II) at time of accessioning based on a predefined part-type dictionary that is loaded into a user file in the software. While there can be exceptions owing to a limited scope of practice (e.g., dermatopathology), in general, these part-type dictionaries are an unreliable basis for accurate billing code assignment in terms of final claim preparation and release. The CPT and/or HCPCS-II codes and units of service on the claim must be supported by the final pathology report, so if these codes are assigned via LIS part-type dictionary at the time of accessioning, they absolutely must be validated (and changed as indicated) in comparison to the final pathology report prior to finalizing the patient account and releasing the claim to the responsible party.

2. *CPT/HCPCS-II Code Determinations*: We have stressed at various points in this chapter that the final pathology report is and must be considered the exclusive source of support for all professional and technical charges for each patient case. Accurate and complete charge coding per case can only be accomplished after the responsible pathologist has signed out the report. Any charges that may be entered into the laboratory information or patient accounting system prior to case sign-out (e.g., part-type at time of accessioning or special stains based on pathologist order) should be considered tentative, pending validation once the case is complete.

Someone must carefully evaluate each pathology report at the time of or immediately after sign-out to determine the billable services, accurate billing code per each service, and units of service. That someone might be the pathologist who worked on the case, another pathologist assigned responsibility for performing this task for the group as a whole, a specially trained medical secretary or lab technical person, or a professional coder. Obviously, whoever performs this function must have in-depth knowledge of the coding taxonomy, rules, and nuances as they pertain to anatomic pathology and related physician and laboratory services. Furthermore, they must be motivated to attend to this task with the care for accuracy and completeness that is required.

Deciding who should be responsible for assigning billing codes to your cases is as much personal preference as anything else. In general, particularly for smaller private practices, the pathologists often take responsibility for the coding. But with larger practices and in teaching environments, allocating this responsibility to thoroughly trained professional coders usually works best. (It is difficult to attain a uniform level of knowledge, skill, and commitment at the physician level when you are dealing with more than six or eight pathologists.) An arrangement that we have found to be ideal when pathologists play a major role in the charge determination process is for one or two professional coders to validate all codes and units as a final fail-safe measure. Nonetheless, we generally like to see pathologists involved in the process because that is an important way by which they come to know enough about the coding rules such that they can thoroughly document billable services in their medical reports.

Key Concept
CPT code assignment is the professional responsibility of the pathologist, but in groups larger than about eight, maintaining current knowledge and facility with coding nuance can be problematic, so development of a coding specialist may be useful.

A critical task that cannot reliably be performed at the pathology report sign-out stage is billing code translation needed to fulfill a particular payer or insurer requirement. Medicare rather frequently demands that certain specific pathology services be coded differently than what is prescribed by the American Medical Association's (AMA) CPT codebook (for example, at the date of this writing, a prostate needle biopsy case must be reported to Medicare as one unit of HCPCS-II code G0416 instead of as multiple units of 88305.) These billing code translations and adjustments can be accurately determined only upon verification of the patient's insurance, and said verification typically is not available until after case sign-out. Therefore, provision must be made at the billing office or commercial billing agent stage of processing for determining and making these code translations and adjustments. Of course, Medicare is not the only payer implicated by this observation.

3. *Procedure Code Modifier Determinations*: A few procedure code modifiers such as "26" (professional component only), "TC" (technical component only), and "GC" (teaching physician) are knowable in advance and fixed for a given practice environment such as a hospital. These few modifiers frequently are set up in the patient account profile for automatic posting by the software as manual intervention is not necessary and would be a waste of valuable staff time.

Other procedure code modifiers, particularly those denoting "separate procedure," are driven by differential case factors such as the insurer, specific combinations of procedure codes for a given date of service, and number of units for any one procedure code. Whether a procedure code modifier(s) is required for a particular case, and which of several possible modifiers that may be, rarely is or can be known with certainty at or prior to the time of case sign-out. Hence, procedure code modifiers of this type should not be taken into account prior to the billing office stage of work. In general, we recommend that procedure code modifier determinations be made exclusively by professional coders just prior to the release of patient charges to the claim-filing module of the revenue cycle system.

4. *ICD Diagnosis Code Determinations*: ICD diagnosis coding is an arcane science that usually consumes a significant and disproportionate amount of time case-by-case. For these reasons, we recommend that the ICD diagnosis coding function be assigned to professional coding staff instead of the pathologists associated with a practice or laboratory. The principal exception to this recommendation pertains to specialist cases where the universe of relevant diagnoses is small such that the practitioner can refer to a concise crib sheet to accurately code most cases. The specialties to which this exception may apply are dermatopathology, clinical pathology, hematopathology, renal pathology, neuropathology, and cytopathology. A major advantage of the specialty crib sheet approach is that the diagnoses associated with these cases not infrequently are somewhat nuanced or ill-defined such that the physician is in a much better position than a professional coder to identify reasonable diagnosis codes for these cases.

5. *Other Data Element Considerations*: Most other data required to file a "clean claim" will be readily available to the billing office or commercial billing agent from the patient face sheet, the pathology report, and files maintained by the office or agent. For example, the office or agent should maintain a file of common referring physician names with their NPI numbers, another file with the name and NPI number of each performing physician in the group practice or at the lab, and yet another file with the name and CLIA number associated with each practice site. Of course, a mechanism must be in place to update these files as quickly as possible whenever a data element changes, including additions and deletions.

Revenue Cycle Policies

Case: Billing and Collection Policies

All the groundwork for your revenue cycle management system appears to have been laid. But you have a nagging feeling that something important has been overlooked. Then it hits you: Policies! The many patients you serve daily must be treated uniformly and fairly, and that means policies must be in place to guide your business office or commercial billing agent. Similarly, the business people that represent your practice must know how you feel about dealing with insurers and other outsiders. Now you are ready to formalize the policies that will govern and guide the daily operation of your revenue cycle management system by implementing suggestions such as those set forth below.

Discussion: Reasonable and appropriate billing and collection policies are essential to consistent and equal treatment of all patients.

A well-run practice or laboratory is founded on and guided by a core set of sensible policies such as the following:

- *Usual and Customary Charges*: Your usual and customary charges should be set based on fair market value. In general, that means the standard fee for each billable service will be set just a few dollars more than the highest-allowed charge by the insurers with which you regularly do business. There is no sense charging a great deal more than that, because it will only make your contract write-off amounts that much greater. Furthermore, you do not want to appear unfair to self-pay patients.
- *Indigent Care Allowances*: Pathologists and laboratories regularly maintain an indigent care allowance policy that takes self-pay patient ability to pay into account. For example, patients with an annual income less than 100% of the federal poverty level might be granted a 100% charity allowance, with the discount reduced as the level of income increases. Hospitals often are willing to share the indigent care information they obtain from individual patients with their hospital-based physicians.
- *Bad Debt and Other Write-Offs*: A small-balance write-off policy is standard practice for physicians and laboratories; for example, a patient balance of $10 might be written off automatically as it would cost more to bill and collect that amount. Patients should be sent at least three statements under normal circumstances, and then the account should be referred to a collection agency if no response is received from the patient. There is no sense carrying likely bad debts in your account receivable balance. The collection agent should be instructed regarding how aggressive you want it to be when attempting to collect accounts on your behalf.
- *Courtesy Allowances*: Courtesy allowances, especially those involving referring physicians, their family members, and their employees, can be a major source of compliance concern. You are best advised to work with your legal counsel and compliance consultant when setting up the courtesy allowance policy for your practice or laboratory.

- *Electronic Claims and Receipts*: It is standard of practice today that physician and laboratory claims be filed electronically, and the vast majority of government payers and private insurers are well-equipped to accommodate electronic claims. Furthermore, it is a good idea for your billing office or commercial agent to be set up to receive payment electronically, as well as to accept credit card payment from individual patients.

Your billing and collection policies will expand and change over time. With experience you will find that the core policies set forth above do not cover all the circumstances that your operating environment demands. Furthermore, state and local laws as well as federal standards will change, and that may influence the creation of a new policy for your practice/laboratory or a change in initial policy. Independent advisors, including your local legal counsel, should be consulted from time to time to ensure that all requisite policies are considered and properly framed. Important input can also be obtained via national conferences and webinars, such as those sponsored by the APF.

Management Reporting

Case: So How Are We Doing?

Dr. Charles Roubaix, the new president of Mountain Pathology Associates, was enjoying the opening reception at the annual meeting of the APF. He was meeting experienced leaders of practices like his own. But wow, the discussions were making him wonder about his own practice. Bernie, head of a large practice in New England, said his billing costs were under 5 %. Jim, from the far West, argued that the national billing company he used increased collections by 11 % over his prior in-house operation. George, from the Midwest, bragged that he had reduced days of A/R by nine after hiring a new business manager. Fortunately, the wine and finger food were good because Charles was a bit nervous. "Am I supposed to know these things about my practice? And how might I benchmark our performance and perhaps improve metrics?"

Discussion: There is a core set of revenue cycle management reports that you will want available to you on a monthly basis. These are essential to monitoring key elements of the system as well as its overall operation. Timeliness of management reports is critical, because you want to identify problems as early as possible to effect solutions well before things get out of hand.

Your practice is up and running after much planning and hard work. The fundamental revenue cycle system appears to be functioning smoothly and effectively. But how will you monitor its functionality on an ongoing basis? What metrics and benchmarks should you look at—and how often—to ensure that the system continues to operate in a proficient manner? We will give you key suggestions in this concluding section, based on our years of experience.

- *Operating Budget/Income Statement (See Section "Practice Structures", Chap. 1)*: An operating budget covering both projected net revenue (gross charges less discounts, allowances, and bad debts) and operating expenses (including physician base salaries and benefits) is essential to managing a pathology practice or laboratory. A budget is the roadmap that lets you judge month by month ("mile by mile") whether you are on course or straying into dangerous territory.

- *Revenue versus Receipts*: Gross revenue is the amount that is potentially collectible given the services you have furnished and your initial estimate of the unit value of each different service you provide. Of course, most government payers and private insurers will not pay your full usual and customary charge per procedure: They will demand an often significant discount. But you need to know the gross charges versus receipts per month for each major payer to ensure that payers are keeping their promises and that your billing office is promptly and properly filing claims with those payers. Similarly, bad debt, charity allowance, and other write-offs need to be monitored month by month to ensure that they are within expectations. You may also decide at some future date that your usual and customary charges are too high or too low based on the collection rates showing up in the monthly report.

- *Days of Revenue in Accounts Receivable*: An account receivable is a legal claim against an insurer or patient for services rendered and a promise of payment. Nonetheless, you cannot pay yourself or your employees until account receivable balances are converted to cash. (Yes, a bank might lend you money using your accounts receivable as collateral, but that can only go on for a short period of time.) Your objective is to convert patient account balances to cash as quickly as possible, say 28–40 days on average. Once the objective is set, it must be monitored against actual performance, and that is where the metric "days of revenue in accounts receivable" comes into play. The metric is calculated by dividing the gross account receivable balance by the average gross revenue per day—the account receivable balance and the gross revenue per day figures can represent the activity for individual payers, or they can represent all payers and patients in the aggregate.

- *Physician Productivity*: Monthly and year-to-date procedure volume information is very helpful in monitoring overall practice/laboratory performance as well as productivity at the individual physician level. The overall data is needed to determine if the entity is expanding or contracting, and the physician-level data is needed to determine if everyone is pulling their fair share of the total load. Of course, allowances should be made in advance for productivity adjustments that take into account such matters as practice/laboratory administrative duties, hospital medical director duties, practice specialty (e.g., dermatopathology versus general surgical pathology), and so on (see Appendix A, Case 1).

- *Charge Denial Rate*: You need the ability to break down payments and denials by payer and CPT code. A payer or insurer may deny one or more charges on a claim simply as a way to hassle you, but more often the denial means your billing office or commercial biller did not observe a required procedure code modifier, failed to take a quantity limit into account, or otherwise did not actually file a "clean claim" the first time around. (Medical necessity denials attributable to insufficient or nonconforming ICD diagnosis coding are an increasing source of charge rejection by payers and insurers at this time.) It is very important to monitor the absolute and relative number of charge denials by type and in total on an ongoing basis. These metrics will give you early warning if you have a training or motivation problem involving your billing personnel (or commercial billing agent) or an issue with a particular insurer that may require legal counsel intervention.

As your practice or laboratory matures, you will gain valuable experience and understanding regarding the management information that is helpful in maintaining the financial viability and effectiveness of the entity. You will also learn over time what allocation of management report information works best for your practice or laboratory; for example, what material is to be considered by the physician owners versus what data is best left in the hands of the practice or laboratory business administrator. Finally, you will gain insight into the format of management reports that is most meaningful to you and the other physician owners; for example, at a basic level, whether charts and graphs are preferable to more traditional numbers-oriented reports. Independent advisors might be retained from time to time to assist in refining the management reports and process.

Chapter 5
Applying the Knowledge

Michael L. Talbert

Implications and Strategies Driven by the Current System or "Why Are Things the Way They Are?"

Case: Exploiting Payment Anomalies

Dr. Carol Smith has completed an anatomic pathology/clinical pathology (AP/CP) residency and is 3 months into her surgical pathology fellowship. Her husband has a specialized job and would have difficulty moving. Dr. Smith has narrowed her job search to her current metropolitan area. Two jobs are available, and Dr. Smith has interviewed for both positions. The first position would be at an independent gastrointestinal (GI) pathology lab where she would sign out endoscopic biopsies approximately 8 a.m.–3 or 4 p.m. Monday through Friday with no night call or weekend work. The second position would entail joining three other pathologists covering a 300-bed hospital. Dr. Smith would do predominantly AP but also direct the microbiology laboratory. She would work 8 a.m.–5 or 6 p.m. with one in four nights and weekends on call. Weekend call would include about 8 h of work, including performing autopsies, if needed.

While the second job clearly involves more work in a higher acuity environment, the first job would pay approximately 20 % more per year with similar amounts of vacation. How could this be?

Discussion: While the higher acuity more general practice may offer a partnership opportunity and potentially be more stable, business models develop to exploit inefficiencies and inequities in the payment systems. As such, a pure outpatient biopsy lab focused on diagnostic biopsies can produce more revenue per pathologist than a more general practice environment, enabling a pathologist to potentially earn more while working less. However, the two work environments would be very different, and the more general environment may prove more interesting or more professionally fulfilling than the outpatient biopsy lab.

If we consider how physician services are compensated, much can be understood regarding business and practice trends over the recent decades. The bulk of physician services for Medicare patients are compensated through Medicare Part B and determined using submitted Current Procedural Terminology (CPT) codes. The

M. L. Talbert (✉)
Department of Pathology, University of Oklahoma Health Sciences Center, 940 Stanton
L. Young Blvd., BMSB 451, Oklahoma City, OK 73104, USA
e-mail: michael-talbert@ouhsc.edu

© Springer International Publishing Switzerland 2016
L. A. Hassell et al. (eds.), *Pathology Practice Management*,
DOI 10.1007/978-3-319-22954-6_5

situation is analogous for physician services provided for patients covered by Medicaid and private insurance. As such, the bulk of physician services are covered by relatively set payments per service provided, with the caveat that there be corresponding International Classification of Diseases (ICD) codes submitted to justify the provided service(s). This has led to a number of somewhat predictable trends.

Payment Per Service Rewards More/Additional Services

While physicians often discuss ethics, professionalism, the Hippocratic oath, and other lofty selfless concepts, the simple fact is that, in many settings, the more services you do, the more you are paid. Whether this is an explicit goal or an unrecognized bias for an individual or a group, there is an undeniable human tendency to want more. There is also often a disconnect between the cost of a service and its overall value. The decision to perform a second or third different confirmatory immunohistochemistry stain when one might suffice to support a diagnosis may not withstand the rigors of evidence-based medicine but may be rationalized based on feeling even more secure with a diagnosis or providing support for a strongly favored diagnosis should the first stain prove to be negative or noncontributory. This more subtle overuse of services that may be billed can also be driven by the sense of defensive medicine. For example, a pathologist may perform mucicarmine and immunohistochemical stains for keratin, carcinoembryonic antigen (CEA), leukocyte common antigen ("would not want to miss lymphoma"), and vimentin ("do we not always order vimentin to show that at least something stained?") for an otherwise straightforward diffuse infiltrating adenocarcinoma of the stomach with signet ring cells using the internal reasoning of, "if this ever went to court, I would want stains to support my diagnosis." In doing this, payments for this case could increase several fold, all in the name of "good medicine." The subtle or overt driver to perform more services on the physician side may be compounded by the lack of opposing drivers on the patient side. The patient may have a limited or, in many cases, no co-pay for the additional service(s). Plus the patient is already relying on the physician to do what is needed and not do what is not indicated.

This combination of drivers, even when physicians are well meaning, can bias toward additional services in any specialty or practice setting. Efforts have been made to mitigate these drivers through utilization review, utilization targets, capitation, and particularly more recently, the use of pricing pressures on the patient side, such as increased co-pays, high deductible policies, and in-network pricing.

Utilization controls through utilization review are simply denial of payments for services provided based on preestablished criteria that are sometimes unknown to the provider (so-called black box). These criteria can be based on factors such as age, number of services provided, or the specific ICD code provided among a host of other reasons. In some cases, payment may be obtained following submission of additional data/documentation regarding medical necessity, an action involving additional work and expense. Utilization targets may also be in the form of total expenses per patient per time period or episode of disease. For example, with capitation, there is a fixed payment per covered beneficiary for a specified time period with the provider or group of providers now financially incentivized to provide fewer services and hence retain a greater share of the fixed payment. Numerous variations on this approach exist. For instance, primary-care providers may "take risk" (i.e., accept the fixed payment up front, not knowing which services a group of covered beneficiaries will require), and subcontract with pathologists or independent laboratories typically at discounted prices or laboratory services could be "carved out" by the insurance company, which then may contract with, for example, a national laboratory. Some arrangements may also include certain "withheld" portions of the per member per month payment that constitutes the provider's risk of exceeding a utilization or total cost target such that an insurance company holds a percentage of the monthly payment that is released to the provider(s) only if patient expenditures do not exceed an established target. A pathology group may be involved in a number of these arrangements and will most probably have contracts with multiple insurance plans besides participating with Medicare and Medicaid. Understanding how each arrangement works is key, and the variety of payor contracts and hospital contracts a group may possess can create significant differences in pathologists' income between similar-sounding groups (e.g., six pathologists covering two hospitals).

Co-pays and high deductibles attempt to decrease utilization by incentivizing greater patient involvement in the care purchasing decision. If a patient must pay 20% of a bill or the first US$4000 of health care for a year, he or she may be more likely to question the provider about the benefits and necessity of a service before its provision. An offshoot of this is the move to "inform the consumer" through price transparency, with the idea that a patient may choose a less expensive provider if they know the price up front. Yet another variation along these lines is so-called reference pricing where an insurance company may cover up to a certain amount for a procedure, such as hip replacement, thereby incentivizing the patient to seek a provider charging the covered "reference" amount or less to avoid additional out-of-pocket expense.

On balance, these efforts probably do have some effect, but they also play out in the popular press and political discussions. Capitation is criticized as incentivizing physicians to withhold care for money, while utilization review by insurance companies may be characterized as insurers coming between doctors and their patients to limit care and maximize their profits. More recently, the effort to do pre-utilization control at the national level was attacked as creating "death panels." Our freewheeling, do-it-all system where the providers (including hospitals) do well, the insurers do well, and the patients bear limited direct liability for receiving one more medical service predictably drives up utilization and overall costs and is difficult to change without fundamentally adjusting the drivers themselves.

Some Services May Become More Attractive from a Reward Standpoint

Case: Some Services May Become More Attractive from a Reward Standpoint

Dr. Michael Smith, the new chairman of the Southern University pathology department, was preparing for his first round of annual faculty evaluations. To evaluate clinical productivity of his subspecialty surgical pathologists, he asked the departmental business administrator for a spreadsheet showing relative value units (RVUs) by pathologist and collected revenue by pathologist. A listing for three of the pathologists is shown in Table 5.1.

Dr. Smith scratched his head and thought, "Wow, they are so different. It looks like Dr. Free is not earning her clinical salary. I thought my anatomic pathology director said they had similar workloads."

How can this be?

Discussion: Though the RVU system was intended to normalize work effort and hence payment, with the relatively limited number of surgical pathology CPT codes, services under certain codes can vary substantially in difficulty and time required leading to variations in payment for work performed. In this example, the dermatopathology specialist is signing out large numbers of relatively simple skin biopsies and excisions under CPT code 88305. The breast pathologist, in contrast, does a mix of breast biopsies (CPT 88305), excisions (CPT 88305 and 88307), and mastectomies (CPT 88307 and 88309), each of which, on average, requires multiples of the work required for a skin biopsy/excision, even accounting for the differences in RVUs assigned to the higher codes for the breast pathologist. While the skin pathologist may be fairly compensated per service, the breast pathologist is relatively undercompensated for surgical pathology professional services.

For the pediatric pathologist, total RVUs fall somewhere in between. However, for the pediatric pathologist, on average, there may be more services provided for patients covered by Medicaid which, depending on how Medicaid payments are set in the state, can result in relatively different average payment per RVU as compared to collections of pathologists primarily providing services to a typical adult patient population of Medicare/Tricare/Champus, commercial insurance, Medicaid, and self-pay.

Therefore, given these variations in work, RVUs, and payment schema, the three faculty members could be doing similar amounts of work but collecting very different payment amounts. This example demonstrates how certain subspecialty areas can be more lucrative and illustrates why you must be cognizant of a wide variety of variables when considering issues of workload, pay, and fairness.

A typical business makes a profit by producing a product or providing a service for less than what the product or service costs to produce, creating a so-called profit margin. Bigger margins are typically better, and total profit rises as volume rises for products or services that have a positive margin. Margins and hence profits rise when costs are reduced, and often the cost of providing a unit of service or making

Table 5.1 Table for case: some services may become more attractive from a reward standpoint

Pathologist	Specialty	RVU	Collections (US$)
Dr. Jones	Dermatopathology	11,000	425,000
Dr. Howard	Pediatric pathology	5500	250,000
Dr. Free	Breast pathology	3100	100,000

RVU relative value unit

a product drops as volume rises, the so-called economy of scale. Applied to pathology, the margin on an 88305 diagnostic biopsy professional service is hopefully positive but depends on many factors: the time required to examine the biopsy, the efficiency of the pathologist, the efficiency of the sign-out process, the cost of billing, the efficiency of collection, the cost of the practice setting, the value of an 88305 on a negotiated fee schedule for patients with a negotiated fee schedule type payment arrangement, and even if the patient has coverage at all. The margin can be improved by improving any of these factors. Similarly, increases in volume may drive efficiencies or enable greater investment in the system to provide automation and better computerization.

While there are over 8000 different CPT codes, one weakness of this system for defining services is the difference in efforts and expenses to provide different services that may be described by the same CPT code. As an extreme example of this breadth in pathology, an 88305 professional component may describe a relatively straightforward skin biopsy of a basal cell carcinoma or a difficult breast needle core biopsy of a complex sclerosing lesion. Yet, the payment for each service would be the same if the patients had the same insurance payment scheme. An experienced pathologist could diagnose several basal cell carcinomas in the time required for the breast core biopsy, resulting in a skewing of payments on a time basis even if the breast biopsy required additional CPT codes for immunohistochemical stains. There are similar differences in the technical component. Embedding, cutting, and staining a nine-block transurethral resection of the prostate (88305-technical component, 88305-TC) is much more work and, hence, expense than performing the technical component on a simple single-block skin biopsy.

These apparent discrepancies between effort and payment have led to a sort of arbitrage effort to capture "easy" specimens while avoiding, at least on a relative basis, more difficult specimens. So we have seen the growth of large, sometimes venture-funded laboratories that focus on outpatient biopsies, along with the trend toward insourcing pathology services by non-pathologist-owned clinical practices, especially for skin, GI, and genitourinary specimens. This has been done to exploit the relative differences in effort required to provide services under a single CPT code, to effect economies of scale, and to take advantage of the gradual rise in the technical component over the decade and a half before 2013. Predictably, the model came under much reexamination when the 88305-TC was reduced by 53% January 1, 2013. (Once again, this showed the power of payment schema to impact how and where health care is delivered. When trying to understand the health system, it is often useful to start with understanding how the money flows.)

The result has been that the hospital-based pathologist has felt under siege, not necessarily controlling the flow of cases and now relying on the more difficult and time-intensive specimens while providing frozen section coverage and overseeing a 24/7 laboratory service. Also predictable was the 20-year push for hospital-based pathologists to gain control of "the means of production" by taking over the provision of histology services from the hospital. This allowed the hospital to exit a service they had limited interest in while the pathologist could then focus on improving specimen flow, increasing investment to improve pathologists' productivity, and possibly combining multiple smaller histology labs to gain economy of scale. It also provided an otherwise hospital-bound pathology group with a platform to expand its outpatient reach aided by enhanced informatics among other flexibilities and to expand test menus to increase immunohistochemical stains and add molecular testing.

> Using RVUs for a set of procedures as a comparative measure is conceptually a powerful idea, but for procedures with a VERY broad range of effort such as the CPT code 88305, it has introduced perverse incentives and misleading conclusions relative to underlying relative effort and cost that plagues pathology practice today.

Not all of these resulting effects have been negative. Centralization of specimen types can allow for greater practitioner specialization, more standardized and focused evaluation protocols and reporting, and enhanced informatics. All of these translate into potentially better patient care and provider service. Successful primarily hospital-based pathology groups have been able to grow outreach, better integrate patient care over a region, and develop greater specialization and depth of expertise. The trade-off has been discontinuity of care with biopsies leaving the practice area where resections and other treatments are done, creation of multiple smaller condo and pod labs staffed by a single and sometimes part-time pathologist, and a disincentive to practice in the inpatient environment—a critical role for pathologists. And predictably, the incentives of an "in-house lab" for urologists (and others) have been shown to lead to increased numbers of biopsies when compared with urology practices that do not profit from having histology and pathology "in house" [1, 2].

Case: Consolidating Histology Services

Mountain Pathology Associates (MPA) is a 15-pathologist practice in the upper Midwest that serves the regional tertiary care referral center and five smaller hospitals in the region. MPA had had some success in the office-based market, usually with physicians who felt strong alignment to an MPA-served hospital, but a national commercial laboratory provided the majority of outpatient clinical and anatomical services with a slick reporting system and regular courier service.

Mountain Pathology pathologists felt frustrated by the sophistication of technical component services provided by the various hospitals. While each hospital had a histology laboratory, some had only limited immunohistochemistry menus. To make matters worse, between the six hospitals, there were three anatomic computer systems, none of which interfaced with physician offices. At a strategic retreat, MPA pathologists determined that they must control their means of production and update their IT capabilities to compete with the national commercial laboratory. Also, several pathologists worried that the limitations in their technical component support were making it difficult to recruit new fellowship-trained pathologists from cutting-edge programs.

Over the ensuing weeks, with the help of a national consultant, a plan was designed. The smaller hospitals were approached about getting out of the histology business. In essence, the pathology group would buy the equipment and hire the personnel with the goal of centralization. MPA promised a new anatomic information system and would use couriers to move tissues and slides. Hospitals would be billed for patients covered by federal payors, and economically, the hospitals would see a neutral outcome when comparing the new setup with net revenues from running their own histology labs. In return for working with the pathologists, the hospitals could expect faster turnaround times through use of an expanded immunohistochemistry menu and better reporting through use of a new AP system. It was felt that all practitioners would like the new arrangement. Four of the five small hospitals agreed to participate in the project, and thus, Opus Diagnostic

Services (ODS) was born. Within 6 months, much of the promise was realized, and within the first year, ODS was profitable and adding additional services. At this point, the fifth small hospital histology laboratory was folded in, and finally, after 18 months, the tertiary care histology lab was absorbed by the now booming ODS. By this time as well, the immunohistochemistry menu was 50 % larger than the menu at the tertiary care histology lab, and substantial additional outpatient AP volume had been added. While the new entity ran more efficiently, no personnel were laid off as they were needed to handle the new business. Volume had grown so much that a new pathologist had been recruited, and a second recruitment was beginning.

Discussion: The success of a pathology practice depends in part, if not substantially, on the quality and degree of technical component support. Gaining control of histology and secretarial functions can lead to substantial improvements, create opportunity for growth, allow for advancements in information technology, and reorganize the competitive landscape in a region.

Case: GI Biopsy Problems

Dr. Phil Mayes put down his pen and looked up from the numbers on the legal pad. "This is going to be ugly," he sighed. The three big gastroenterology groups in the metro area had just announced a merger and Phil's pathology group had been asked to "bid on" the new combined group's endoscopy center business. While the GI group preferred to open their own histology laboratory with a contracted pathologist as medical director, the group was also looking for some form of bundled pricing of pathology professional fees. They wished to develop novel pricing schemes and expand market penetrance and reach. The GI group announced a 7-day response time for proposals and indicated that they were soliciting proposals from other pathology service providers.

All this created quite a dilemma for Dr. Mayes and his group. They risked loss of their current business, but in meeting the goals of the GI group, while it might mean a growth of GI biopsy business, the incremental gain would be limited and overall could be negative once the additional professional effort was factored in. At this point, Dr. Mayes resolved to phone two other pathology group leaders from different parts of the country that he had become friends with through national meetings. He hoped to talk through the situation and see what ideas the others had; perhaps they had faced similar situations.

Discussion: The outpatient biopsy market is much more fluid than the inpatient market. CPT codes and their professional components do not distinguish between inpatient and outpatient markets even though inpatient cases are typically more difficult and an inpatient practice entails much more of a 24 h/7 days a week approach. While a stable outpatient biopsy business can be very lucrative to a pathology practice, control of the market can be difficult as other practices and even other specialties devise strategies to reap some of these potential gains.

References

1. Mitchell J. Linkages between utilization of prostate surgical pathology services and physician self-referral. Medicare Medicaid Res Rev. 2012;2(3). doi: http://dx.doi.org/10.5600/mmrr.002.03.a02.
2. Mitchell JM. Urologists' self-referral for pathology of biopsy specimens linked to increased use and lower prostate cancer detection. Health Aff. 2012;31(4):741–749. doi:10.1377/hlthaff.2011.1372.

Chapter 6
Current Major Trends and Considerations for the Future

Michael L. Talbert

Case: Proving Our Value

Dr. Gina Pizotti took her second deep breath as she finished reviewing Midwestern Pathology Associates' (MPA) most recent monthly financials. Anatomic pathology monthly revenue had fallen by US$5000 compared to 1 year ago. Losing the local dermatology practice's biopsies to a national lab had created a deficit that was hard to fill. Payments for other anatomic services were at best flat, and there seemed to be limited prospects for additional new business. A total of US$60,000 a year—that was US$10,000/pathologist—was a tough revenue shortfall when everyone was working so hard.

The medical directorship contract would be up for renegotiation in 8 months. The hospital claimed to be struggling to stay in the black, and Dr. Pizotti had heard that some of the other clinical medical director contracts had simply been eliminated. As president of MPA, Dr. Pizotti felt responsible for keeping incomes at least level.

Discussion: This is not a unique scenario and illustrates the challenge for many pathology practices. Part B revenue has become harder to grow, and payment per service has not been rising significantly. Many practices are looking at new approaches to being paid. With hospital margins under pressure in many settings, simply expecting the hospital to increase directorship payments is typically not viable. Many pathologists are looking at possible gainsharing models where pathologist-led initiatives at cost reductions or other positive outcomes could be directly compensated. Some pathology groups are simply documenting such interventions in anticipation of future contract negotiations with the idea of showing value and either negotiating increasing payments or avoiding potential cuts. In the MPA example, perhaps the blood bank director had implemented a new blood product utilization review system that saved US$50,000 over the past year, or perhaps a new molecular platform in microbiology reduced broad-spectrum antibiotic usage and reduced the length of stay in patients with certain infections. Capturing such "clinical vignettes" and quantitating their impact could be invaluable at contract discussion time, especially if the gains were, in total, quite significant. And, for those interventions for which gains were sustained over time, the gains would be like an annuity and accrued year after year. Of course, as in many other areas of life, the question is often, "what have you done for me lately," so this approach would be an ongoing process, much like documenting process improvement.

Much of the challenge of leading the financial aspects of a pathology practice lies in adapting to national and local trends. While we currently seem to be in a time of

M. L. Talbert (✉)
Department of Pathology, University of Oklahoma Health Sciences Center,
940 Stanton L. Young Blvd., BMSB 451, Oklahoma City, OK 73104, USA
e-mail: michael-talbert@ouhsc.edu

© Springer International Publishing Switzerland 2016
L. A. Hassell et al. (eds.), *Pathology Practice Management*,
DOI 10.1007/978-3-319-22954-6_6

very rapid change in pathology as well as the rest of medicine, the change is occurring unevenly across the country, and responses have varied region to region. Looking out over the next several years, multiple trends must be considered:

1. The rise of value-based purchasing/pay for performance and the expansion of quality incentive programs such as the Physician Quality Reporting System (PQRS) with transition to the Merit-Based Incentive Payment System (MIPS) in 2019
2. The growth of accountable care organizations (ACO), bundled payments, and similar new arrangements of providers
3. Continued downward pressure on payments for pathology and laboratory services
4. Challenges in the workforce—numbers, training, and adaptability
5. Potential influence of technologic disrupters, for example, insourcing with digital pathology, in vivo microscopy, enhanced biomarkers for primary diagnosis and monitoring, and increasing point-of-care testing options
6. For academic pathologists, continued uncertainty in funding for graduate medical education (GME) and research

Two of the more interesting trends are the growth of value-based purchasing/pay for performance and ACOs, trends that are partly driven by the Affordable Care Act (Patient Protection and Affordable Care Act, a.k.a., Obamacare) but which have also been embraced by private insurers with numerous "demonstrations" and experiments in different markets. With value-based purchasing, the payor, for example Medicare or a private insurance company, will vary payment for a service or services based on some factor in addition to justification of medical necessity. For example, for a few years, pathologists enjoyed the possibility of a small percentage increase in their overall payments from Medicare for successful participation in PQRS, which is now a penalty for failure to participate. Similarly, hospitals may have a small payment variation based on certain measures for common conditions such as congestive heart failure and diabetes or patient satisfaction scores. Currently, most pay for performance is based on process measures, but it is expected that, with time, the focus will shift to true outcome measures such as risk-adjusted mortality or other measures of health, and efficiency measures, such as adjusted length of stay. For pathologists, that may pose a distinct challenge. PQRS is now based on specific pathologist actions in defined service scenarios using intermediate process measures. How we pathologists will demonstrate an effect on patient outcomes is unclear, though it would seem that laboratories that have embraced a Lean culture and are reaping the process improvement results may have evidence of efficiency improvements they can share with their institutions. Practice leaders should therefore closely follow this trend and ponder how their professional efforts affect the continuum of care and outcomes for both outpatients and inpatients.

A similar dilemma exists with ACOs. An ACO is a group of providers, typically physicians or physicians and hospitals, that provides health services for a defined population. Currently, the aim is to share savings versus the expected expenditures. In this model, the effort will be towards population health, keeping people out of the hospital, and managing chronic disease. Once again, the role of the pathologist, how pathologists will show value and how pathologists will be paid, remains to be determined and may be shaped by pathologists themselves. As such, pathologists must work hard to remain relevant in the process and perhaps seek to lead in any ACO discussions and potential ACO formation within their own practice environments. Individual practices and organized pathology should be keenly interested in gathering outcome and impact data from their interventions to bring to these discussions. A similar challenge exists with clinically integrated organizations (CIO).

The discussion above implies at least some move towards payment models other than fee-for-service. A pathologist or pathology group that is part of an ACO for at least a portion of their practice could be compensated on some form of internal fee-for-service model, on a salary basis, or perhaps by a different arrangement. If pathologists are able to adapt and bring value by reducing unnecessary testing, improving and accelerating the workup and diagnosis of patients, facilitating outpatient management of chronic disease, and ultimately by showing measurable impact on patient outcomes, they should seek some form of value-based compensation lest they risk being further commoditized to the level of a "purchased service." In valuing such gains, however, pathologists should not fall prey to single sum benefits based on achieved savings, especially when those savings may be recurring year after year. Looking out 10 years, the changes will be gradual, and it is hard to believe that a component of typical fee-for-service does not still exist in a decade. As such, there will most likely be a prolonged period with multiple major payment schemes and continued evolution of payment schemes to reward outcomes. This evolution will most likely differ from region to region and will itself offer opportunities to arbitrage between the differing systems depending on the skills and experience of a practice and where the most attractive margins may appear.

The recent Medicare Access and CHIP Reauthorization Act of 2015's consolidation of incentives into the MIPS signals the next level of changes, at least for Medicare. Other payors will likely continue to evolve similarly. While rulemaking and implementation should be carefully followed, the general trend and outline are clear: Existing incentive programs will be rolled together and more strongly coupled to alternative payment mechanisms. While the recent legislation maps some Medicare payment factors out more than 10 years, pathologists and pathology practices must continue to appropriately position themselves in their local environment.

At present, there is downward pressure on payment rates for pathology and laboratory services. In 2013, we saw Medicare cuts to payments for the histology technical component and molecular testing. In 2014, there were changes in how immunohistochemistry and fluorescence in situ hybridization (FISH; which Medicare deemed to be overvalued) were reimbursed. In 2015, Centers for Medicare & Medicaid Services (CMS) further restricted coding for prostate biopsies as prostate biopsies were targeted as an overutilized service. This downward pressure shows no sign of abating, which will continue to drive pathologists to focus on efficiencies and productivity as well as to seek alternative payment methods such as those described above.

Similar downward pressures exist in funds for the research and education missions for academic institutions. Overall, National Institutes of Health (NIH) funding has been nearly flat, and situations such as the "sequester" have reduced funding across all grants. Other sources of research funding such as industry and foundations have not increased to close the gap and, in many cases, have been under pressure themselves. With funding success for the individual NIH grant in the single digits and the decline in clinical revenue pressuring the historic cross subsidy of clinical funds into the research operation of most academic centers (the grants themselves do not entirely pay for the research mission and infrastructure), many academic centers are scaling back on research, requiring higher funding productivity or salary and indirect cost coverage on grants, or eliminating programs. Much of the same story exists with funding for GME, that is, residents and fellows. Payments to hospitals have been reduced and discussion continues in political circles regarding further cuts. Paradoxically, this contrasts with increases in numbers of medical schools and medical school class sizes in response to current and projected physician shortages. We have more training positions to grant medical degrees but are not increasing the corresponding postgraduate training positions; in fact, in typical schizophrenic political fashion, pressure towards the opposite is occurring. How this plays out for individual practices is difficult to predict. A relative shortage of pathologists would put upward pressure on wages and further differentiate successful practices (they will be able to recruit) while structural changes in health care and pathology in particular could result in a surplus of pathologists or, more likely, create a subset of pathologists who do not have the skillset or mindset and ability to adapt to the changing environment. Clearly, pathology training programs will also need to continue evolving to produce graduates capable of success in the changing environment.

In the challenging environment described above, pathologists also must be cognizant of the two-edged sword of technological change. While a new technology such as in vivo microscopy or next-generation sequencing can provide new service opportunities for pathologists and also potentially help pathologists differentiate themselves from competitors, poorly deployed new technology or an inability to afford new technology can place a practice at a competitive disadvantage. Furthermore, while it is relatively easy to evaluate a new technology's impact on similar types of practices, as described by Harvard Business School's business guru and best-selling author Clayton Christenson [1, 2], some of the most disruptive changes originate outside a particular industry. So a new technology or business model such as outsourcing pathology professional services via the cloud to a third world country with lower wages (difficult or impossible now but not inconceivable in the future) could radically and suddenly alter the pathology practice playing field.

Case: Better Information Technology

Dr. Bessin leaned back from the scope with a sense of satisfaction. He had worked for some 6 months programming his "digital sign-out assistant," and it had performed flawlessly as he signed out 30 colon biopsy cases. He had completed the cases in about half the time required without the digital assistant and without a secretary. Dr. Bessin smiled and thought aloud, "I wonder if I can get the digital assistant optimized for large resection specimens."

Discussion: Pathology is an information specialty—the correct diagnosis presented in an actionable format delivered how and where needed…in the appropriate time frame. Thus, information technology (IT) is vital to nearly all aspects of our practices. Pathologists should actively consider potential IT strategies and upgrades for their practices and be prepared to invest in improvements. While in-depth consideration of IT strategies, technology, technology evaluation, and IT purchase are beyond the scope of this book, areas for consideration, and this list is not exhaustive and will continue to grow over time, would include:

- Specimen identification and tracking: Bar codes and radio-frequency identification (RFID) tags have replaced hand labeling of specimens and in doing so, have increased patient safety (fewer lost or mislabeled specimens) and allowed for scanning and better tracking with increased efficiency on the front end (pre-analytic) stages of operation.
- Enhanced accessioning: Better electronic health record (EHR) and laboratory information system (LIS) connectivity have reduced reliance on paper requisitions, enhanced information flow, decreased challenges in handwriting interpretation, and improved the downstream billing process.
- Process control: Positive specimen identification at each step in the diagnostic process has yielded impressive gains in productivity when coupled with techniques such as Lean and Six Sigma. We know of several situations where groups have either programmed their own process control systems (envision a bar code scanner at every touch point in the surgical pathology process) or purchased systems that have led to substantial and sustained improvement in surgical pathology case throughput by identifying bottlenecks, mapping the peaks and valleys of specimen flow, and identifying unwanted variation in procedures.
- Gross description: Tools such as gross templates, voice recognition, and integrated digital photography have greatly improved grossing throughput and allowed for error reduction and simplification as compared to the rambling descriptions of old.
- Microscopic diagnosis: Facilitating the pathologist's work may provide the "biggest bang for the buck." From digital dictation and voice recognition to templates and preformatted reports to online tools and ancillary test ordering, many practices have steadily increased pathologist productivity by focusing the pathologist on the high-value activity of examining slides and making diagnoses. As total digital pathology becomes a reality, we anticipate continued gains and practice differentiation. These particular gains are an imperative; pathology professional component payments have, on the whole, declined over the past two decades when accounting for inflation and, most likely, at best, will continue to lag inflation.
- Photography: Digital imaging has become ubiquitous (think Google glass), easily manipulated, and easily stored. Documentation for medical, teaching, research, medicolegal, or marketing purposes has been greatly simplified.
- Reporting: Better IT for reporting may be a hot area over the next several years as we focus on making our progressively more complex reports easily understood while retaining the entire diagnostic, prognostic, and treatment-oriented data set. Concepts such as the integrated disease report that is essentially redone sequentially as additional studies become available are being piloted. A few practices have worked to combine pathology and radiologic information into a single "diagnostic report."
- Consultative decision support: Managing population health and maximizing the utility of testing while limiting waste of resources in a world of very complex test menus requires the development of sophisticated decision support tools, algorithms, and real-time access to pathologist consultative expertise. Leading practices and institutions have developed disease-management teams equipped with appropriate IT tools to avoid improper use of laboratory tests and improve reflex-testing schemes.
- Report delivery: As our health system complexity continues to grow and providers are progressively more afloat in a sea of information, a clear, concise report delivered to the right person(s) at the right place on the right device in an appropriate timeframe has become even more important. Flexibility in report delivery complicates IT challenges but can provide a distinct competitive advantage. Patient-accessible reports are a growing trend and can bring pathologists much closer to their patients.
- Data mining: With the growing emphasis on outcomes, bundled payments, and caring for defined populations, data mining has grown in importance. Whether at the practice level, the

hospital level, or population level, pathologists must be involved in the process. Pathology and laboratory testing produces numerous discrete data sets on patients and represents much of the objective data in a patient's medical record. Uses range from quality improvement and practice standardization to measuring cost of care and providing outcomes data. As insurers look to further control costs, novel arrangements will create new methods of data sharing with insurers.

- Billing: Billing systems continue to mature, and electronic filing and remittance continue to boost productivity and reduce errors. The growth of novel arrangements such as bundled payments may stress current billing capabilities or may provide a boon.
- Marketing: Digital media such as Facebook, Twitter, YouTube, and the like are radically altering fundamental communication—that is, how messages are sent and received. What this means for pathologists and their customers, patients and providers, remains to be seen. Perhaps your practice will create a new paradigm.
- Quality assurance: Whole-slide imaging can greatly facilitate case sharing both across a practice and across the globe. While computer-based diagnosis of surgical pathology seems a few years off, digital tools such as neural networks and measuring tool suites can aid pathologists in assuring patient safety.
- Overall practice management: It is now possible to measure many more aspects of a practice than even 10 years ago. Whether specimen transit time, collections per submitting provider or patient zip code, time spent by a single histologic slide on a pathologist's microscope stage or time from receipt to opening of a report by a clinician who constantly complains about turnaround time, IT is clearly revolutionizing practice management. Overall, opportunities abound for major improvements in productivity, quality, patient safety, and service. What competitive advantage can you create for your practice on this front?

References

1. Christenson. C. The innovator's dilemma: when new technologies cause great firms to fail. Watertown, MA: Harvard Business Review Press; 1997.
2. Christensen CM, Grossman JH, Hwang J. The innovator's prescription: a disruptive solution for health care. New York: McGraw-Hill Publishing; 2008.
3. Nash DB, et al. Population health: creating a culture of wellness. 2nd ed. Burlington, MA: Jones & Bartlett Learning LLC; 2016.

Part II
Financial Management of a Practice

Overview

Case: Time versus Money

Rick, Fred, and George have practiced pathology together for over 15 years in a five-pathologist group. All three are empty nesters and enjoy traveling and outdoor activities. Over lunch one day, Fred opined, "You know, if we hired a sixth pathologist, we could each take another 7 or 8 weeks of vacation each year." George, the most financially conservative one of the three, weighed in, "I guess we would make less money, right?"

Discussion: For independent pathology groups in particular, there is an ongoing dynamic between time and money. Work more, make more money; work less, make less money. While these both philosophical and practical discussions fall under a discussion of group dynamics, such discussions are meaningless without understanding a group's finances. What does hiring a pathologist cost a practice, both initially in the early years of practice and then when the once new pathologist is paid similarly to the senior pathologists? Any calculation would need to include salary, bonus, benefits, professional expenses, malpractice insurance, office expenses, and any additional support. This would indicate a need for well-characterized expense categories and bookkeeping.

An independent private practice is essentially a small business. A department of pathologists employed by a hospital is analogous to a division in a large company. An academic department may range from being like a small business unit with relatively independent financial decision-making and the ability to retain "profits" (excess revenues minus expenses) to something financially resembling the department of employed pathologists where the finances are essentially managed by the larger organization.

That being said, all practice groups, whether independent or integrated into a larger organization, should have an income statement, a budget, and a means of tracking any reserves, while an independent practice should also maintain and use a balance sheet. An *income statement* is a tabulation of revenues and expenses that yields a net gain, loss, or break even for the time period under consideration. A *budget* is essentially a projected income statement in which future revenues and expenses are forecast for a defined time period. The ongoing experience in the form of an income statement is then periodically compared to the budget or forecast which generates variances between actual amounts and budgeted amounts that then should be investigated/explained. A *balance sheet* lists an entity's assets against liabilities to provide insight into the capital situation of a practice. Simple practices will have limited assets and few if any liabilities, typically limited to pending bills. A more sophisticated practice may have more assets and/or a line of credit. More complicated arrangements, such as when the pathologists own a histology laboratory, are often achieved through the use of a second corporate entity (see below) which would have its own income statement and balance sheet, a balance sheet that would then reflect any equipment, computer system, and/or owned laboratory space as well as any debts.

Chapter 7
The Income Statement

Linda McLean and Michael L. Talbert

Case: Income Statement

Dr. Tom Stanton is completing his third year with Mountain Pathology Associates and has been voted in as a partner pathologist effective next month. He has heard stories of six-figure end-of-year bonuses for the partners and has been looking forward to making a major payment on his remaining school loans. However, when the president of the group informed Tom of his successful partnership vote, he was also told that bonuses would be much smaller than usual due to the combination of decreased revenues and increased expenses leading to a much lower net. Tom has felt dazed for 2 days since that conversation and has wondered if he may have joined the wrong group. His wife told him, "Maybe you should learn more about the revenues and expenses. After all, you are going to be a partner."

Discussion: Ultimately, in an independent private practice or practice that controls its own revenues, money available for salaries will reflect the interplay between revenues and expenses. All practices should track revenues and expenses with an income statement and work to optimize the net income through increasing revenues and controlling expenses in a measured, sensible fashion. Tom's wife is correct. Tom should ensure that close attention is paid to revenues and expenses through an income statement and, if he has suspicions that insufficient attention is being paid to these important elements, he should work to rectify the situation and perhaps volunteer to help.

The income statement is the key tool for managing the financial aspects of a practice. Its structure is:

Revenue − Expenses = Net income

Those responsible for monitoring the financial health of a practice (or a lab or any other business) must both understand *and* believe the numbers and hence information provided by an income statement. In the authors' experience, this may require time to understand how parts of the income statement interact and to adjust

L. McLean (✉) · M. L. Talbert
Department of Pathology, University of Oklahoma Health Sciences Center, 940 Stanton
L. Young Blvd., BMSB 451, Oklahoma City, OK 73104, USA
e-mail: linda-mclean@ouhsc.edu

M. L. Talbert
e-mail: michael-talbert@ouhsc.edu

© Springer International Publishing Switzerland 2016
L. A. Hassell et al. (eds.), *Pathology Practice Management*,
DOI 10.1007/978-3-319-22954-6_7

categories to better reflect how the practice is operating. Each month (typically, reporting periods are monthly) as these numbers become available from your accountant or business administrator, one should look at absolute numbers for each entry, whether revenue or expense, and compare numbers with the prior month and budget. It can also be very helpful to smooth out some of the natural month-to-month variability by looking at fiscal year-to-date numbers and comparing them to both prior year-to-date numbers and budgeted year-to-date. Any significant variance should be explained. While you may learn to expect certain levels of variances in numbers such as revenue from Part B billing or supply expenses, any unexpected variances should be investigated. By investigating and explaining variances, one can decide if a variance is a onetime event or portends something more significant. It may also lead one to identify problems such as a client who no longer sends work to you, a change in denial practices by major insurance companies, or an accidental overcharge from a vendor. By identifying and explaining variances in income statement categories, one can better understand the practice, protect the practice by mitigating the impact of the changing environment and more accurately analyze future threats and opportunities.

> Look for the deviations—the outliers in either direction—to get the most from review of your financial statements.

Case: Mountain Pathology Income Statement I

Figure 7.1 shows a simplified income statement for Mountain Pathology Group, an eight-pathologist practice covering two hospitals, a large central hospital and a smaller satellite hospital 6 miles away. Mountain Pathology Group rents space in a business park where their billing and accounting operations are housed. The group employs two general administrative personnel and three billing staff. A part-time accountant keeps the books. They contract for legal advice, tax support, and additional accounting.

Note the overall structure of the income statement: Revenue–Expense = Net income.

Each month the accountant updates the income statement and the two most senior partners review the numbers.

Case: Mountain Pathology Income Statement II

For March (Fig. 7.2), the two senior partners identified five areas (yellow) of potential concern or opportunity to review with the accountant.

Describe possible scenarios for each highlighted item.

1. Although the practice could have been billing for the professional component of clinical pathology (CPC), they had not been. Billing for CPC began in January of the previous fiscal year and revenue began rising in January and February. A year into CPC billing, collections are much higher.
2. Contractual adjustments are the differences between billed amounts for services and money collected. For example, the list price of an 88305 (Current Procedural

Revenue and Expense Statement - Mountain Pathology Group	Jan	Feb	Year to Date (YTD)	Last YTD	YTD monthly average	Last YTD monthly average
Revenue						
Part A - Main Hospital	$27,000	$29,000	$56,000	$55,000	$28,000	$27,500
Part A - Satelite Hospital	$2,000	$2,000	$4,000	$4,000	$2,000	$2,000
Professional service income						
Patient Billing - Clinical Pathology Component	$45,000	$45,212	$90,212	$32,500	$45,106	$16,250
Patient Billing - Part B	$702,000	$699,000	$1,401,000	$1,356,200	$700,500	$678,100
Contractual adjustments, bad debt, patient refunds...	-$375,000	-$385,200	-$760,200	-$705,000	-$380,100	-$352,500
Private autopsies	$8,000	$12,000	$20,000	$17,000	$10,000	$8,500
Other income [veterinary specimens, interest]	$1,256	$2,430	$3,686	$2,600	$1,843	$1,300
Total Income	$410,256	$404,442	$814,698	$762,300	$407,349	$381,150
Expenses	Jan	Feb	Year to Date (YTD)	Last YTD	YTD monthly average	Last YTD monthly average
Pathologists' Salaries	$186,900	$187,900	$374,800	$355,000	$187,400	$177,500
Bonuses	$0	$150,000	$150,000	$120,000	$75,000	$60,000
Administrative & Staff Salaries	$20,833	$20,833	$41,666	$39,500	$20,833	$19,750
Fringe benefits [Payroll taxes, FICA, insurance, pension contribution, workers comp]	$51,933	$89,683	$141,617	$118,335	$70,808	$59,168
Total Salaries	$259,666	$448,416	$708,083	$632,835	$354,041	$316,418
Educational, Conferences, Dues, Subscriptions	$523	$3,200	$3,723	$4,200	$1,862	$2,100
Professional fees - legal, licenses, consults, malpractice	$8,522	$8,563	$17,085	$12,750	$8,543	$6,375
Building expenses						
Rent/Mortgage	$2,300	$2,300	$4,600	$4,200	$2,300	$2,100
Depreciation	$600	$600	$1,200	$1,100	$600	$550
Maintenance - Office, computers, building, etc.	$2,635	$1,625	$4,260	$4,000	$2,130	$2,000
Utilities - phone, IT, pagers, electric, building insurance	$2,744	$2,306	$5,050	$4,200	$2,525	$2,100
Equipment - Office, computers, etc.	$944	$22,300	$23,244	$3,700	$11,622	$1,850
Supplies, postage	$2,700	$153	$2,853	$3,250	$1,427	$1,625
Other - software, mileage	$4,685	$450	$5,135	$7,500	$2,568	$3,750
Total Supplies	$25,653	$41,497	$67,150	$44,900	$33,575	$22,450
Total Expenses	$285,319	$489,913	$775,233	$677,735	$387,616	$338,868
Net Income	$124,937	-$85,471	$39,466	$84,565	$19,733	$42,283
Net Income over Revenue %	30.5%	-21.1%	4.8%	11.1%	4.8%	11.1%

Fig. 7.1 Mountain Pathology Income Statement I

Terminology (CPT) code for a typical diagnostic biopsy) is higher than the Medicare rate or rates contracted with insurance companies. The use of higher rates maximizes income by ensuring a billed rate above what an insurance company may pay (you do not want to leave anything on the table), but has the perverse effect of billing very large amounts to patients with no insurance, many of whom cannot pay despite being responsible for a relatively high bill. Higher rates also result in higher contractual adjustments. For Mountain Pathology Group, contracts were renegotiated and the negotiations were not as successful as in past years. The contractual rates dropped. Additionally, Medicare re-evaluated two of the most used CPT codes and decreased their reimbursement rate.

Revenue and Expense Statement - Mountain Pathology Group	Jan	Feb	Year to Date (YTD)	Last YTD	YTD monthly average	Last YTD monthly average	Need to explain
Revenue							
Part A - Main Hospital	$27,000	$29,000	$56,000	$55,000	$28,000	$27,500	
Part A - Satelite Hospital	$2,000	$2,000	$4,000	$4,000	$2,000	$2,000	
Professional service income							
Patient Billing - Clinical Pathology Component	$45,000	$45,212	$90,212	$32,500	$45,106	$16,250	1
Patient Billing - Part B	$702,000	$699,000	$1,401,000	$1,356,200	$700,500	$678,100	
Contractual adjustments, bad debt, patient refunds...	-$375,000	-$385,200	-$760,200	-$705,000	-$380,100	-$352,500	2
Private autopsies	$8,000	$12,000	$20,000	$17,000	$10,000	$8,500	
Other income [veterinary specimens, interest]	$1,256	$2,430	$3,686	$2,600	$1,843	$1,300	
Total Income	$410,256	$404,442	$814,698	$762,300	$407,349	$381,150	
Expenses	Jan	Feb	Year to Date (YTD)	Last YTD	YTD monthly average	Last YTD monthly average	Need to explain
Pathologists' Salaries	$186,900	$187,900	$374,800	$355,000	$187,400	$177,500	3
Bonuses	$0	$150,000	$150,000	$120,000	$75,000	$60,000	
Administrative & Staff Salaries	$20,833	$20,833	$41,666	$39,500	$20,833	$19,750	
Fringe benefits [Payroll taxes, FICA, insurance, pension contribution, workers comp]	$51,933	$89,683	$141,617	$118,335	$70,808	$59,168	3
Total Salaries	$259,666	$448,416	$708,083	$632,835	$354,041	$316,418	
Educational, Conferences, Dues, Subscriptions	$523	$3,200	$3,723	$4,200	$1,862	$2,100	
Professional fees - legal, licenses, consults, malpractice	$8,522	$8,563	$17,085	$12,750	$8,543	$6,375	4
Building expenses							
Rent/Mortgage	$2,300	$2,300	$4,600	$4,200	$2,300	$2,100	
Depreciation	$600	$600	$1,200	$1,100	$600	$550	
Maintenance - Office, computers, building, etc.	$2,635	$1,625	$4,260	$4,000	$2,130	$2,000	
Utilities - phone, IT, pagers, electric, building insurance	$2,744	$2,306	$5,050	$4,200	$2,525	$2,100	
Equipment - Office, computers, etc.	$944	$22,300	$23,244	$3,700	$11,622	$1,850	5
Supplies, postage	$2,700	$153	$2,853	$3,250	$1,427	$1,625	
Other - software, mileage	$4,685	$450	$5,135	$7,500	$2,568	$3,750	
Total Supplies	$25,653	$41,497	$67,150	$44,900	$33,575	$22,450	
Total Expenses	$285,319	$489,913	$775,233	$677,735	$387,616	$338,868	
Net Income	$124,937	-$85,471	$39,466	$84,565	$19,733	$42,283	
Net Income over Revenue %	30.5%	-21.1%	4.8%	11.1%	4.8%	11.1%	

Fig. 7.2 Mountain Pathology Income Statement II

3. Since the practice's profit margin was high last year, pathologists were given raises. Fringe benefits rose a corresponding amount plus the increased fringe benefit cost reflects rising rates for the group-provided health insurance.
4. The renegotiation of contracts required some additional legal advice.
5. The company computers in the offices needed to be upgraded or replaced in order to handle a new operating system.

Overall, Mountain Pathology Group is doing well. Thanks to the institution of professional component billing in clinical pathology, their revenue is well ahead year-over-year. The group is showing significant net income on a month-to-month basis that will be available for bonuses, which could be paid out at any time. Typically,

Revenue and Expense Statement - Mountain Pathology Group						
Revenue	Jan	Feb	Year to Date (YTD)	Last YTD	YTD monthly average	Last YTD monthly average
Part A - Main Hospital	$27,000	$29,000	$56,000	$55,000	$28,000	$27,500
Part A - Satelite Hospital	$3,000	$3,000	$6,000	$4,000	$3,000	$2,000
Professional service income						
Patient Billing - Clinical Pathology Component	$45,000	$45,212	$90,212	$60,000	$45,106	$30,000
Patient Billing - Part B	$703,000	$698,000	$1,401,000	$1,400,000	$700,500	$700,000
Contractual adjustments, bad debt, patient refunds...	-$395,000	-$402,000	-$797,000	-$775,000	-$398,500	-$387,500
Private autopsies	$8,000	$12,000	$20,000	$16,000	$10,000	$8,000
Other income [veterinary specimens, interest..]	$1,256	$1,450	$2,706	$2,600	$1,353	$1,300
Total Income	$392,256	$386,662	$778,918	$762,600	$389,459	$381,300
Expenses	Jan	Feb	Year to Date (YTD)	Last YTD	YTD monthly average	Last YTD monthly average
Pathologists' Salaries	$198,000	$197,500	$395,500	$355,000	$197,750	$177,500
Bonuses	$0	$150,000	$150,000	$120,000	$75,000	$60,000
Administrative & Staff Salaries	$20,833	$20,833	$41,666	$39,500	$20,833	$19,750
Fringe benefits [Payroll taxes, FICA, insurance, pension contribution, workers comp]	$54,708	$92,083	$146,792	$118,335	$73,396	$59,168
Total Salaries	$273,541	$460,416	$733,958	$632,835	$366,979	$316,418
Educational, Conferences, Dues, Subscriptions	$523	$3,200	$3,723	$4,200	$1,862	$2,100
Professional fees - legal, licenses, consults, malpractice	$8,522	$8,563	$17,085	$12,750	$8,543	$6,375
Building expenses						
Rent/Mortgage	$5,250	$5,250	$10,500	$9,500	$5,250	$4,750
Depreciation	$600	$600	$1,200	$1,100	$600	$550
Maintenance - Office, computers, building, etc.	$2,635	$1,625	$4,260	$4,000	$2,130	$2,000
Utilities - phone, IT, pagers, electric, building insurance	$2,744	$2,306	$5,050	$4,200	$2,525	$2,100
Equipment - Office, computers, etc.	$944	$1,752	$2,696	$3,700	$1,348	$1,850
Supplies, postage, ..	$2,700	$153	$2,853	$3,250	$1,427	$1,625
Other - software, mileage, ...	$4,685	$450	$5,135	$7,500	$2,568	$3,750
Total Supplies	$28,603	$23,899	$52,502	$50,200	$26,251	$25,100
Total Expenses	$302,144	$484,315	$786,460	$683,035	$393,230	$341,518
Net Income	$90,112	-$97,653	-$7,542	$79,565	-$3,771	$39,783
Net Income over Revenue %	23.0%	-25.3%	-1.0%	10.4%	-1.0%	10.4%

Fig. 7.3 Mountain Pathology Income Statement III

independent pathology groups will pay out substantially all net income by year's end to avoid paying taxes on the group's profits. Of course, taxes would then be paid by the recipients of the bonuses when they file their individual tax returns.

Case: Mountain Pathology Income Statement III

What if the two senior partners were given the income statement in Fig. 7.3 rather than the income statement examined above?

What do you see that might need explaining? (Think about this before turning the page and reviewing Fig. 7.4.) Discussion:

Explanations for the highlighted amounts in Fig. 7.4 are:

1. Part A payments for the satellite hospital have increased from US$2000 to US$3000/month. This was due to a renegotiated contract reflecting new medical director services such as overseeing an expanded test menu and responding to strong evidence that Mountain Pathology has been adding value in measurable ways.

Revenue and Expense Statement - Mountain Pathology Group

Revenue	Jan	Feb	Year to Date (YTD)	Last YTD	YTD monthly average	Last YTD monthly average	Need to explain
Part A - Main Hospital	$27,000	$29,000	$56,000	$55,000	$28,000	$27,500	
Part A - Satelite Hospital	$3,000	$3,000	$6,000	$4,000	$3,000	$2,000	1
Professional service income							
Patient Billing - Clinical Pathology Component	$45,000	$45,212	$90,212	$60,000	$45,106	$30,000	
Patient Billing - Part B	$703,000	$698,000	$1,401,000	$1,400,000	$700,500	$700,000	
Contractual adjustments, bad debt, patient refunds…	-$395,000	-$402,000	-$797,000	-$775,000	-$398,500	-$387,500	2
Private autopsies	$8,000	$12,000	$20,000	$16,000	$10,000	$8,000	
Other income (veterinary specimens, interest..]	$1,256	$1,450	$2,706	$2,600	$1,353	$1,300	
Total Income	$392,256	$386,662	$778,918	$762,600	$389,459	$381,300	

Expenses	Jan	Feb	Year to Date (YTD)	Last YTD	YTD monthly average	Last YTD monthly average	Need to explain
Pathologists' Salaries	$198,000	$197,500	$395,500	$355,000	$197,750	$177,500	3
Bonuses	$0	$150,000	$150,000	$120,000	$75,000	$60,000	4
Administrative & Staff Salaries	$20,833	$20,833	$41,666	$39,500	$20,833	$19,750	
Fringe benefits [Payroll taxes, FICA, insurance, pension contribution, workers comp]	$54,708	$92,083	$146,792	$118,335	$73,396	$59,168	5
Total Salaries	$273,541	$460,416	$733,958	$632,835	$366,979	$316,418	
Educational, Conferences, Dues, Subscriptions	$523	$3,200	$3,723	$4,200	$1,862	$2,100	
Professional fees - legal, licenses, consults, malpractice	$8,522	$8,563	$17,085	$12,750	$8,543	$6,375	
Building expenses							
Rent/Mortgage	$5,250	$5,250	$10,500	$9,500	$5,250	$4,750	6
Depreciation	$600	$600	$1,200	$1,100	$600	$550	
Maintenance - Office, computers, building, etc.	$2,635	$1,625	$4,260	$4,000	$2,130	$2,000	
Utilities - phone, IT, pagers, electric, building insurance	$2,744	$2,306	$5,050	$4,200	$2,525	$2,100	
Equipment - Office, computers, etc.	$944	$1,752	$2,696	$3,700	$1,348	$1,850	
Supplies, postage	$2,700	$153	$2,853	$3,250	$1,427	$1,625	
Other - software, mileage	$4,685	$450	$5,135	$7,500	$2,568	$3,750	
Total Supplies	$28,603	$23,899	$52,502	$50,200	$26,251	$25,100	
Total Expenses	$302,144	$484,315	$786,460	$683,035	$393,230	$341,518	
Net Income	$90,112	-$97,653	-$7,542	$79,565	-$3,771	$39,783	
Net Income over Revenue %	23.0%	-25.3%	-1.0%	10.4%	-1.0%	10.4%	

Fig. 7.4 Mountain Pathology Income Statement III with variances highlighted

2. Contractual adjustments increased, in this case due to a Centers for Medicare & Medicaid Services (CMS) cut in Medicare payments that ultimately resulted in decreased net collections.
3. Pathologist salaries are up by an average US$20,000/month. This was due to a US$10,000/year raise for the partner pathologists and the hiring of a new pathologist.
4. Bonus payments year-to-date increased due to higher bonus payments to the partners made possible by better financial performance of the practice.
5. Fringe benefits increased, which was expected due to increased salary/bonus payments. Also, there was a modest increase in the cost of employer-provided health insurance.

Revenue and Expense Statement - Bayou Histology						
Revenue	Jan	Feb	Year to Date (YTD)	Last YTD	YTD monthly average	Last YTD monthly average
Hospital Income	$152,000	$149,000	$301,000	$295,000	$150,500	$147,500
Patient Billing Income	$59,852	$58,666	$118,518	$116,522	$59,259	$58,261
Other income [vetinary specimens, interest..]	$1,256	$1,450	$2,706	$2,600	$1,353	$1,300
Total income	$213,108	$209,116	$422,224	$414,122	$211,112	$207,061
Expenses	Jan	Feb	Year to Date (YTD)	Last YTD	YTD monthly average	Last YTD monthly average
Technologist Salaries	$81,200	$85,000	$166,200	$159,022	$83,100	$79,511
Technologist Overtime	$1,522	$1,644	$3,166	$3,200	$1,583	$1,600
Office Staff Salaries	$20,833	$20,833	$41,666	$39,500	$20,833	$19,750
Fringe benefits [Payroll taxes, FICA, insurance, pension contribution, workers comp]	$25,889	$26,869	$52,758	$50,431	$26,379	$25,215
Total Salaries	$129,444	$134,346	$263,790	$252,153	$131,895	$126,076
Medical Direction	$833	$833	$1,666	$1,666	$833	$833
Educational, Conferences, Dues, Subscriptions	$200	$350	$550	$700	$275	$350
Liability Insurance	$850	$758	$1,608	$1,500	$804	$750
Rent/Mortgage	$8,300	$8,300	$16,600	$15,000	$8,300	$7,500
Equipment Leases	$279	$300	$579	$600	$290	$300
Equipment maintenance and service contracts	$7,852	$4,985	$12,837	$9,822	$6,419	$4,911
Maintenance - Office, computers, building, etc.	$2,635	$1,625	$4,260	$4,000	$2,130	$2,000
Utilities - phone, IT, pagers, electric, building insurance, property tax, etc.	$4,752	$4,699	$9,451	$8,922	$4,726	$4,461
Lab supplies	$29,877	$31,222	$61,099	$59,885	$30,550	$29,943
Proficiency Testing	$125	$131	$256	$262	$128	$131
Referrals	$1,200	$1,400	$2,600	$2,800	$1,300	$1,400
Office supplies, postage, ..	$2,700	$2,650	$5,350	$4,200	$2,675	$2,100
Other - software, mileage, courier, advertising, etc.	$9,785	$8,755	$18,540	$20,111	$9,270	$10,056
Total Supplies	$69,388	$66,008	$135,396	$129,468	$67,698	$64,734
Total Expenses	$198,832	$200,354	$399,186	$381,621	$199,593	$190,810
Net Income	$14,276	$8,762	$23,038	$32,502	$11,519	$16,251
Net Income over Revenue %	6.7%	4.2%	5.5%	7.8%	5.5%	7.8%

Fig. 7.5 Bayou Histology Income Statement

6. There was an increase in total rent from US$1000 to US$1250/month. Unfortunately, the business park location has become very popular and there is a long list of potential tenants wanting to rent space. Mountain Pathology is looking for a lower cost option.

Case: Bayou Histology Income Statement

Bayou Histology Lab is an independent histology lab organized as an S corporation that provides histology services to hospital patients and outpatients served by the Big River Pathology Practice. It was formed through the amalgamation of three hospital histology labs and is owned by the partner pathologists of Big River Pathology. It bills hospitals and patients for histology services. It employs 14 technologists, 6 clerical personnel and accessioners, a supervisor, and a manager. Bayou Histology buys most of its equipment, utilizes We Carry courier services to pick up specimens and deliver slides, and rents space in a centrally located business park. Bayou Histology also handles a limited number of veterinary cases as well as the histology for occasional small research projects for the local university.

Bayou Histology's income statement is seen in Fig. 7.5. For your monthly review, which items suggest a need for further investigation?

Revenue and Expense Statement - Bayou Histology							
Revenue	Jan	Feb	Year to Date (YTD)	Last YTD	YTD monthly average	Last YTD monthly average	Need to explain
Hospital Income	$152,000	$149,000	$301,000	$295,000	$150,500	$147,500	
Patient Billing Income	$59,852	$58,666	$118,518	$116,522	$59,259	$58,261	
Other income [veterinary specimens, interest]	$1,256	$1,450	$2,706	$2,600	$1,353	$1,300	
Total Income	$213,108	$209,116	$422,224	$414,122	$211,112	$207,061	
Expenses	Jan	Feb	Year to Date (YTD)	Last YTD	YTD monthly average	Last YTD monthly average	Need to explain
Technologist Salaries	$81,200	$85,000	$166,200	$159,022	$83,100	$79,511	1
Technologist Overtime	$1,522	$1,644	$3,166	$3,200	$1,583	$1,600	
Office Staff Salaries	$20,833	$20,833	$41,666	$39,500	$20,833	$19,750	
Fringe benefits [Payroll taxes, FICA, insurance, pension contribution, workers comp]	$25,889	$26,869	$52,758	$50,431	$26,379	$25,215	
Total Salaries	$129,444	$134,346	$263,790	$252,153	$131,895	$126,076	
Medical Direction	$833	$833	$1,666	$1,666	$833	$833	
Educational, Conferences, Dues, Subscriptions	$200	$350	$550	$700	$275	$350	
Liability Insurance	$850	$758	$1,608	$1,500	$804	$750	
Rent/Mortgage	$8,300	$8,300	$16,600	$15,000	$8,300	$7,500	2
Equipment Leases	$279	$300	$579	$600	$290	$300	
Equipment maintenance and service contracts	$7,852	$4,985	$12,837	$9,822	$6,419	$4,911	3
Maintenance - Office, computers, building, etc.	$2,635	$1,625	$4,260	$4,000	$2,130	$2,000	
Utilities - phone, IT, pagers, electric, building insurance, property tax, etc.	$4,752	$4,699	$9,451	$8,922	$4,726	$4,461	4
Lab supplies	$29,877	$31,222	$61,099	$59,885	$30,550	$29,943	
Proficiency Testing	$125	$131	$256	$262	$128	$131	
Referrals	$1,200	$1,400	$2,600	$2,800	$1,300	$1,400	
Office supplies, postage, ..	$2,700	$2,650	$5,350	$4,200	$2,675	$2,100	
Other - software, mileage, courier, advertising, etc.	$9,785	$8,755	$18,540	$20,111	$9,270	$10,056	
Total Supplies	$69,388	$66,008	$135,396	$129,468	$67,698	$64,734	
Total Expenses	$198,832	$200,354	$399,186	$381,621	$199,593	$190,810	
Net Income	$14,276	$8,762	$23,038	$32,502	$11,519	$16,251	
Net Income over Revenue %	6.7%	4.2%	5.5%	7.8%	5.5%	7.8%	

Fig. 7.6 Bayou Histology Income Statement with variances highlighted

Please identify line items for further investigation before moving on to Fig. 7.6. Explanations for highlighted amounts in Fig. 7.6 are:

1. The workload began to increase so a new technologist was hired and began work on February 1.
2. Additional space was rented to handle the increased workload and rent increased by US$800/month.
3. Service and parts were needed for a nonfunctional tissue processor and since there was no service contract in place, the costs were quite high.
4. Building insurance, IT, and electricity costs increased due to the additional space that was added.

Chapter 8
More Complex Arrangements

Michael L. Talbert

Case: An Anatomic Pathology (AP) Lab Buy-In

Dr. Hal Green was excited to be offered a partnership track position with Midwestern Pathology Associates, the strong regional pathology group serving most of his home state. The pay was good, and, if all worked well, Hal would be offered partnership after 3 years. Hal was excited because Midwestern was slowly growing, and they owned their own histology and cytology labs, as well as controlling the extensive courier network and what he had been told was a first-rate billing operation. The partners had referred to the 80 support personnel as Midwestern Diagnostic Services (MDS), and one partner had bragged about the periodic dividends paid by MDS to the partner pathologists. Hal was told he would have the opportunity to buy in to MDS once he was a partner. The partners seemed excited by this, so Hal assumed it would be a good thing. What should Hal be asking?

Discussion: Unless he was planning to work at Midwestern Pathology for only a year or so, Dr. Green would want to know more about MDS prior to signing his employment agreement. He should ask about the relationship between the two entities and whether a buy-in to MDS was required of him as a partner or was optional. Dr. Green should also have a rough idea of the value and finances of MDS and how shares would be priced. For any buy-in, a pathologist should understand how it might be structured, whether financed out of salary or outside money (i.e., a loan) and whether as a onetime deal or structured over several years. Finally, Dr. Green should understand the rough business plans and prospects for MDS over the coming years as well as how he might sell the shares upon leaving the group or retirement.

Thus far, we have dealt primarily with a straightforward independent practice that would typically be a professional corporation, but there are an infinite variety of complexities that may be desired to exploit an opportunity, increase flexibility, grow market share, or enable the pathologists to achieve a different financial or structural objective. For example, for over two decades, many pathology groups pursued control of histology laboratories to serve their practices in a more efficient manner, to create a vehicle to expand services such as adding molecular-based testing for the human papillomavirus, to potentially return profits to the partners, or to combine histology labs to achieve economies of scale. While this strategy was

M. L. Talbert (✉)
Department of Pathology, University of Oklahoma Health Sciences Center, 940 Stanton
L. Young Blvd., BMSB 451, Oklahoma City, OK 73104, USA
e-mail: michael-talbert@ouhsc.edu

© Springer International Publishing Switzerland 2016
L. A. Hassell et al. (eds.), *Pathology Practice Management*,
DOI 10.1007/978-3-319-22954-6_8

made less attractive by significant cuts to histology technical component (TC) payments on January 1, 2013, how would this best be achieved? One could, depending on state laws, hire non-pathologists into a professional corporation, but this could create problems with retirement plans since there are limits on retirement plan contributions of highly compensated employees, depending on retirement plan options and participation among lower-paid individuals. Some groups elect to start other companies, often as C-corporations or S-corporations, as vehicles to house histology laboratories. Partner pathologists would typically be shareholders, and a buy-in program would exist for new pathologists or for pathology group members who attained partner status. A buyout process would also often be used for shareholders who left the practice. Absent a buy-in process, the histology lab shareholders could become a minority of the pathology group and, similarly, absent a buyout process, a significant fraction of the shares of a strategically important histology lab could be held by retired pathologists or their spouses (on their death or even potentially on divorce). Using strategies such as these, independent pathology groups have owned clinical laboratories, anatomic pathology labs, billing operations, and even couriers. One could also use such vehicles to do joint ventures with another pathology group or even a hospital. Such a vehicle could also be sold, such as the sale of a clinical laboratory to a regional or national laboratory. From a practical standpoint, these arrangements are potentially very advantageous to the pathologist but do require careful attention to legal and tax issues. Human resource (HR) issues can also multiply in a company owned by pathologists. It is prudent to structure the entity to minimize pathologist interference in day-to-day activities by pursuing a strong and clear management structure, solid HR support, and professional accounting.

These arrangements also must be evaluated as one is contemplating joining a practice (How do things work? Am I expected to buy in?), when one is leaving a practice (What is the buyout process? How are the shares valued?), or when practices are looking to merge or combine in other ways.

> Key relationships to understand within a practice are those between the practice and various essential supporting and related entities. Buy–sell arrangements, methods of valuation, sources and distribution of income, and their impact on decisions need to be examined for alignment with the goals of the practice members.

Case: Thinking Ahead

Coastal Pathology was a growing 12-pathologist group serving 5 hospitals 20 years ago when they outfitted and opened a combined histology and cytology laboratory by consolidating the anatomic pathology labs of the 4 smaller hospitals. Each of the pathologists invested US$10,000 to purchase equipment and start up Coastal Diagnostics. Over the ensuing years, both Coastal Pathology and Coastal Diagnostics grew. Coastal Pathology added 4 additional hospitals and over 100 physician offices while growing to 26 pathologists. Coastal Diagnostics grew as well and added in-house courier and billing services. Coastal Diagnostics developed an enviable immunohistochemical staining menu and routinely performed reference studies for pathologists outside of Coastal Pathology. The latest venture added fluorescence in situ hybridization (FISH) studies for tumor workups, and next-generation sequencing was under consideration. Coastal Diagnostics was a strong financial success and paid annual dividends that had long exceeded the original investors' initial investment. New pathologists had been allowed to buy in for progressively rising amounts upon obtaining partnership in Coastal Pathology. Valuations of Coastal Diagnostics were done annually by the existing shareholders and typically undervalued what the shares would bring in a sale to a national corporation. Everything seemed successful, and the somewhat lower share price enabled new partner pathologists to purchase shares.

After 20 years of much celebrated success, the pathologists realized some problems with the arrangement. Given the relative undervaluation of shares relative to the generous dividend payments, retiring pathologists held their shares such that much of the company was no longer held by active pathologists, but rather shares were concentrating in the possession of retired pathologists, their surviving spouses, or their estates. Compounding this, new partner pathologists were less interested in purchasing shares since a full buy-in to Coastal Diagnostics had grown to resemble an entire year's base salary. The alarm bells rang even more loudly when Coastal Diagnostics received an unsolicited offer to purchase the company that valued it three times higher than it had been valued at its most recent annual valuation.

How could this challenge have been avoided?

Are there alternative structures that may have been more practical?

Case: Merging Apples and Oranges

Oak Tree Pathology was a regional powerhouse with an over 15-year history of creating successful ventures. The pathologists owned a separate anatomic pathology laboratory providing TC services and medical billing. Oak Tree Pathology wanted to expand into the western half of its state and began discussions with a larger hospital-based practice that was in a leadership transition. The antitrust issues seemed surmountable, and some form of combination or alliance would produce a level of expertise that would rival a major academic medical center. Following some introductory discussions, a small group with representation from both practices aided by consultants signed nondisclosure agreements and began to exchange data. Both parties were surprised to find out how successful the large but relatively simple single hospital-based practice was in comparison to the complicated multihospital, multi-entity Oak Tree Pathology. It quickly became evident that the more financially successful single hospital-based practice had no interest in embracing a high degree of complexity with its attendant risks. The workgroup could not construct an apparent win-win that would allow the groups to operate together, and discussions were amiably terminated.

Discussion: Sometimes complexity is just that—complexity. All novel ventures or additions to a practice beyond the simple core of practicing pathologists should be carefully thought through and much thought given to possible future scenarios including issues created by future changes in payment rates, practice patterns, technology, and the like.

Chapter 9
Practice Sales and Mergers

I Married into the Smith Family; Why Am I Living with the Taylors?

Karim E. Sirgi

Overview

We are all influenced, while growing up, by stories of fictional and real people falling in love, starting a family, and living happily ever after. Ingredients of a happy and successful marriage are transmitted from generation to generation irrespective of culture and ethnicity. Finding the right life partner is an aspiration for most boys and girls around the world; our inherited and acquired social behaviors revolve consciously or unconsciously (one could also say, clumsily or otherwise) around finding and retaining that ideal mate. It is somewhat surprising that the same amount of memory transmission, education, planning, and strategizing is not extended to finding the right business partner or mate considering that most of us spend much more awake time outside the house and away from our family.

Case: Pathology Practice Sales and Mergers Are a Fact of Life

After the moderately intense high school years, competitive college journey, grueling medical school grinder, and specialty and subspecialty residency and fellowship finishing touches, it is time for Saleem to find a "real" job. Similar to finding a mate, criteria of job search happiness and success are considered and interview dances are scheduled. He sets his eyes on an attractive privately owned pathology practice of 12 pathologists, owning and controlling a state-of-the-art multispecialty technical laboratory and enjoying strong contractual relationships with major hospitals and surgery centers, in an attractive metropolitan area with rich urban cultural opportunities and easy access to spectacular outdoor activities. All associates are on a relatively short partnership track and partners wholeheartedly embrace an egalitarian and all-inclusive culture. Through the years, the group has struck a nice work/lifestyle balance and all members enjoy a generous amount of days and weeks off. Saleem brings to the table a subspecialty very much needed by the group with a potential for business growth in areas never seriously explored before by them. In this flirting phase both ask each other all the right questions and each party provides the "right" answers. It is a match made in heaven and the union is consummated 9 months later at the completion of his fellowship year: He has officially joined the happy and thriving Smith family! A couple of years later, while still on a partnership track, the partners are approached by the Taylor family in-

K. E. Sirgi (✉)
LambdaX3 International, 4949 South Syracuse St., Suite 300, Denver, CO 80237, USA
e-mail: ksirgi@lambdax3.com

© Springer International Publishing Switzerland 2016
L. A. Hassell et al. (eds.), *Pathology Practice Management*,
DOI 10.1007/978-3-319-22954-6_9

terested in corporate merger. Rumors are flying within the group and his near-idyllic professional situation has the potential to dramatically change. A year later, Saleem finds himself a member of the Smith–Taylor, or Taylor–Smith or Smitay or Taysmit family: Welcome to the world of mergers and acquisitions in pathology!

Pathology Practice Models

Similar to real families, pathology practices come with different models of affiliation, hierarchy, contribution expectations, wealth distribution, succession roadmaps, and other critically important practical and cultural considerations that insure their longevity and success (and occasionally their failure and demise). Although one does not usually expect a business family to exist as long as a family of blood-related individuals, both types of families share many of the same characteristics of success and failure in given societal and cultural environments.

1) *The academic practice model:* The institutional hierarchy is well established at all academic levels. Pathologists are employees of the university or of a university established and controlled professional entity. Salaries are commensurate with academic rank and achievement. Mergers and acquisitions are usually initiated at the institutional level and pathologists, similar to other members of the medical staff, benefit or suffer from the result of such activities without much control of or input into the process or final outcome.

2) *The private practice model*

   a. *Owned by a group of partners:* Pathologists are usually hired on a track leading to partnership and consequent ownership after a number of years that varies from group to group (usually between 3 and 5 years). Governance of these groups is also variable but usually delegated to a board of directors composed of current partners with or without participation from senior management or membership from successful professionals and leaders recruited from outside the group. Professional and technical relationships with hospitals and other clients are established under the corporate name of the group.

   b. *Owned by a sole or duo of proprietors:* This model was common many years ago but still exists in some parts of the country. Contracts to provide professional and technical pathology services are specifically assigned to one or two group owners or under the name of corporations entirely owned by them. In this practice model, all pathologists of the group are employees of the owners who make all decisions for the group. The hierarchy of command is rarely in doubt in such practice models.

   c. *With or without ownership of a laboratory technical operation:* Either models a or b above may include ownership of a technical laboratory operation with various degrees of routine and esoteric complexity.

3) *The hybrid model:* Although the majority of pathologists working in academia are employees of the institution, there are also rare examples of privately owned and academically based pathology practices blessed (or burdened) by a hybrid

responsibility of business ownership and academic achievement. Their practice model is akin to model 2(a) above.

4) *The hospital or group employed pathologist*: Pathologists are often employed by hospitals, hospital systems, or multispecialty groups. In those settings, there is limited independence and the future of the pathologists is tied to the larger entity. Mergers/acquisitions are not uncommon and the pathologists are usually, but not always, incorporated into any new entity.

5) *The big commercial laboratories, with a national presence:* These laboratories are usually publically owned and traded. As such, they are led by executive teams with broad experience in the laboratory industry and are staffed by technical and medical professionals with a vast array of specialty and expertise. Although physicians and PhDs assume the directorship of various departments, the executive team and their board of governors unequivocally assume the business governance of these corporations.

6) *The commercial laboratories with a specific area of esoteric expertise:* Many of these laboratories are at the start-up stage of their business evolution. Their ownership, staffing, and governance are akin to (5) mentioned above with various opportunities for employees to share in stock options.

Mergers and Acquisitions (M&A)

Although mergers and acquisitions are often mixed in their diminutive M&A denomination, each of these terms brings with it specific meanings with profound legal, practical, cultural, and emotional implications.

Merger

Boiled down to its simplest essence, a merger is a union of two corporate entities that have decided to pursue business as one. Beyond the legal and tax identity unification, it is really the blending and assimilation of cultures between two (or more) distinct organizations that determine the long-term success of that effort.

Acquisition

As the term implies, one organization acquires the properties and assets of another one in this type of transaction. There is a selling and buying process that takes place with the usual resulting relinquishing of governance control to the buyer. Although well understood in the business world, this last point may be difficult to accept in a world of physicians accustomed to owning and controlling their medical practice.

Why Merge/Sell?

Many factors have converged during the past 20 years to encourage physicians, including pathologists, to seek association within larger professional groups:

- Ever-increasing complexity of medical specialties and the need for ready access to subspecialists.
- The need to improve negotiation and contractual positions with payers and large health-care providers (getting a "seat at the table").
- Economies of scale for technical and professional talents.
- Improving purchasing power with suppliers.
- Broadening geographic reach and coverage.
- Increasing ability to organize care along specialized service lines, with its implications on overall quality of care delivery.
- Bettering chances of attracting the brightest and best talents for all levels of the organization (professional and technical staff).
- Enhancing deployment of best operational and professional practices to a broader enterprise.
- Accessing more capital for better space and equipment.
- Initiating and participating in R&D projects.
- Engaging in a defensive move in order to neutralize one or more competitors.

Optimists look at an M&A activity and envision positive outcomes that could potentially result from joining forces between two complementary organizations. Pessimists and cynics focus only on the material aspects of that effort, with dollar signs and complex spreadsheets and pro formas dominating the conversation.

> Pearl of wisdom: When approached by potential partner organizations, be wary of those that focus predominately or solely on goals of short-term financial rewards (even if substantial), not supported by a vision of gradual growth, quality achievement and excellence in service delivery.

The M&A Journey

Mergers between professional organizations of pathologists can and do happen irrespective of practice size or setting, as long as two or more organizations bring to the table complementary skills and assets capable of building a unified organization that cumulatively brings to the table more positives than the sum of either one of the constituent companies. This is referred to as synergy.

Acquisitions, on the other hand, usually happen between an acquiring organization that has much more financial means and clout than the acquired one, for any number of the reasons enumerated in the paragraph above.

Whether considering a merger or an acquisition, it is safe to compare many of the steps involved in either processes to a (usually) well-orchestrated courting experience between two parties exploring the potential of a long-term union, including:

a. The initial contact:

Interested parties may approach your organization from all sorts of expected and unexpected sources; be prepared to recognize the subtle and not so subtle signs that may indicate an exploring and/or interested party:

- A casually inquisitive conversation at a local or national meeting.
- A vendor for a larger organization inquiring whether you had considered a potential association with a competitor to further the growth of a market product (e.g., "would you be willing to work with us on expanding the business of uropathology in this market?").
- A national laboratory referring more and more of its local and regional business to your specialists (of course, one could also assume that their national capacity for handling that business has been saturated and/or that local physicians are demanding that their cases be sent to you based on your reputation of service excellence).
- Known brokers of laboratory consolidation making a direct inquiry about your intentions for strategic growth.
- Direct approaches by well-funded start-up companies searching for a physical laboratory presence (a.k.a., CLIA certificate) for their concept and planned expansion.
- Direct inquiry from a competitor on whether "it is time for us to work together and join forces in this crazy world?" (It does not get any clearer than that!)

b. The first meeting:

The initial signal has been sent (I saw you and I am interested to know you better) and it is now followed by "can we meet?" The meeting can be as casual as having a coffee in house or at an outside facility between a couple of representatives from each organization, or as formal as bringing key players from both organizations to a conference room for structured conversations and presentations. *How information* is exchanged during these first meetings will be as critical as to *what* is exchanged. Again, borrowing analogies from the courting process between two human beings, the impact and potential future reward of saying "I like you" is very much dependent on the emotional and situational setting in which that declaration was made.

I still vividly remember participating, many years ago, in the very first meeting that would eventually lead to a merger between my group and another local one. Leaders of both organizations, following a few introductory phone calls between key players, had arranged the meeting. A few minutes into the meeting, one pathologist nicely summarized for the attendees all the reasons that justified a merger between the two groups (the initial oh-so-good "we like you, we complement each other, and we would love to get to know you better"). Another pathologist from the same group immediately felt compelled to bring a clarification to the statement of his partner: "We like you but we are not sure why and the burden is really on you to convince us that we are justified in thinking that maybe perhaps we like you." Needless to state that his statement was a serious mood killer; it led to an almost immediate adjournment of that meeting. It then took a full year of healing for the two groups to meet again, after some of the original players had been discretely "excused" from attending follow-up meetings.

1. Who should attend the initial encounter?

Although there is no magic answer or set formula to this question, think of people who are good at *bidirectional* communication: Your organization is going to need people who can not only communicate well with the outside party but also can internally bring back to the group the positives, negatives, and potential risks and benefits identified during the initial meetings. You may have a pathologist that presents great to the outside world but has strained relationships with his partners. On the other hand, you may also have a well-liked partner who feels out of his comfort zone in less familiar external situations. The initial meeting is not meant to iron out technical details of a future association; it should really be focused on introducing one organization to the other, building trust, and exploring, in very general terms, whether synergies exist to bring the two parties together for future more in-depth conversations.

Case: Cultures and Chemistry Matter

> Years ago, Magnum Pathologists, PC approached another group of local pathologists with whom they thought they had hospital system affiliation synergies. On one side of the conversation was a group known for its egalitarian philosophy, and on the other side was a group known for its autocratic leadership style. Magnum Pathologists had selected for the initial conversation one of the junior partners known for his gentle demeanor and very methodical approach to business matters. The other group had chosen their all-powerful leader known for his "take-no-prisoners" approach to business negotiations. The gentle, methodical partner was immediately perceived by the other side as "weak and indecisive." Magnum Pathologists immediately perceived the other party as bullying and non-compromising; the merger conversation literally died after one meeting: Personal chemistry matters!

2. Expanding the initial contact team into a steering committee:

After the initial few encounters between representatives of both groups, the decision to pursue M&A discussions or not with the other party will need to be made. Even if one party has decided that the time is not right to pursue such discussions, it is always a good idea to leave the door open.

The author knows of a group for which one of the two mergers happened after initial conversations had been interrupted for more than a year. Many years later, after two further successful mergers, a national organization acquired the technical operations even after the advance had been kindly dismissed almost 12 months before.

In any case, once the decision to pursue the M&A discussions is taken, it is advisable to enrich the initial exploratory team with members who can bring specific technical and professional expertise to the process.

On the professional practice side:

- Staffing and work distribution philosophies
- Partnership track record and roadmap
- Subspecialty work allocation

- Work/lifestyle balance
- Governance style and philosophies
- Organizational culture

On the administrative/technical side:

- Organizational structure
- Administrative talents present and needed
- Technical services needed and offered
- Human resource matters (pre- and post-merger/acquisition).

On the financial/legal side:

- Financial health of either organization
- Valuation of either organization
- Current and post-merger/acquisition legal corporate structure
- Taxation structural considerations
- Governance documents

c. About attorneys:

Although legal, financial, and tax specialists may not be needed during introductory conversations between the two entities, their presence or, at a minimum, the constant availability of their counsel will be *absolutely crucial* to the advancement and success of the M&A effort. Corporate and tax attorneys will elevate the conversation to levels of sophistication and complexity you never thought possible. At some point, you will find yourself listening to attorneys on both sides discuss in English, legal, and tax technical concepts that may as well have been written in a Martian dialect. In those instances, do not get discouraged: Get yourself a big bowl of popcorn, sit back, and enjoy the show. It is a necessary process resulting from innumerable legislative measures enacted that very few of us mere mortals truly understand. As a matter of fact, having witnessed attorneys on both sides of these M&A efforts contradict themselves and each other, I am now convinced that nobody really understands how the system works … but it somehow works! In any case, attempting an M&A without the counsel of tax and legal corporate specialists may as well be considered corporate suicide.

A word of caution is in order however about legal matters directly affecting the *daily practice* of medicine and pathology: Listen to the counsel of your legal and financial experts but do not abdicate to them the hundreds, if not thousands, of decisions that will have to be made in order to bring the two organizations together. In a hospital and in private group settings, I have often seen physician groups passively attend to legal structural matters critical to the success of their future practice and willingly delegate practical decisions to their hired experts. It is beneficial to remember that these experts work for you and that your colleagues and you will have to live and work many years with decisions made during these crucial meetings.

For example, I am aware of a situation where during a group's second merger and first acquisition experience, the attorneys were "pushing" hard for a very restrictive, almost punitive, version of a noncompete clause to include in future professional contracts. The pathologists, in turn, pushed back harder and ended up with a version more in tune with the group's values and culture. Many times over subsequent years, the pathologists had an opportunity to appreciate the well-founded appropriateness of their active "resistance."

In addition, attorneys love boiler-plate clauses affecting vacation time, part-time status, outside activities allowed by the group, disability allowance, and many others to be included in professional contracts: Just make sure those legal employment and practical clauses match your organization's vision, culture, and values. If not, push back within the confines permissible by local, state, and federal laws.

d. Is there such a thing as overcommunication?

The simple answer is no! It is common for both parties to enter this process with a serious level of anxiety and even suspicion. These emotions are not only outwardly directed but are also inwardly based. The outside parties considering joining forces have not had a chance to really know each other and therefore establish a minimum level of comfort and trust. In addition to the discomfort or lack of trust with outside parties, the following internal parties will most certainly be wary of the ongoing M&A discussions:

- Pathologists at various stages of the partnership track journey and/or of their career.
- Management of technical staff employed by the group.
- Technical staff employed by the group.
- Hospital management of institutions covered by the group.
- Laboratory staff of hospitals covered by the group.
- Clients of the group.
- Community leaders affected by the M&A activity.

Of course not all the stakeholders above will need to get the same level of confidential information, and not all communication will need to be disseminated at the same time. It will, however, be of critical importance to have in place a communication strategy that will include, at a minimum:

- Identification of various audiences that will be recipients of communication.
- The various levels of confidential information that will be communicated to each party.
- The timeliness of the various communications.
- The parties responsible for disseminating the information.

This last point is particularly important to emphasize, as the communication needs to be disciplined, authorized by the leadership and consistent. Individual members attending negotiations should not feel empowered to disseminate sensitive information without prior clearing by the appropriate channels of leadership. The popular adage of "loose lips sink ships" is very true in such a setting. Often, confidentiality agreements are used to define and restrict flow of information.

However, maintaining absolute secrecy of M&A discussions is an illusion as M&A exploratory activities are hugely disruptive for all parties involved and will certainly not go unnoticed by minimally observant players, even if national-security level secrecy safeguards are put in place. In order to avoid uncontrollable false rumors and innuendos, put in place a sound communication strategy as early as possible during the M&A process.

Case: Open Communication Pays Off

> After my previous pathology group agreed to sell its technical laboratory operation to an upstart national outfit, after long months of negotiation and before we signed on the bottom line of the final documents, we made sure to approach the various hospital administrations with whom we had established a long-standing, successful relationship to inform them of what we were planning to do and why we thought it was the right thing to do for the overall availability and quality of our services. In doing so, we also made it very clear that we wanted to insure a smooth transition post acquisition and invited their input and feedback at all levels of the upcoming process. Before approaching these administrators, my previous pathology group had also internally identified key hospital players from whom we would consider a "veto" vote on the upcoming acquisition. Although we did not offer such a veto vote during their conversations with any of the key hospital administrators, we did make it very clear numerous times during the meetings with them that the intention was not to present them with a "fait-accompli" and that our primary concern was enhancing the quality and availability of premiere diagnostic services to the patients we had both been entrusted to care for. My previous pathology group received a unanimous vote of support from every hospital administration approached and from all the other key stakeholders. The legal counsel of one of the two major hospital systems that we covered also commended us for the transparency of communication, and recognized and appreciated our willingness to give them a silent vote on behalf of the physicians and patients we cared for. She positively contrasted this approach with that of another group who had sold their entire operation to a national reference laboratory and had sent them a team of attorneys, after the fact, to present them with a "take it or leave it" already signed deal; needless to say that she believed that our more open, proactive approach was conducive to further consolidating an already solid relationship, and carrying it forward into the future.

e. Ingredients of M&A success:

With my former group, I was intimately involved in bringing together three independent and privately owned pathology groups through two separate merger efforts. Although the legal and financial aspects of these mergers were complex and challenging, the post-merger assimilation of processes and cultures at all levels of the organization was truly what defined the majority of our challenges on a daily basis. For many years, we politely referred to these challenges as "growing pains."

Any attorney and tax specialist worth their salt can provide you with a list of technical, legal, and financial processes needed to achieve the technical aspects of a union between two groups of professionals. The real ingredients of success, however, truly reside in the innumerable intangible variations of intra- and intergroup cultural differences, and the willingness of both groups to work out those cultural differences for the greater good of the contemplated larger group.

If you ask a purely technical person how to prepare a pasta dish, their natural answer would be to dip spaghetti in boiling water and, maybe, add to it some canned tomato sauce. Ask the same question of an Italian grandma and she will pour into it hundreds of recipe details transmitted to her from generation to generation. The pasta and the boiling water is what attorneys and tax specialists will provide you upfront. The hundreds of recipe details are what the cultural fiber of each group will bring to the table for a long-lasting, memorable, and successful experience. Examples of such recipe ingredients include:

- Workload/income/lifestyle balance
- Governance style and philosophy
- Work distribution preferences
- Respect for subspecialty specificities and variances
- Appetite for business entrepreneurship, that is, risk tolerance
- Demographic diversity (age, gender, ethnicity, and religion)
- Comfort with practice settings such as hospital versus outpatient based practices
- Desire for geographic integration of practices
- Experience with managing technical personnel
- Allowances for extracurricular activities and moonlighting
- Allowance for part-time employment and impact on partnership status
- Tolerance and guidelines for differential compensation
- Recognition, support, and reward for leadership activities
- Minimum continued medical education requirements
- Adaptability to practice pattern changes

In my experience, it is not unusual for two groups contemplating the benefits of a merged larger group to spend much more time on the pasta and boiling water at the expense of the hundreds of critical cultural recipe ingredients that will really determine the long-term success and flavor of the final product. Grandma would certainly frown on such an approach!

Practice Valuation—Time to Talk Money!

No business courting process, as intense and culturally compatible as it may be, ever leads to an acquisition without an exchange of assets that makes financial sense for both parties. Assets can be tangible such as cash, buildings, and equipment for example, or intangible such as intellectual property, practice reputation, diversity, and depth of expertise and technical know-how. The buyer is looking to purchase a business with an ongoing income stream *and* built-in potential for future growth, and the seller is looking at being compensated fairly for building up the business and bringing it to that critical point of acquisition desirability.

a. Why are investors even interested in acquiring laboratories?

Although regulatory and reimbursement pressures are constantly rising in the health-care industry, M&A activity in the diagnostic laboratory sector has remained strong through the years.

- The laboratory industry fundamentals are solid and stable.
- Private equity groups are attracted by the noncyclical nature of the laboratory industry: Laboratory testing drives some 70% of medical decisions made (but represents only a small percentage of health-care expenditures).
- Laboratory testing can affect sectors of the industry not related to the direct provision of health care, such as the pharmacologic and research sectors.

- The laboratory market remains extremely fragmented with remarkable opportunities for consolidation in both the independently owned and hospital-based diagnostics spaces, representing a third and a bit less than two thirds of the total market, respectively (minor components are physician office labs and other) [1].
- Molecular diagnostics and its impact on personalized medicine have the potential to create market growth opportunities not even imagined today.
- Hospitals are increasingly interested in selling their laboratory business.
- Retiring baby boomers are increasingly looking at cashing out on independent businesses they helped create and grow.

b. Determining fair market value:

Establishing a fair valuation of a pathology practice is probably the most sensitive aspect of an M&A process. When courted for their medical practice, pathologists (and physicians in general) have a natural tendency to look at their practice with the eyes and mind of a proud parent amazed at the charm, intelligence, and uniqueness of their child. Business people, on the other hand, bring to the process a healthy dose of objectivity; they are concerned with such items as cash flow, market presence, contracts in place, potential for growth, accounts receivables, operational efficiency, information technology infrastructure, geographic reach, debts incurred, general state of the economy, regulatory pressures, pending litigations, revenue cycle, and competition. Whereas physicians are focused on highlighting their level of education and expertise, the fanatical loyalty of their customers and their dedication to patient care made legendary in their community, their business counterparts are focused on such nonsexy items as gross revenue, return on investment (ROI), and earnings before interest, tax, depreciation and amortization (EBITDA).

The stage of establishing a fair market value to the company is not for the faint at heart as it involves principles borrowed from the art and science of business, corporate and taxation law, and finance. This is *the* stage where having a crack team including the talents of a corporate attorney, tax specialist, savvy business manager, real-estate appraiser, laboratory equipment appraiser, and even an investment banker, is going to pay huge dividends for the group and the fairness of the overall M&A process. Having these specialists on hand can also help defuse some of the contentiousness usually associated with this critical phase of the process.

c. Valuating "Goodwill" (also known as "Blue Sky"):

The goodwill component of a business is that part of the business value *over and above* the value of its identifiable assets. Having a fantastic reputation in town but an unprofitable business does not necessarily qualify the group for financial rewards of goodwill. Employing the best super-specialists in the region in a group that is consistently burdened by debts not supported by appropriate cash flows also does not qualify that group for a goodwill premium. Goodwill is an added value to an overall successful business, not a convenient band-aid to an ailing operation.

Although intangible in its nature, goodwill is not theoretical or unreal. What has the potential to make it unrealistic, if not unreal, is the attitude that both parties often bring to the table: Pathologists and other physicians usually have an overinflated impression of their practice goodwill and value, whereas business buyers and hospital administrators are often dismissive of it to the point of even not recognizing it at all. There is no doubt that M&A negotiations can be undermined and even completely interrupted by such extreme views of the goodwill element. Although there are objective accounting and financial formulas for evaluating the goodwill element that a practice brings to the table, the common sense element is often the ingredient missing from the goodwill calculation equation.

d. Valuation rule of thumb:

From a technical accounting point of view, there are three basic approaches to valuating any business, including a laboratory operation:

- The income approach: What is the present value of expected future cash flows?
- The market approach: How much has the market previously paid for a similar acquisition?
- The cost approach: What is the value of all tangible assets purchased (therefore excluding all intangible assets)?

Based on industry experience, laboratory acquisition prices (therefore valuation) have been based in the past 5–10 years on paying a multiple for one of two accounting parameters:

- Net revenue: 1.5–2.5 multiple
- EBITDA: 6–17 multiple

The broad range of multiples shown above truly demonstrates the unique nature of each acquisition, and the resulting additive synergies and competencies that it brings to the purchasing company. The multiple mentioned above also assumes purchase of the totality of the controlling interest in the company. Of course, various models of ownership and post-purchase governance exist with a resulting impact on the final purchase price.

True Story During advanced stages of the negotiations for the sale of our technical laboratory operation, the buyers and our previous group's board of directors gave a presentation to the pathologist partners and described in detail the ultimate purchase amount and each partner's share of that amount. The presentation was held at a fancy restaurant and, at that stage of the negotiations, the mood was overall supportive, as our board of directors had done a good job at keeping the partners informed at various stages of the process. The numbers described by the buyers did not come as a surprise to that audience. Weeks later, the chief negotiator for the buyer's team asked for an urgent audience with our board: It turned that the entire valuation of the company had to be redone on a different accounting basis; one party had used a cash method of accounting for the initial valuation and the other had used an accrual method of accounting. Based on the revised numbers, the initial valuation had been decreased by multiple millions of dollars. Does it not remind you of the US-European space probe that traveled 461 million miles but was destroyed by flying too deep into the Martian atmosphere because of incorrect trajectory calculations due to designers using the imperial system of units and a navigation team the metric one? [2] Needless to say that a lot of message massaging was then needed to explain this mother of all snafus to the partners!

What Else Should you Consider?

My previous group grew through multiple mergers and one large acquisition. At the end of those three activities, we became a group of 30 pathologists covering multiple hospitals and surgery center sites, delivering general and highly subspecialized pathology services organized along specialty service lines, and extended our technical and professional reach to multiple states around the country. Although the end result was something we were all very proud of, we could probably have proceeded differently along our M&A journey(s). Retrospectively, I would probably have designed the following additional safeguards:

a. Getting to better know each other:

A trial period pre-M&A would have been very nice for our various pre-merged groups. Through various escalating common activities, we may have been better able to test the validity of the merger assumptions, evaluate the cultural chemistry between the three groups, and address identified incompatibilities and/or obstacles, thus minimizing post-merger "growing pains" and heartburn.

Examples of such pre-merger activities would have included:

- Exchange of pathologists across group lines.
- Deployment of pathologists in geographies and practice settings representative of their future settings.
- Meaningful social events bringing the groups together in various settings (with and without spouses, with and without critical nonphysician staff, at work facilities and off-work settings).
- Exchanges of leadership talents (physician and nonphysician staffs) to various critical areas of the operation or, at minimum, leadership dyads to observe and compare leadership styles and philosophies.
- More extensive open conversations between all members of the groups, not just the leadership or designated steering committees.
- Identifying nay-sayers on both sides and inviting them to serve across company lines; then reevaluate their position vis-à-vis the M&A effort.

b. Building a grace period into the post-merger noncompete clause:

In spite of due diligence, the end result of a merged group can be unattractive to individual members of the original groups. By no fault of their own, they may find themselves wedded to a new family in which they did not seek membership in the first place (remember the title of this chapter!). Instead of severely limiting their practice choices with other groups in town, these unhappy members should be encouraged to seek alternative employment without holding over their head the specter of restrictive and/or punitive noncompete agreements. Of course, non-solicitation clauses should still prevent departing pathologists from actively recruiting business away from the abandoned company.

c. Establishing a prenuptial agreement: Is there a roadmap out of this union?

Establishing upfront a "way out" of an unhappy corporate relationship is an interesting proposition with supporters and detractors.

Supporters will argue that no union should be irreversible. The emotional and financial damages of an unsuccessful merger and forced cohabitation could be disastrous for the corporation as a whole and for many of its individual discontent members.

Detractors will argue that members, especially those who were not entirely in favor of a merger in the first place, will never be "all-in" if a way to deconstruct the corporation was built into the merger documents. The idea is that these members will work hard on finding, if not causing, the appropriate conditions and timing to elicit those articles that would lead to the end of the merged entity. Detractors argue that a corporate prenuptial would in effect establish a perpetual non-commitment to the merged entity.

I once was strongly on the side of the anti-prenuptial camp for the reasons explained in the paragraph above. However, I believe that my position has changed and that I would not be that strong of an opponent to a pre-merger or pre-acquisition corporate prenuptial today, with an important nuance: Rather than focusing solely on articles of deconstruction, I would argue for a detailed roadmap defining *criteria of success* for an M&A, based on a list of objective and subjective parameters. Not meeting these objectives after predefined intervals of time (1, 2, and 3 years for example), would trigger escalating corrective measures ultimately leading to pre-agreed upon corporate actions (buy-back, corporate separation, decentralization, etc.). Today, I would also argue that not having these measures in place has the potential to lead to uncomfortable if not unsuccessful long-term forced cohabitation.

In Conclusion

Disruptive changes affecting health care in the USA are encouraging physician groups, including pathology groups to seek strength (and shelter) in numbers. Having experienced multiple mergers and one major acquisition with my previous group, I can unequivocally vouch for the wisdom of that approach: At the end of our first two mergers, we ended up covering nine hospitals in two competing healthcare systems; in addition to a strong hospital base, we had the busiest privately owned outpatient laboratory operation in a multistate radius. We were able to organize complex diagnostic services (hematopathology, pediatric pathology, bone and soft tissue tumors, dermatopathology and others) in service lines able to attract the brightest young and more experienced talents from around the country. Many, if not most, of our services rivaled those offered by local and national academic institutions. The blip of our presence on the national diagnostic radar screen grew to the point of being recognized by most of the "usual suspects" interested in laboratory acquisition and consolidation. We became the object of assiduous courting for acquisition on an almost monthly basis. We ended up selling our technical laboratory operation at great profit for the partners, to a start-up outfit in search of a platform laboratory operation for a planned national growth. At the same time, we were able to keep a 100% independent and self-governed private corporation of pathologists in charge of its own decisions and destiny. None of the above would have happened if we had not engaged in M&A activities at various phases of our corporate existence.

True Story 1: Size Matters

In 2006, UnitedHealthcare and Hospital Corporation of America (HCA) got into a serious national contract dispute that resulted in a temporary exodus of united insured patients to competing local hospitals. This could have caused a major disruption to my group's workloads and, consequently, cash flow, except that, through the results of two successive mergers, my group was now based at nine local hospitals almost equally divided between the two giant local hospital systems. The exodus of a group of patients from one hospital system to the other caused no disruption to us except for the temporary internal reallocation of technical and professional resources from one side of the operation to the other: Size and geographic presence matter!

True Story 2: Size Matters Again

Also in 2006, two of the busiest local groups of urologists merged to build the largest full-service urology center in the Rocky Mountains region. In doing so, they moved the totality of their outpatient services from the various hospitals they covered and consolidated the bulk of their hospital-based surgeries to a much smaller number of local hospital sites. Here again, our sheer size and breadth of service lines expertise allowed us to capture the totality of their new facility-based pathology work through an independent professional contract and almost all of their hospital-based work through our coverage of their newly consolidated hospital presence: Merged larger groups have a better chance at capturing opportunities resulting from disruptive health-care developments!

References

1. G2 Intelligence. U.S. clinical laboratory and pathology testing 2013–2015. Market analysis, trends, and forecasts. Kennedy Information, LLC; 2013.
2. Hotz RL. Mars probe lost due to simple math error. Los Angeles Times; (1 Oct 1999).

Part III
Contracting

Chapter 10
Payor Contracts

Case: The Devil Is in the (Contract) Details

Community Pathology, P.C. provides professional pathology services for the patients of its local hospital and has an active outreach practice and a technical component histology laboratory that performs technical component services for the outreach clients. It typically bills its professional services for hospital patients with the-26 professional modifier and bills on a global basis for the outreach services.

Community Pathology, P.C. has been asked by its hospital to participate with Good Health Plan, a managed care payor in the region. The pathology group receives a sample participating provider agreement that is titled "Hospital-Based Physician Agreement." The contract explains that covered services include the "physician services provided by Group to hospital inpatients and outpatients." The Good Health Plan representative explained that all pathology groups in the state have the same contract, and the plan makes payment for all services provided by pathology groups.

In addition, the fee schedule exhibit states that "Good Health Plan will pay Group for its Covered Services in accordance with the Good Health Plan fee schedule." There is a current fee schedule included in the package, and the Good Health Plan representative informed Community Pathology, P.C. that the plan's fee schedule is typically 120% of the Medicare physician fee schedule, which is similar to other managed care plans in the community. However, the contract itself does not include a minimum guaranteed fee schedule nor does it reference any guaranteed payment rate.

Under the proposed terms, would Good Health Plan reimburse Community Pathology, P.C. for its professional and technical component services to outreach (nonhospital patients)?

Does the contract guarantee the pathology group payment at 120% of Medicare, or can Good Health Plan change its fee schedule at any time?

How should contract be modified to ensure that Community Pathology, P.C. receives payment for its global outreach services?

If Community Pathology, P.C. bills for professional component of clinical pathology services, should specific payment for these services be addressed in the contract?

J. P. Wood (✉)
McDonald Hopkins LLC, 956 Main St., Dennis, MA 02638, USA
e-mail: jwood@mcdonaldhopkins.com

© Springer International Publishing Switzerland 2016   125
L. A. Hassell et al. (eds.), *Pathology Practice Management*,
DOI 10.1007/978-3-319-22954-6_10

Most pathologists in private practice will negotiate many managed care and other third-party payor contracts during their careers. Some of these contracts may be directly between the pathology provider and the payor, and others may involve an intervening contracting entity, such as a physician-hospital organization (PHO), an independent physician association (IPA) or an accountable care organization (ACO). At times, the pathologist may not have much negotiating leverage with the payor, yet even in these situations, it is important to understand the terms that are offered by the payor and evaluate whether participation in the contract is beneficial. This chapter provides a comprehensive roadmap of the principal contracting components that a pathology provider can follow when evaluating a managed care contract and/or negotiating with the managed care entity.

Initial Contracting Considerations

Prior to negotiating or entering into any managed care contract, a pathologist should ask why he or she (or his or her group practice) wishes to enter into the contract. Perhaps the contract is necessary to maintain the pathologist's current patient base or to expand it? The contract might be required by an affiliated hospital or important referral source.

Next, the pathologist should define his or her contract expectations. If the pathologist does not sufficiently define his or her expectations prior to negotiating the contract, those expectations may not be met or may not even be addressed during contract negotiations. Moreover, if the pathologist discusses expectations with his or her practice or negotiating team in advance of contract negotiations, the pathologist can determine if his or her expectations are realistic, or need to be revised, based on the experiences of the other pathologists or team members in negotiating with managed care entities.

To support financial expectations during contract negotiations, pathology providers should conduct a thorough financial analysis of practice and business operations. Simply stated, a pathology provider needs to understand, and share with its negotiating team, the financial specifics of its operation, including the fixed and indirect costs associated with its services. Having this information will assist the pathology provider to determine what reimbursement rates are necessary and appropriate in contract negotiations.

Pathologists should consider how important the contract is to their business interests. If the contract is not important, the pathology provider can be less flexible in contract negotiations. If the contract is critically important, more flexibility may be required. Pathologists should remember that physicians who refer patients to them are usually contractually required to send managed care patients to participating providers. For convenience, such physicians may choose to send all of their referrals to participating providers. Therefore, a pathologist's failure to participate in a managed care contract may preclude the pathologist from receiving not only a physician's managed care referrals but also such physician's nonmanaged care referrals.

Always know why you are signing (or not signing) a contract.

Preparing for Negotiation of a Managed Care Contract

A pathology provider should have a plan of negotiation prior to negotiating any contract and especially contracts with managed care entities that usually employ very sophisticated and experienced negotiators.

As a preliminary matter, a pathology provider should not assume that the provider must sign the standard managed care contract as there is almost always room for negotiation. Prior to negotiating a managed care contract, the pathology provider should do the following:

1. Assemble an appropriate contract team including provider representatives, and legal and financial representatives, among others. The importance and complexity of the contract should determine the composition of the team.
2. Determine who will negotiate the contract and avoid multiple contact points. The contract negotiator should be provided with written negotiating parameters.
3. Require that the managed care entity appoints someone who has decision-making authority to negotiate the contract on its behalf.
4. Identify problem areas in current managed care contracts and consider how they can and should be corrected and addressed in new contracts.
5. Identify the "must have" and "deal breaker" positions in new contracts before negotiations begin and prioritize requested amendments.
6. Attempt to negotiate the contract on your home turf.
7. Set a timetable for contract completion.

Key Managed Care Contract Provisions

The following material outlines the key managed care contract provisions that should be considered by pathologists during the review and negotiation of the contract. These are not listed in the order of importance, but rather in the order that they typically appear in a managed care contract. This list can be used as a checklist for contract review.

Proper Parties to the Contract/Relationship to Each Other It is important that the contract be executed by the proper party for the pathology practice. If the provider is a corporate entity (e.g., professional corporation or association, limited liability company, general corporation, or partnership), the contract should be with the corporate entity and not an individual. If not all members of the corporate entity (e.g., members in a group practice) want to participate in the managed care contract, the contract should specifically identify the participating physicians.

The managed care contract should provide that both parties are independent contractors and that the pathology provider has no liability or responsibility for the acts or omissions of the managed care entity. In addition, the contract should specify that the managed care entity will not exercise control or direction over professional judgment. If the managed care entity owns or operates its own facilities (such as the health center of an health maintenance organization (HMO)), the contract should provide that the provider is not liable for injuries to patients due to a defect in the facilities.

Defined Terms The pathology provider should review all defined terms, especially the definitions of "Payor" and "Covered Services" or their respective equivalents, because these definitions can have substantive effects upon the contractual relationship. The term "Payor" should not extend to additional plans or payors without the pathology provider's prior written consent, as this could be used to extend the contract to "silent PPOs" (Preferred Provider Organizations) who utilize the agreed upon fee schedule without the pathologists' knowledge.

The term "Covered Services" should not be subject to unilateral alteration by the payor without the pathology provider having the ability to terminate the contract on reasonably short notice. The definition of Covered Services can be particularly relevant to pathology providers who wish to bill and receive payment for their professional component of clinical pathology services as well as to providers who wish to bill and receive payment for esoteric testing and molecular/genetic testing.

Some payor contracts are drafted to cover only inpatient and outpatient services, some are drafted to cover only nonhospital (outreach) services, some contracts only cover clinical laboratory services, and other contracts cover only anatomic pathology services. Some contracts cover only technical component services and others cover only professional component services. Therefore, it is imperative to clarify the definition of Covered Services to ensure that the pathology provider will be paid for the full range of its services.

Materials Incorporated by Reference If the contract addresses exhibits, quality assurance guidelines, provider manuals, or any other form of reference that the pathology provider is required to follow, a copy must be analyzed in advance and filed with the contract. If any exhibits, quality assurance guidelines, provider manuals, or any other form of reference are addressed in the contract, the contract should specify that the contract itself will control if any of these documents are inconsistent with the contract, that a copy must be given to the provider in advance if any of these documents are modified, and that the provider has the right to terminate the contract prior to the effective date of any modifications of such materials.

Credentials and Qualifications The contract should clearly set forth (i) credentials and other qualification requirements for pathologists, (ii) accreditation and/or the certification requirements for facilities, and (iii) that the managed care entity will preserve and require employers and other third parties to protect the confidentiality of confidential/proprietary information, except where disclosure is required by law or a third-party contract. The pathology provider should delete requirements that are not applicable to the service being provided by the provider.

Pathologists should be wary of the provisions that require the provider to notify the managed care entity of incidents of possible malpractice. Disclosure regarding incidents of possible malpractice could be viewed as an admission of malpractice in subsequent litigation. It is important that any contemplated disclosures of possible malpractice should be reviewed in advance with legal counsel.

Services Provided To adequately assess the managed care contract, it is critical to determine what services are covered under the contract. This can be accomplished by reviewing the schedule(s) of benefits contained in the subscriber contracts. The pathology provider should determine whether the contract requirements will require the provider to expand operational capabilities or materially alter normal business operations. Pathologists should be aware of and object to the following:

1. provisions that give the managed care entity the power to unilaterally amend the schedule of covered services without giving the pathology provider the right to terminate the contract at least on reasonably short notice
2. language that requires services to be provided at a level of quality higher than that which is generally required (which could significantly increase liability exposure)
3. blanket requirements to provide 24 hours per day services, 7 days a week
4. provisions that require unreasonable turnaround time
5. provisions that require the pathology provider to continue rendering services upon the insolvency or termination of the managed care entity or termination of the contract

Utilization and Peer Review The pathology provider should review all utilization protocols, policies, and procedures in advance of signing the contract. If any utilization protocols, policies, and procedures cannot be followed by the pathologists due to the type of services being provided, these items should be deleted from the contractual obligations. The pathology provider should also determine whether the utilization and peer review protocols, policies, and procedures of the managed care entity blend with the provider's utilization management and peer review programs (e.g., claims submission deadlines, electronic claims submissions). The contract should specify the provider's rights for alleged violations of policies and procedures, including appeal rights. Appeal to an outside arbitration panel is preferred.

It is important to determine the pathologist's obligations regarding referrals and authorization guidelines and the precertification of services (i.e., how does the pathologist determine if necessary authorization/precertification is obtained, how will the pathologist actually obtain authorization/precertification, and what is the risk to the pathologist if necessary authorization/precertification has not been obtained?). The pathology provider should attempt to negotiate language that explains that pay-

ment will not be denied due to another participating provider's or patient's violation of utilization protocols, policies, or procedures (e.g., failure to meet a billing
deadline).

Fee for Service Payment Terms If payment is made to the pathology provider on
a fee-for-service basis, the contract should clearly identify the fee schedule to be
utilized and attach a copy of the minimum fee schedule as an exhibit. It is best to
avoid language that applies the payor's internally developed fee schedule, as such
fee schedule could be modified by the payor at any time. The managed care entity
should not be able to unilaterally reduce the fee schedule, at least not unless the
provider has the right to terminate the contract on short notice.

The contract should address whether payment will be made for the professional
and/or technical components of all services. If the pathology provider performs
both components, the contract should confirm that payment will be made for both
components. The contract should also explain whether payment covers all categories of patients, or only hospital inpatients and outpatients. Increasing numbers of
private payors limit their standard "pathology" contracts to only hospital inpatient
and outpatient professional services, and the contracts do not cover nonhospital
professional services or any technical component services.

Caution should also be given to language that could permit the managed care
entity to unilaterally impose payment edits, similar to Medicare's correct coding initiative edits, that could limit the number of reimbursable units of service, or impose
other payment restrictions such as rebundling edits.

If pathology providers expect payment for professional component of clinical
pathology services, they should specify the payment terms in the contract.

It is important to remember that prompt payment is part of the consideration for
the provider's agreement to accept discounted fees. Payment by the payor to the
pathologist should be tied to the date the properly completed bill is submitted and
not the "approval" date (the latter is largely up to the managed care entity). The
agreement should specify when a claim will be considered "properly completed"
(i.e., what form must be used and what information must appear on it). The pathology provider may wish to negotiate late payment penalties.

If significant administrative responsibilities are assumed with respect to a managed care contract, such as substantial credentials review or utilization management, the provider may want to seek compensation for these services from the managed care entity.

The pathology provider should attempt to delete "most favored nation" clauses.
A "most favored nation" clause requires the provider to give the managed care entity the more favorable financial terms agreed upon between the provider and any
other payor. Generally, a "most favored nation" clause should only be triggered by
financial arrangements with substantially similar plans (e.g., same type of plan,
same patient volume, and same geographic area).

The method of billing the managed care entity should be reasonable and compatible with the current system. The pathology provider should review the specific information that must be disclosed for billing purposes and the specific billing forms.

Other payment considerations include determining if there is a default reimbursement for new codes and tests that may be added in the future and if the managed
care entity can downcode or bundle claims unilaterally. The pathology provider
should also review restrictions on billing for non-covered services and confirm that
such services may be billed to the patient without the necessity for a signed advance
beneficiary notice.

Capitated Payment Terms If payment is made to the pathology provider on a capitation or other "at-risk" method, the contract should specify the payment rate, the
payment schedule/time frame, and any exceptions to or limitations on payment. The
rate should be subject to renegotiation upon specified events. The managed care
entity should not be able to unilaterally reduce the payment rate unless the provider
has the right to terminate the contract on short notice.

Under risk payment contracts, it is also critical to specify the "stop-loss limit."
The stop-loss limit is the limit of liability of the provider and is usually tied to a set
dollar amount per member, per year. The pathology provider should negotiate an
annual aggregate stop-loss limit for all members assigned to the provider to protect
against numerous expensive individual cases.

For capitated payment contracts, the pathology provider should also consider negotiating a "safety net" provision, whereby payment is made on a capitation basis,
but with a guarantee that the aggregate capitation payment will be "no less than" a
specified discounted fee-for-service amount.

The pathology provider should watch provisions that permit the managed care
entity to adjust deductibles, coinsurance, and copayments downward without an appropriate adjustment upward in the capitation rate. Lower deductibles, coinsurance,
and copayments mean higher utilization.

ACO Shared Savings If a pathology provider is participating in an ACO or other
shared savings programs with a payor, the provider may wish to explore its own
"shared savings" model with the ACO. For example, the pathology provider could
determine a baseline of pathology expenses for the prior year. To the extent that
the pathology provider is able to manage utilization, educate physicians regarding
proper ordering of tests, assist physicians in timely interpretation of test results, etc.,
it may be able to lower overall expenditures by the ACO or other payor. The compensation provision would then provide for payment of a portion of these savings
to the pathology provider.

Liability Insurance The pathology provider should confirm that the insurance or
self-insurance requirements under the managed care contract are fair and can be met
without significant additional expense. If the provider is self-insured, the contract
should specifically permit self-insurance. The pathology provider should beware
of contracts that limit insurance to "occurrence" policies. Claims-made insurance
should also be an option.

The provider should not agree to insure against all losses and liabilities. Instead,
coverage requirements should be subject to standard policy exclusions and limitations. The pathology provider should also ensure that it does not agree to insure in-

dividuals or situations that are not covered under its policy. For example, language requiring the payor to be added as an additional insured party to the pathology provider's policy should be deleted.

The managed care entity should be required to maintain adequate professional liability insurance, general liability insurance and, if a risk-bearing entity, reinsurance.

Indemnification and Hold Harmless Provisions The pathology provider should carefully review any indemnification provisions with its insurer. Most insurance policies do not cover contractual indemnification provisions. Possible substitute language is: "Each party shall be responsible for its own acts and omissions to the extent it would be responsible under statutory or common law, and nothing contained in this Agreement shall impute or transfer responsibility for the acts or omissions of one party to the other party."

The pathology provider should beware of provisions that impose liability on the provider beyond that which would exist under applicable law (e.g., liability for acts/ omissions of third parties). In addition, the pathology provider should avoid provisions that shift liability to the provider or make the provider solely responsible for medical care decisions (e.g., unduly shift all responsibility for patient care decisions to the provider).

Reporting, Record Retention, Disclosure, and Facility Inspection The managed care contract should specify what information and records have to be maintained and disclosed (e.g., internal financial information). Record disclosure should be made subject to all applicable laws, regulations, and ethics codes. The pathology provider should not be required to maintain records longer than the provider's standard retention period.

The pathology provider should ensure that record disclosure is limited to the records of subscribers of the managed care entity unless broader disclosure is required by law or by federal or state agencies. The provider should not be required to disclose proprietary business information, or, if such information must be disclosed, the managed care entity should be required to protect its confidentiality and refrain from using such information except where disclosure is required by applicable law.

The pathology provider also should confirm that the managed care entity or provider has proper release forms (including the Health Insurance Portability and Accountability Act (HIPAA) authorizations) in place before releasing a copy of any patient records to a managed care entity.

Use of Name The contract should explain the managed care entity's policy regarding the use of the provider's name in the managed care entity's marketing and promotional materials. The pathology provider may wish to request the right of prior review, and preferably, the right of prior approval, of marketing and promotional materials that reference the provider.

Termination of Contract It is important for the pathology provider to identify how the contract can be terminated. If the contract can be terminated "without good cause," the provider should confirm that the termination rights are reciprocal and balanced. Similarly, "with cause" (or for "good cause") termination language should be reciprocal and balanced between the parties. If there is a provision for "with cause" or "good cause" termination, the term "with cause" or "good cause" should be defined.

The pathology provider should obtain the right to terminate the contract upon a certain amount of notice, preferably not to exceed 90 days, so that a "bad" contract can be terminated quickly. The provider should watch for provisions that permit such notice termination only at the end of a term, as these will lock the provider in for each term of the agreement.

The managed care entity should not be permitted to terminate the contract for the acts or omissions of a single professional. The contract should provide for termination action only against the individual professional.

The pathology provider should obtain the right to terminate the contract immediately if the managed care entity fails to make payment, files for bankruptcy, or becomes insolvent.

Dispute Resolution The managed care contract should describe the procedure for resolving disputes and the venue for resolution of disputes. The contractual language should give the provider the right to present its argument and to hear the opposing arguments/evidence. The provider should also have at least one level of appeal to an independent third party. Some contracts refer to the dispute resolution procedures of the American Health Lawyers Association or the American Arbitration Association, and both are acceptable alternatives.

The pathology provider should beware of dispute resolution procedures where the managed care entity has final authority to resolve disputes. Instead, the provider should push for the right to submit disputes to an independent body such as an arbitration panel. The provider should also avoid restrictions on the provider's ability to litigate against the managed care entity or engage in a class action or arbitration. It is advisable to delete provisions that state that the contract is governed by the laws of another state, or that the venue for dispute resolution is in another state.

Other Provisions The contract should specify how notices have to be sent under the contract (e.g., by certified mail). It is preferable to require notice to be sent in a format in which a receipt is confirmed (such as certified mail or overnight courier delivery), rather than regular mail, general mailings, or Web site notices. Managed care contracts are increasingly specifying Web sites as permissible means of providing notice, which can be problematic for the pathology provider. No provider has time to constantly review a managed care entity's Web site.

Amendment and modification to the contract should be mutually agreed, in writing, and with prior notice. At a minimum, the contract should contain the right to terminate if key terms are amended or modified.

The contract should explain the parties' rights, if any, to assign the contract. The pathology provider should avoid provisions that permit the managed care entity to assign the contract without the provider's consent. The provider may wish to have the right, however, to assign the contract to its affiliates or successors without the managed care entity's consent.

The foregoing are not the only legal provisions in a typical managed care contract, but these items represent common provisions that should be considered by pathologists when evaluating and negotiating a managed care contract. The method of billing the managed care entity should be reasonable and compatible with the current system. The pathology provider should review the specific information that must be disclosed for billing purposes and the specific billing forms.

> Be wary of any aspect of an agreement, such as any internally produced fee schedule, that may be unilaterally modified without mutual assent.

Case: Recoupment or Recourse?

Suburban Pathology Associates, LLC is a participating provider with Statewide Health Plan. Out of the blue, Suburban Pathology Associates, LLC receives a recoupment notice from Statewide Health Plan, explaining that Statewide Health Plan has determined that Suburban Pathology Associates, LLC has been overpaid US$225,000 for its pathology services and if Suburban Pathology Associates, LLC does not repay the amount in full within 30 days, Statewide Health Plan will withhold the sum from all future payments due to Suburban Pathology Associates, LLC for services rendered to subscribers of Statewide Health Plan.

Can Statewide Health Plan issue an overpayment notice under the agreement and, more importantly, can it recoup the alleged overpayment by withholding amounts from future payments?

What are Suburban Pathology Associates, LLC's appeal rights under the participating provider agreement? Is there a short time frame to file an appeal?

Case: Recourse Following a Payment Change

City Pathology, Inc. is a pathology practice focused on the outreach marketplace. It has a particular focus on dermatopathology, but also provides other pathology services for nonhospital outreach patients. City Pathology, Inc. has its own technical component histology laboratory and therefore can provide global (professional and technical component) services. It signed a participating provider agreement many years ago with Big Health Plan. After years of being paid favorable rates by Big Health Plan, City Pathology, Inc.'s collections from its global services billed to Big Health Plan fell by 50%. Upon inquiring with Big Health Plan as to the reason, the Big Health Plan representative explained simply that Big Health Plan not only has reduced its payment rates, but it will only pay providers such as City Pathology, Inc. for professional services. Only National Laboratory can bill and be paid for technical component services on a going forward basis.

What recourse does City Pathology, Inc. have under its participating provider agreement with Big Health Plan?

Does the agreement address unilateral changes to payment rates by Big Health Plan?

What is the description of covered services in the agreement? Does the description cover technical component services?

Chapter 11
Hospital Contracts

Jane Pine Wood

Case: A Sudden Threat

Community Pathology, P.C.'s contract with City Hospital is up for renewal. There is a new CEO at the hospital. The new CEO allegedly was recruited to improve City Hospital's financial bottom line and cut expenditures, and the pathologists have heard that he refused to make Part A payments to the pathologists at his former hospital.

When Community Pathology, P.C. receives the renewal contract from City Hospital, there are several major changes from the existing contract. All Part A payments have been eliminated. The contract states that the group is prohibited from billing for its professional component of clinical pathology services. The contract charges the practice rent for its use of the laboratory offices for professional interpretations. In addition, the contract gives the hospital the right to bill globally for the hospital technical component services and the pathologists' professional component services, with the hospital determining the amounts to be paid to the pathologists for such globally billed services.

When Community Pathology, P.C. expresses concerns to the new CEO, he responds that "If you don't like it, then I'll just put this contract out to bid to other pathology groups."

What are the compliance issues raised under the new contract? Can Community Pathology, P.C. agree to accept zero Part A payments in exchange for the exclusive contract?

Does the hospital have any exposure under the fraud and abuse laws for the actions of the CEO? Do the members of the hospital's board have any personal exposure?

What steps can Community Pathology, P.C. take, both before receiving the new contract and after receiving the new contract, to better position itself for negotiating with City Hospital?

Hospital Contract Negotiations for Pathologists

The negotiation of a pathology practice's hospital contract generally is one of the practice's most critical tasks. The dynamics of the relationship between a hospital and its hospital-based pathologists continue to change and become more complex. Payment amounts from hospitals are generally declining. In addition, third party payor reimbursement methodologies are changing, with more accountable care organizations, shared savings, bundled payments, and capitation. Both of these trends result in efforts by hospitals to exert more control over managed care contracting for pathology services.

J. P. Wood (✉)
McDonald Hopkins, LLC, 956 Main St., Dennis, MA 02638, USA
e-mail: jwood@mcdonaldhopkins.com

© Springer International Publishing Switzerland 2016
L. A. Hassell et al. (eds.), *Pathology Practice Management*,
DOI 10.1007/978-3-319-22954-6_11

Other trends include greater restrictions on outside activities by pathology practices as hospitals attempt to retain volume, shorter contract terms, and more contracts subject to competitive bidding.

Pathology practices must carefully plan the negotiation of their contracts with hospitals not only to maximize the Part A compensation from the hospital but also to avoid undue restrictions on their medical practices and outside activities. The parties must be mindful to avoid the compliance issues that would arise from a contract in which the hospital receives, directly or indirectly, inappropriate remuneration from the pathology practice.

Negotiation Preparation

The process of preparing for the negotiation should begin many months in advance of the expiration date of the current contract. A game plan should be established that would include at least the following preparatory steps:

1. Review the terms of the current contract of the pathology practice with the hospital and determine if any problem areas exist from the pathology practice's standpoint or from the hospital's perspective. Have there been any tacit amendments to the contract that have not been memorialized in writing? Have any promises been made by the hospital of any future accommodations or contract modifications?
2. Determine the strategic plan of the hospital. What is the hospital's current and projected financial condition? Is the hospital in merger or affiliation talks with other health systems? How well is it doing in attracting managed care plans or the business of other third parties? Is the hospital planning any projects off site in which the pathology practice could be involved? Are any professional services which could be provided by the department being routinely sent to outside providers?
3. Check with the other hospital-based groups in the hospital. What has been the general experience of the anesthesia, radiology, or emergency room groups in their negotiations? A word of caution is needed here. Agreements on the part of nonintegrated hospital-based groups related to what they will accept as fees, or prices, or collective activity that involves a boycott, refusal to deal, or the threat of either, can violate federal and state antitrust laws.
4. Determine how the pathology practice is perceived by the hospital or the medical staff. If the perception is in any way negative, how can the pathologists act to change negative perceptions?
5. Determine how dependent the pathology practice is on the level of hospital financial support it receives. To what extent (and how) could the pathology practice deal with various levels of change in that support?
6. Determine what opportunities may exist in the next few years to provide services at locations other than the hospital, including other hospitals and freestanding medical facilities.

In short, groups need to "do their homework" before entering into contract negotiations with the hospital. Information and preparation is critical. Financial information and comparative data can be extremely valuable in negotiations or in responding to questions raised by the hospital personnel.

> Preparation for contract negotiations is a critical part of the process, and best started before the ink is dry on the last contract.

Selling the Value of Pathology Services

As explained above, it is critical for pathology practices to educate their hospitals about the value of the services provided by the pathologists. As a first step, pathology practices should explain, in detail, the various types of pathology services that they provide, including anatomic pathology services, professional component of clinical pathology services, blood banking services, autopsy services, graduate medical education services, research services, outreach services, etc. The pathologists should ensure that the hospital administration understands the significant commitment of time and expertise required to provide these services, especially those services for which the pathology practice cannot bill payors or patients (i.e., services for which the sole source of compensation is the hospital).

If the pathology practice has one or more pathologists with specialty expertise, this pathology specialization and its relation to the provision of specialized services by the hospital and its medical staff should be emphasized. For example, one or more pathologists with hematology expertise offer significant support to the provision of oncology services at the hospital. A pathologist with pediatric specialization is vital to a hospital that prides itself upon its pediatric services. Without such pathology expertise, the hospital and members of its medical staff would not be able to provide the same level of specialized hospital and medical services.

The pathology practice should explain that quality pathology services are directly related to more satisfied medical staffs and patients, which means that the hospital is less likely to lose referring physicians and patients to competitors. Quality of care is increasingly an important issue to some payors, and the expertise of the pathology services can have an impact on the hospital's ability to secure preferred managed care contracting.

Pathologists can effectively market the clinical laboratory and anatomic pathology services offered by hospitals to physician offices, surgery centers, nursing homes, and other health-care providers, and often are the single most important factor in a client's selection of pathology and laboratory services. It is advisable for pathologists to assess the dollar value of the outreach services provided by the hospital, and explain to the hospital the critical role that the pathologists play in securing this business and retaining it.

Quality pathology services reduce the risk of malpractice liability for hospitals and attending physicians. If hospitals are interested in cutting costs and are looking for the "lowest cost" provider of pathology services, the hospitals may be increasing their exposure from a liability perspective. Pathology practices should remind budget-minded hospitals that courts have held hospitals legally responsible for the negligent selection of hospital-based physicians, and the more prudent approach for hospitals is to pay a reasonable amount to secure the services of competent and trained pathologists. In addition, pathologists also can assist hospitals in reducing their liability exposure through their supervision and oversight of hospital laboratory personnel.

Pathologists play a key role in controlling costs in hospital laboratories. If the hospital treats its pathologists fairly and looks for "win–win" scenarios with its pathologists, then the pathologists will be much more attentive to controlling laboratory costs while maintaining quality services. During contract negotiations, it is advisable for the pathology practice to educate the hospital about the steps taken by the pathology practice to control expenses in the laboratory to the financial benefit of the hospital.

Another important benefit that the pathology practice provides to the hospital is with respect to the accreditation and certification of hospital laboratories. Pathology practice is responsible for not only providing medical direction as required by the Clinical Laboratory Improvement Amendments of 1988 (CLIA), the College of American Pathologists (CAP), and the Joint Commission, but also providing the supervision and oversight of all of the technical services provided by the hospital's laboratory personnel.

With the increasing importance of shared savings under accountable care organizations, bundled payment methodologies and other payor incentives to provide cost-effective care, the pathologists' professional component of clinical pathology services are critical to the financial success of the hospital. These are the services that pathologists provide that contribute to the efficient operations of the hospital laboratory, including interactions with clinicians to assist in the selection of appropriate tests for patients, monitoring ordering of tests to detect inappropriate or unnecessary test ordering, implementing cost control measures in the laboratory, establishing and enforcing policies that are designed to promote quality and timely services, etc.

Legal Compliance

It is critical to review the legal compliance issues that arise in contract negotiations between hospitals and pathologists. Remuneration between a hospital and pathologists may implicate the Medicare and Medicaid anti-kickback law, particularly if the pathologists are required to pay direct or indirect remuneration to the hospital (or otherwise provide a benefit to the hospital) as a condition of providing services to the hospital's inpatients and outpatients.

The Office of the Inspector General (OIG) has explained that a hospital's demand for compensation from its hospital-based physicians is suspect under the anti-kickback law (Department of Health and Human Services, OIG Management Advisory Report: Financial Arrangements Between Hospitals and Hospital-Based Physicians, pp. 3–4, January 31, 1991). This OIG report specifically discusses no, or token, reimbursement to pathologists for Part A services in return for the opportunity to perform and bill for Part B services at that hospital. The OIG's Compliance Program Guidance for Hospitals also cautions against arrangements with hospital-based physicians that compensate the physicians less than fair market value for their services, including no, or token, Part A compensation for pathologists (OIG's Compliance Guidance for Hospitals, footnote 25, February 1998). By refusing to pay adequate compensation to pathologists for their Part A services or by conditioning the contract upon the provision of direct or indirect benefits or remuneration from the pathologists, hospitals and their individual administrators and trustees may violate the anti-kickback law, thereby subjecting themselves to criminal and civil penalties. The pathologists may share in this compliance risk if they agree to the terms.

Key Contractual Provisions

Parties to the Contract

If the pathologist is practicing through a professional corporation, partnership, or limited liability company, the contract generally should be with the entity and not with the individual. Any payment by the hospital should be made to the entity to avoid tax problems.

It is preferable from the pathology group's standpoint to have each professional employee of the group acknowledge in writing that he or she is bound by the terms of the contract and any extension, modification, or replacement contract. This is important because the hospital contract may contain provisions, which affect vested rights of the employee, such as termination of hospital privileges upon termination from the pathology group. The terms of the pathology group's employment agreements should match obligations under the hospital contract.

The contract should be carefully written to extend to successor entities (including purchasers) and assignees due to the increasing number of hospital consolidations and combinations.

Relationship of the Parties

The contract should state that the hospital will not exercise direction or control over the practice of medicine by the pathologists. In addition, the contract should provide that the pathology group is not liable for injuries to patients due to a defect in hospital facilities.

It is advisable to state that the employees, agents, and other independent contractors of the hospital are not the employees, agents, or independent contractors of the pathology group and that the physician group has no liability or responsibility for their acts or omissions.

Qualifications of Professionals
Pathologists should be mindful of provisions that permit the hospital administration to circumvent the medical staff credentials review procedure, such as "All pathologists rendering services at hospital are subject to the prior and continuing approval of hospital's CEO."

The hospital contract should permit the provision of services by both board certified and board eligible pathologists. As a compromise, if the hospital demands board certification, there could be a grandfathering of certain pathologists and a transition period during which pathologists are allowed to pass their boards.

Services Provided by Pathology Group
Coverage requirements should be specified in the contract or the pathology group should only commit to providing adequate coverage in accordance with sound medical principles as determined by the group, in consultation with the hospital. The contract should distinguish between "on site" and "on call" coverage periods.

The pathology group should object to language that requires services to be provided at a level of quality higher than that which is generally required. An example of such language is "Pathology Group shall provide services at the highest level of quality." Such language sounds laudatory, but could increase the liability exposure to both the hospital and the pathologists.

The pathology group's obligation to provide services should be conditioned upon the hospital's obligation to provide adequate equipment, space, services, and personnel in accordance with all applicable licensure and accreditation standards.

The obligation to participate in committees and in educational programs should be subject to a reasonableness standard and should be consistent with the bylaws, rules, and regulations of the medical staff, as well as applicable regulatory requirements. The specific committees on which the pathology group wants to serve should be specified.

Managed Care Contracting
The hospital's ability to obtain a managed care contract may depend to some degree on whether its pathologists also participate under the contract. Managed care payors often pressurize hospitals to "deliver" their pathologists as providers under the managed care contract. Therefore, pathologists should be wary of provisions which give the hospital the right to require the pathology group to enter into alternative delivery system or managed care contracts. An example of such a provision is "Pathology Group shall execute such agreements as may be necessary to become participating providers in such third-party reimbursement programs as hospital may from time to time direct." It is advisable to include language that gives the pathology group the ability to decline to contract with payors who offer unreasonable terms.

Exclusivity
The pathology group should be given the exclusive right to provide professional pathology services at the hospital. The contract should stipulate reasons for the exclusive contracts, such as standardization of procedures, more efficient scheduling, and more efficient use of facilities. Such legitimate reasons for an exclusive

arrangement can help defend against an antitrust challenge. If other providers in the hospital perform certain services that would typically be considered as pathology services, it is important to limit the exceptions to the exclusive arrangement as specifically as possible.

The contract should state that the hospital does not have the right to "outsource" the department's services without the pathology group's permission. An exclusive contract can be destroyed if the hospital is able to unbundle the work and give portions of it to outside parties. Watch provisions that limit the exclusive to services at the hospital.

It is preferable for the exclusivity provision to extend to each facility of the hospital (or any subsidiary, parent, or affiliate of the hospital) to the extent such facility can be adequately staffed by the pathology group. This could be in the form of a right of first refusal.

Departmental Operations

The method for selecting the department director and successor department directors should be specified in the contract. All department directors should be members of the pathology group. Identify the initial department director. The duties of the director should be specifically delineated.

The contract should state that the bylaws, rules, regulations, and policies of the hospital cannot be altered in any manner which materially increases the obligations of the pathology group under the contract without the group's consent.

Services Provided by the Hospital

The contract should identify the space and utilities to be provided by the hospital, the type of equipment and supplies to be furnished by the hospital, the personnel to be provided by the hospital, etc. These items should be sufficient for the proper and efficient operation of the department and be consistent with generally accepted standards. All items and services provided by the hospital should be consistent with the requirements of CLIA, CAP, and the Joint Commission, as well as all other applicable licensing and accrediting bodies.

The pathology group probably will want the right of prior input regarding the hiring, firing, etc. of nonprofessional personnel in the department. The hospital may resist any restrictions upon its relationship with its employees, particularly because the hospital remains ultimately liable for its employees.

Compensation for Services

The contract should specify the amount and/or method of payment for both professional services and administrative services. Typically, the pathology group's compensation for its professional anatomic pathology services and professional clinical consultative services is its collections from billing patients and their third-party payors for the services. The pathology group may also receive compensation for professional component of clinical pathology services provided to patients covered by private health plans through such direct billing. However, compensation for professional component of clinical pathology services for patients who are beneficiaries of government health plans, for medical director services, and for other designated administrative services (in the aggregate, commonly referred to as "Part A services") should be paid by the hospital to the pathology group. As noted above, the failure of the hospital to pay fair market value for these Part A services can present a serious compliance issue under the Medicare and Medicaid anti-kickback law for both parties.

The Medicare program provides for reimbursement for the professional component of clinical pathology services to Medicare beneficiaries through Medicare Part A Diagnosis Related Group (DRG) payments to hospitals, rather than through Medicare Part B payments to pathologists. When the Medicare program decided to shift the reimbursement for professional component services from Medicare Part B to Medicare Part A, the Centers for Medicare & Medicaid Services allocated payment for professional component services into its DRG calculations. The current Medicare reimbursement methodology for professional component of clinical pathology services presumes that the hospital will reimburse the pathologists directly for these services. Therefore, the hospital does receive money from the Medicare program for these services and should remit payment to the pathologists.

The contract should explain whether the Part A payment from the hospital is intended to cover professional component of clinical pathology services only for Medicare and Medicaid hospital patients, or also for some or all patients covered by private payors. This is especially important if the pathology group bills or wishes to commence billing for professional component of clinical pathology services to private patients. Pathologists will want to protect against interference with the right to bill for the professional component of clinical pathology services. This can be done in several ways, including becoming educated about professional component billing, educating other pathologists in the group, proactively educating the administration and the medical staff, monitoring and keeping track of any patient questions and/or complaints, developing a formal policy for addressing patient questions and complaints, and avoiding hospital contract provisions that prohibit professional component billing. The contract also should require the hospital's cooperation in the development of appropriate notification language for the hospital administration as well as registration forms.

The contract should require renegotiation of the compensation provisions in the event changes in law, regulation, or health plan policies restrict or alter the pathology group's right to bill for professional services.

> Avoid any trace of "kickback" allegations by ensuring that both parties have recognized fair market value for all goods, services, and space.

Billing
The contract should specify the pathology group's right to direct bill for services. In addition, the hospital should be required to supply in a timely manner all information required by the pathology group to bill and collect for professional services.

The manner in which the fees for professional services will be determined should be specified. It is obviously preferable if fee determination is left to the discretion of the pathology group. If the hospital demands veto power or the right to set the fees, an objective standard should be utilized, such as comparability to fees charged by other pathologists in the community and/or at comparable hospitals.

The hospital should be required to maintain the confidentiality of the pathology group's fee schedule. If the hospital receives a request for fee information, it should only release the fee information in question and not the entire fee schedule unless it has the prior consent of the pathology group. A procedure should be established for handling such fee information requests.

Global Billing

Global, bundled, or other packaged billing/pricing is expected to increase over the coming years, and, in response, many hospitals are including language in contracts to address such billing. Pathology groups should attempt to restrict the ability of the hospital to bind the group to global billing. At the very least, the hospital contract should state that global billing can only be offered by the hospital if it has been requested by the payor, meaning that it cannot be initiated by the hospital (at least, not without the consent of the pathology group). It is vital that the group be guaranteed a voice in bargaining with the managed care payor to adequately protect the group's interest. In addition, the hospital should agree that it will not disclose the global bill provision to payors.

Liability Insurance

Pathologists should review the liability insurance requirements to confirm that the required insurance levels are appropriate and can be met without significant additional expense. It is important not to agree to insure against all losses and liabilities. Instead, coverage requirements should be subject to standard policy exclusion and limitations. In addition, language should be reviewed to confirm that coverage requirements do not include individuals or situations that may not be covered under the pathology group's policy. This includes "additional insured" language, because the pathology group's policy may not permit adding other entities, such as the hospital, as an additional insured.

If the pathologist has a claims-made policy, the hospital will probably require tail coverage in the event of termination of such policy or if a pathologist leaves the group. This is because insurance coverage under a claims-made policy ends when the insurance policy is terminated or when a pathologist leaves the group. Tail coverage provides insurance coverage for claims which arise after the termination of coverage under the claims-made policy. Often, tail coverage is free of charge if termination of coverage under the policy is due to retirement, disability, or death.

The hospital should be required to maintain adequate professional liability insurance or self-insurance on itself and its employees and agents and adequate comprehensive public liability insurance or self-insurance. The hospital also should maintain liability insurance covering the pathology group and its members with respect to their administrative, research, and teaching functions.

Indemnification Provisions

An indemnification provision is one in which the indemnifying party agrees to pay the other party any dollar amounts that the other party "is out of pocket" as a result of the indemnifying events. For example, if the pathology group agrees to indemnify and hold harmless the hospital for any losses as a result of acts or omissions of the group, then the pathology group must pay the hospital any amount spent or incurred by the hospital in the defense and/or settlement of claims that might arise from the acts or omissions of the pathology group, such as malpractice actions based on errors in the laboratory. Such provisions typically are not covered by the pathology group's malpractice insurance. Therefore, it is important to confirm coverage in writing with the insurance carrier.

Professional liability insurance carriers will usually suggest that such language be eliminated, and recommend substitute language such as "Neither party shall be liable for the acts or omissions of the other party or for the acts or omissions of the employees, agents or other independent contractors of the other party."

The hospital may require that a pathology group indemnify and hold harmless the hospital to the extent that reimbursement is denied due to an improper act of the group. Such indemnity should be limited to the group's proportionate share of responsibility for reimbursement denial, the hospital should give prompt notice to the group of such a denial and take all reasonable steps to challenge it, and the group should be permitted to participate in the challenge. Also, the provision should be reciprocal, so that the hospital agrees to indemnify and hold harmless the group to the extent the group's reimbursement is denied due to an act or omission of the hospital.

Records
Each party's obligations with respect to medical and billing records should be addressed in the contract. Medical records should be distinguished from specimens, slides, etc. The pathology group's right of access to hospital/patient records should be stipulated and should survive the termination of the agreement.

Termination
As a general matter, it is preferable to permit termination for good cause only. If there is a provision for "good cause" termination, the term "good cause" should be defined. A "cure" period should be provided, so that the breaching party has a period of time (typically 15–30 days) to cure the breach and avert termination of the agreement.

If termination is permitted without cause upon a certain period of notice, it is important to understand that the term of the contract (and the period of the exclusivity) is essentially only as long as the notice period. If the hospital has tax-exempt bond financing, Internal Revenue Service (IRS) regulations also may limit the term of the contract.

It is advisable to avoid provisions which permit the hospital to terminate the pathology group for the acts or omissions of a single pathologist. The contract should provide for termination only if the pathology group does not remedy the situation.

Restrictive Covenants
Pathologists will want to avoid noncompetition clauses if at all possible, or at least negotiate a noncompetition clause as narrow and specific as possible with respect to services, duration, and geographic scope.

The group will want to be permitted to engage in outside activities so long as such activities do not interfere with the pathology group's responsibilities under the hospital contract. If there are restrictions on outside activities, such restrictions should cover only true competition, and should be reasonable as to time period and geographic area. Often, a quid pro quo for such restrictions is a right of first refusal to provide services at any new facility of the hospital or a subsidiary, affiliate or parent of the hospital.

The preceding list is not a comprehensive list of every hospital contract provision, but most hospital contracts will address these issues. This discussion can be used as an initial checklist for a review of a proposed (or even an existing) hospital contract.

Case: A New Laboratory

City Pathology, Inc. provides pathology services to Major Medical Center pursuant to an exclusive services contract. City Pathology, Inc. wishes to expand its outreach (nonhospital) work and in connection with such expansion, plans to open its own technical component histology laboratory. City Pathology, Inc. is considering adding some limited clinical laboratory or even molecular pathology services to the laboratory operations as well. City Pathology, Inc. has secured space for the laboratory several blocks from Major Medical Center, Soon afterward, the CEO of Major Medical Center storms into the offices of the pathologists and demands to know why City Pathology, Inc. is taking steps to open a competing laboratory in violation of the restrictive covenant in its contract with Major Medical Center.

What does the contractual agreement with Major Medical Center say about competition? Will the new laboratory actually compete with Major Medical Center?

Can the hospital contract be amended to provide a limited carve-out for City Pathology, Inc.'s contemplated activities?

Chapter 12
Pathologist Employment Contracts

Amelia B. Larsen

Case: The Noncompetition Conundrum

Dr. Pathologist has moved back to her hometown. She has received a job offer from Suburban Pathology Associates, LLC. She is thrilled as she wants to take the job with Suburban Pathology Associates, LLC and start a long career in her hometown, close to her family and never have to move again. Dr. Pathologist has received Suburban Pathology Associates, LLC's employment agreement that she must sign in order to take the position.

What sort of items should Dr. Pathologist be on the lookout for in reviewing her employment contract before signing it and agreeing to take the position?

Realistically, what sorts of things should Dr. Pathologist consider negotiating with Suburban Pathology Associates, LLC concerning her employment agreement?

Key Contractual Provisions

Parties to the Employment Contract

The employment contract should clearly identify the parties and the exact nature of their employment relationship. The nature of the employment relationship can have significant impact on personal rights or responsibilities in relation to the employment. Employment relationships are typically classified either as an employer/employee relationship or the individual is an independent contractor for the employer. An employer/employee relationship typically exists when the employer has a significant amount of control over the work of the employee in terms of hours, including vacation time, location, equipment used, and fees charged. Conversely, an independent contractor completes work on a contractual basis with the employer and is subject to less control by the employer.

The distinction between an employee and an independent contractor is important in determining what the employer must provide to the employee. In an employer/employee relationship, the employer is responsible for taking taxes out of the employee's compensation. Furthermore, the employer must make payments for

A. B. Larsen (✉)
McDonald Hopkins, LLC, 600 Superior Ave., Suite 2100, Cleveland, OH 44114, USA
e-mail: alarsen@mcdonaldhopkins.com

© Springer International Publishing Switzerland 2016

L. A. Hassell et al. (eds.), *Pathology Practice Management*,
DOI 10.1007/978-3-319-22954-6_12

workers' compensation, unemployment insurance, disability insurance, and social security on behalf of the employee. Employers are also required by law to comply with minimum wage and overtime requirements, provide for lunch and rest breaks, and provide benefits for those employees who are eligible under the employer's benefit plan. On the other hand, if you are employed as an independent contractor, the employer will not take any taxes out of your compensation and the independent contractor is responsible for remitting taxes from that compensation. Additionally, an independent contractor will not be eligible for unemployment benefits, since nothing will have been paid into the unemployment fund on their behalf.

However, employers wanting to structure their practices with independent contractors rather than employees need to be careful. Following the economic recession in 2008, many employers have been seeking to find creative ways of decreasing their expenses. One way employers have sought to cut costs has been to classify workers as independent contractors rather than employees—by doing so they are no longer responsible for providing health-care benefits and employment taxes. However, since this is a way of avoiding taxes, the classification of workers has become highly monitored by the Internal Revenue Service (IRS) and the Department of Labor. If an employer is found to have misclassified its workers as independent contractors rather than employees the employer becomes vulnerable to an imposition of fines, penalties, and back-taxes, which has the potential to cost an employer large sums of money. Factors which the IRS and the Department of Labor will look to in determining whether certain individuals have been misclassified include the permanency of the employment relationship, a longer or open-ended commitment indicates an employer/employee relationship; whether the employer provides tools or reimburses the worker for work related expenses, if so it is indicative of an employer/employee relationship; whether the employer provides any sort of training or instructions on how the work should be performed, if so the worker will be classified as an employee; and whether the worker realizes a profit or loss for the work being performed, if so the worker is more likely to be classified as an independent contractor.

One of the most important impacts of the type of employment is who will be held liable in the event of a malpractice claim. If you are an employee, rather than an independent contractor, the employer can be vicariously liable for medical malpractice suits. However, there are still some instances where the employer will be liable even if you are an independent-contractor.

Finally, while one of these employment relationships may sound more preferable over the other, the parties must also consider whether the law in your state prohibits the corporate practice of medicine which would consequently prohibit a corporate employer (an employer whose owners include nonphysicians) from hiring a pathologist as an "employee." Be sure to find out what the law in your state relating to the corporate practice of medicine says prior to negotiating any employment contract. Please refer to the Section *Special Considerations for Employment by Referring Physician Practices* at the end of this chapter for information about special considerations that should be taken into account when defining the employment relationship in the instance of a pathologist who is employed by a referring physician practice (i.e., dermatologist, urologist, or gastroenterologist).

Term

The duration of an employment contract can provide employment stability. However, the longer the term of the employment contract, the more thought that must be given to the proper compensation over the course of the term—both the amount of compensation and the type of compensation (i.e., salary, bonus increases, and equity interest purchase rights). It is common to have a situation where the entering pathologist will be offered only a probationary contract having a fixed term of 12–24 months. In this case, it is appropriate for the pathologist to ask for a representation regarding a future contract. The pathologist can ask for an outline of the terms of the future contract. However, typically the employer will not commit to any future contract.

Please refer to the Section *Special Considerations for Employment by Referring Physician Practices* at the end of this chapter for information about special considerations that should be taken into account concerning the term of the employment contract relationship in the instance of a pathologist who is employed by a referring physician practice (i.e., dermatologist, urologist, or gastroenterologist).

Coverage Obligations and Outside Opportunities

The employment contract may dictate how the pathologist's work coverage will be managed. The pathologist should consider whether responsibility for coverage on nights, weekends, and holidays, if applicable, is shared equally. Most employment contracts will set a minimum amount of hours the pathologist is expected to work, but often will not set a maximum number of hours. The pathologist may want to consider whether he or she will be allowed to participate in certain career-related activities that are not directly related to the employer, such as medical-legal testimony, speeches, and writings. If the employment contract does allow the pathologist to engage in such extracurricular professional activities, it should also address how the resulting income from these activities will be handled—will the employer or the employee be entitled to the income?

Office Locations

Since many medical practices now operate from several different office locations in order to cover larger geographic areas, the employment contract should address the employer's expectations for the pathologist as to which office(s) the pathologist will work from. Even if this is not expressly stated one way or another in the employment contract, it is something that the pathologist should be aware of prior to signing an employment contract. If it is not addressed in the employment contract the pathologist may want to inquire as to whether his or her primary work location could be changed without consent. The pathologist and the practice also need to make sure the pathologist is compliant will all legal requirements and is licensed or certified to practice in each of the locations at which he or she will be working. If one location happens to be across state borders, the pathologist will need to be aware of whether he or she is legally able to practice at that location.

Office Space

Now that the parties have agreed upon where the pathologist will be working, he or she should also consider the conditions of the actual office space itself. While it is not common, the employment contract could include a requirement that the employer provide suitable office space, supplies, equipment, and personnel. The pathologist may want to ensure that the employment contract provides that he or she has access to any necessary medical equipment.

Compensation

The employment contract should be specific as to what compensation will be paid to the pathologist, how often it will be paid, and when it will be paid. If compensation is based on a formula, that formula should be specified in the employment contract. It is important to consider whether the employment contract should include a provision addressing raises. If the contract is for a term that is longer than a year, or includes language which causes it to automatically renew, it is advisable to address raises.

The compensation portion of the employment contract should also specify what employment-related expenses the pathologist is responsible for, and how he or she will be paid. Employee business expenses are generally not deductible on the employee's personal tax return. Employers generally provide pathologists with paid time off to obtain needed continuing education and, within limits, any expenses associated with this education. Some employers may also reimburse the pathologist for other reasonable professional expenses including training, medical staff dues, professional journals, etc. If the employer chooses to cap the amount of money it will reimburse for such expenses, the pathologist should inquire as to whether that cap will increase during the term of the agreement. The pathologist may also want to consider whether the reimbursement cap is similar to that given to other pathologists in your area.

Bonus

It is common for employment contracts to include bonus provisions. Best practice would be to include a mathematically certain formula that is reasonably attainable.

The pathologist should be wary of formulas that provide significant discretion to the employer. It is also advisable to consider whether the bonus formula in the employment contract is similar to what is provided to other new pathologists in the area.

Fringe Benefits

With respect to employee benefits, the pathologist may want to request, and may be entitled to under the Employee Retirement Income Security Act (ERISA), a copy of the Summary Plan Description describing the employer's benefits. ERISA is a federal law that governs the standards for pension plans provided to employees in private industry. ERISA is intended to protect the interests of benefit plan participants by requiring disclosure of financial and other information of employer benefit plans to the plan beneficiaries; establishing a standard of conduct for those managing the plans; and providing for appropriate legal remedies. The pathologist will want to ensure that there is no gap in any coverage, especially health insurance. While disability insurance may be provided, it may not be sufficient to meet the pathologist's needs in the event of a disability. In addition, disability insurance provided by the practice has a taxable payout benefit, in contrast to a disability insurance that is purchased individually by the pathologist. Also, the parties should consider whether the employer will provide options that allow the pathologist to pay for certain expenses, such as dependent care expenses, using pretax dollars. Keep in mind that absent a contractual restriction, all of these group policies could be terminated or modified at any time, leaving the pathologist with only personal policies. Finally, the pathologist should consider what his or her options are with regard to pension or profit sharing plans.

Malpractice Coverage

The malpractice insurance coverage section of the employment contract is one of the most critical areas. The contract should detail the types and limits of malpractice liability coverage that the employer will provide. The pathologist should be careful in considering whether the malpractice coverage provided is adequate. The employment contract should detail who will pay for the coverage. The parties need to consider whether the coverage is occurrence or claims made. If an insurance policy provides for occurrence coverage, it means that the policy coverage dates cover any occurrence giving rise to a malpractice claim during that period. Therefore, under an occurrence coverage policy, if the policy period has concluded but someone brings a claim for something that occurred while the policy was still in effect, the policy will cover that claim. Conversely, claims-made insurance coverage will only cover the claim when both the occurrences giving rise to the claim and the filing of the claim occur within the coverage period. With a claims-made insurance plan, the coverage will continue as long as premiums are paid. When the practice ends, the claims-made policyholder will need to obtain "tail" insurance which will cover any claims made after the end of the practice. If the malpractice coverage is a claims-made policy, the pathologist should ensure that the employment contract addresses who will be responsible for the "tail" insurance. The "tail" insurance coverage is typically a one-time payment. "Tail" insurance is often the pathologist's responsibility; however, the pathologist may be able to negotiate with the employer to provide "tail" insurance coverage in some instances or, if not, may be able to have a future employer pay for such coverage. Malpractice insurance is always something that the parties to the employment contract should address with extreme care, as there can be significant expenses associated with malpractice claims and insurance coverage.

If the pathologist leaves one practice for another and is covered under a claims-made policy, he or she will have to ensure that there is no gap in the coverage. If a switch is made from one employer to another, the pathologist can typically move coverage from one carrier (used at the old employer) to another carrier (used at the new employer). If this is not an option, the pathologist can also obtain "tail" insurance for the old employer's claims-made policy.

Claims-made and occurrence malpractice coverage options each have their advantages. One benefit of the claims-made coverage is that it offers more flexibility; since the coverage must be renewed every year to remain in effect, the pathologist can increase limits or add new coverage that was not available at the start of the policy. With a claims-made policy, when such increases or additional coverage options are added, those changes will also apply to all past years, going back to the start of your coverage. On the other hand, occurrence coverage has the advantage that it is permanent—once the policy is purchased the pathologist does not have to worry when a claim is brought, as long as the policy was in effect at the time of the incident giving rise to the claim.

As far as the costs associated with these two coverage options, an occurrence coverage policy is typically more expensive than a claims-made policy. In the first few years of the policy, claims-made coverage will be much cheaper. However, as time goes on, the premiums of claims-made policies will increase as the policy will now cover a longer time period where an incident could have occurred and it can take several years from the time an incident occurs to the time it becomes a claim. In regard to cost, the pathologist should also consider the cost of the "tail" insurance needed when concluding practice under a particular claims-made policy. A "tail" insurance plan on average costs 175 % of the last year's claims-made plan premium. Thus, if the pathologist has a claims-made policy for several years and must buy a "tail" plan when that policy is terminated, the total cost of coverage will begin to approach the rate of a comparable occurrence policy. Nonetheless, a claims-made policy will typically cost 35 % less for a claims-made policy plus an unlimited tail insurance plan than an occurrence coverage plan for the same period of time. Additionally, many claims-made policies will provide a "tail" policy for free in the event of death, disability, or permanent retirement. This option can make the cost of the claims-made policy considerably cheaper.

Vacation, Disability, Maternity/Paternity, and Sick Leave

The pathologist should be aware of the Family Medical Leave Act (FMLA), a federal law that protects employees' rights to take certain types of work leave. FMLA ensures that employees are given time off from work, without the risk of losing their jobs, for certain qualified medical leave absences, including personal or family illness leave, family military leave, and leave for pregnancy or adoption of a child. It is important that the parties come to an understanding regarding which types of leave the pathologist is entitled to during the term of the employment. This understanding includes specifying which types of leave the employer will pay for, and, if applicable, at what level they will be paid. If the employment contract is for 2 years or more, the contract should address whether vacation, meeting, and sick leave will increase over the term of the contract. The parties should come to an agreement in the employment contract as to whether leave for continuing education will be counted as vacation or not. The pathologist should inquire about the employer's policy on maternity and paternity leave. The employment contract should address leaves of absence—are they allowed and what are the related policies. Finally, the employment contract should suggest whether any unused time will be eligible to be carried forward into future years of the contract.

The contract should include a reasonable definition of disability and include provisions detailing how long salary and benefits will continue in the event of a disability. The contract should specify who will make the disability determination. This determination should be made by an outside physician or an unbiased expert. This provision in the employment contract should provide for any applicable procedure available to challenge the determination of disability.

Termination

Generally employment contracts give both parties a reasonable amount of prior notice in order to terminate the contract. It is common that the employment contract will allow the employer to reserve the right to terminate the pathologist immediately for good cause as determined in good faith by the employer. A prudent prospective pathologist employee would try to have provisions which would limit for-cause terminations to material breaches of the contract after a "cure" period. The cure period would mean that the pathologist would be informed of the concern giving rise to the employer's claim that a for-cause termination is appropriate, and be given a reasonable period of time to fix, or cure, that concern before the employer can actually terminate the employment.

The employment contract should also address the pathologist's rights in the event that a termination of employment occurs. This sort of provision would address how and when accrued salary and bonuses will be paid. The employment contract should provide what rights are available to the parties in each of these termination situations: (1) either party terminates the contract voluntarily, (2) either party terminates the contract for cause (as allowed for in the contract), (3) breach of the employment contract by either party, (4) change in the law, which changes the employment contract's efficacy, or (5) the contract simply expires.

Noncompetition

Health-care employers have become increasingly interested in including noncompete provisions in employment contracts. For pathologists a noncompete provision will require the pathologist not to compete with the employer's business during the term of the agreement or for a time after the expiration of the agreement. Obviously, such noncompete provisions are not favorable to the pathologist employee. In some states a noncompete provision in an employment contract is not enforceable (i.e., California and Massachusetts). Some other states will only allow enforcement of noncompete provisions dependent on several factors including limited geographic scope, a limited period of time, and a limited range of prohibited work activities. Examples of limiting the range of prohibited work activities include restrictions on practicing in a certain practice area within the same market as the previous employer, or prohibiting the former employee's ability to contact any of the previous employer's patients or clients within so many years of leaving the employer. Another potential protection the pathologist may demand could be to limit the event which would trigger the efficacy of the noncompete provision to instances of good cause termination by the employer or notice termination by the employee.

A noncompete contract provision may or may not be important to a pathologist in negotiating an employment contract depending on how connected he or she is to the practice location. It is also important to be aware of the potential consequences of violating a noncompete provision, which include potential forfeiture of whatever money remains due under the employment contract, an injunction forcing the pathologist to leave his or her new employer, or an imposition of liquidated damages. Liquidated damages apply when the employment contract specifically provides for them, establishing that in the event the noncompete provision is breached, the employee will be responsible for paying the specified amount.

Confidentiality

Many employment contracts require the pathologist-employee to keep information, such as financial statements, confidential. The confidentiality provision of the employment contract is not favorable to the pathologist employee, and thus their goal would be to limit the scope of this provision. For example, the confidentiality provision should allow the pathologist to disclose confidential information to certain advisors such as their attorney or accountant.

Future Ownership

A pathologist who is joining a practice may want to discuss future ownership possibilities, if he or she decides to join the practice. Typically, the employer will not commit to ownership in its initial employment agreement.

Assignment

An assignment provision to an employment contract could potentially allow the employer to assign its rights to the contract to another entity or individual. This is particularly important in today's health-care market, where practices are being sold with an ever-increasing frequency. It is in the pathologist's best interest to ensure that the assignment provision requires the employer to obtain the pathologist's consent prior to assigning the contract to another entity or individual.

All-Inclusive

The all-inclusive portion of an employment contract essentially states that the terms agreed to by the parties in the contract are intended to reflect their entire agreement regarding employment of the pathologist with the employer. While this may seem like a minor and insignificant part of the employment contract, each party should carefully consider the potential weight of the all-inclusive provision of the employment contract. If the contract does not contain all promises that each party relied upon when deciding to enter into an employment relationship, those promises will not be a part of the deal, and thus will have no legal effect. If there is a promise that was relied on by either party, they should ensure that it is included in the final employment contract, or else they will have no legal recourse as to the omitted promise.

Hospital Recruiting Agreement

Some employers request a hospital to assist in the funding of a new pathologist, and the new pathologist is required to execute a recruitment (or income subsidy) agreement with the hospital. These agreements should be reviewed very carefully. Many require repayment of the subsidy by the new pathologist. Even if the subsidy is forgiven over a period of years, the new pathologist will be responsible for the income taxes allocable to the forgiven amounts. In addition, such agreements often have substantial service obligations and bind the pathologist to the community for a number of years.

Special Considerations for Employment by Referring Physician Practices

There are additional compliance considerations for pathologists who are employed by referring physician practices such as dermatologists, gastroenterologists, and urologists. A federal law, known as the Stark law, set certain limitations for pathologists who are employed by a referring physician practice. The Stark law requires that the referring practice enter into a written agreement with the pathologist who will be performing the professional interpretations for the practice. This agreement must comply with the Stark exception for personal services or the Stark "bona fide" employment exception (described in detail below). If there is an independent contractor agreement with a pathology practice rather than an individual pathologist, each interpreting pathologist must also sign an acknowledgment of the terms of the agreement. The personal services exception requires that:

1. The arrangement is in writing, signed by the parties, and specifies the services that will be covered by the arrangement
2. The arrangement covers all services that will be provided
3. The term of the agreement is at least 1 year
4. The agreement specifies the compensation, which must be set in advance, consistent with fair market value, and not determined in a way that takes into account the volume or value of referrals
5. The services contracted for do not exceed those reasonably necessary to accomplish the legitimate business purposes of the parties
6. The services and arrangement do not violate any other State or Federal law [42 U.S.C.A. § 1395nn(e)(3)]

The "bona fide" employment exception requires that:

1. The employment is for identifiable services
2. The compensation is consistent with fair market value, is not determined in a way that takes into account the volume or value of referrals and would be commercially reasonable, even if no referrals are made to the employer
3. The compensation is set forth and paid pursuant to a written agreement [42 U.S.C.A. § 1395nn(e)(2)]

To explain further, regardless of whether the pathologist is hired as an employee or as an independent contractor, the compensation paid for the professional component services must reflect fixed, fair market value rates in an arms-length transaction. If the pathologist is a bona fide W-2 employee, the dermatology or other practice may pay the pathologist a percentage of collections for the professional interpretations. If the arrangement is an independent contractor arrangement, a percentage based compensation structure is highly discouraged under the Stark law and instead, the compensation should be a fixed amount, either monthly, per diem, hourly, or per interpretation. The independent contractor pathologist should not be at risk for collection of any amounts.

As provided above, the Stark law contract requirements include various vague terms, such as "fair market value," and "commercially reasonable." In order for the parties to remain protected, they should execute documents contemporaneous with the employment contract to prove fair market value and commercial reasonableness at the time the contract was created. In doing this, the parties are protecting themselves from any changes which may occur to the meaning of these terms after they enter into the employment contract.

Case: Changing the Employment Relationship

The independent eight-person practice of Valley Pathology has been struggling with the issue of practice overhead for some time, and the recent economic downturn has provoked a bit of conflict between the partners about which health plans to provide and how extensively they will fund education and retirement benefits. One of the partners comes forward with a proposal to shift the nature of their relationships with the practice from employees to independent contractors. He argues this would allow the practice to get out of the business of vetting health care and retirement plans and managing reimbursement for various professional expenses, and allow much more independent variation on the part of the partners as to how they want to spend these monies, thus allowing them to lower practice overhead, take home more money, and determine which benefits are of importance to them.

Is this a good idea? Is it legal?

Case: A Malpractice Nightmare

City Pathology, Inc. is a pathology practice with a claims-made malpractice insurance plan. In January, one of the City Pathology's employees, Dr. Pathologist, provided a report containing a transcription error. The error resulted in Pattie Patient undergoing an unnecessary surgical procedure in February. In May of the same year, Dr. Pathologist left City Pathology, Inc. for a new position with Country Pathology, Inc. City Pathology, Inc. promptly removed Dr. Pathologist from coverage under its plan when he left the practice. Similarly, Country Pathology, Inc. promptly added Dr. Pathologist to its occurrence malpractice insurance plan, with his coverage beginning on his first day of work. Dr. Pathologist did not obtain any insurance on his own during his transition from City Pathology, Inc. to Country Pathology, Inc. as he assumed he was covered by the practices' plans. In July of that same year, Pattie Patient sued Dr. Pathologist.

Does City Pathology, Inc.'s claims-made malpractice insurance plan cover Dr. Pathologist for Pattie Patient's lawsuit?

Does Country Pathology, Inc.'s occurrence malpractice insurance plan cover Dr. Pathologist for Pattie Patient's lawsuit?

What could Dr. Pathologist have done differently to ensure he had malpractice insurance coverage for Pattie Patient's lawsuit?

Part IV
Human Resources

Chapter 13
Human Resources (HR) Management

Lewis Hassell, Krista Crews and Linda McLean

Introduction

One of the most complicated and vexing areas of managing a practice of any kind arises from the interactions of people—whether pathologists, nonphysician laboratorians, or billing and administrative personnel. The billing process follows certain rules that are complicated and constantly changing, sometimes without notice. Calculating workloads is arithmetic (albeit controversial), but once a logical formula is established, measurement and comparison can occur. Human behavior, however, regularly balks at rules and confounds logic—a somewhat foreign and disturbing environment for some individuals. This chapter deals with a few of the major human resources (HR) functions within pathology organizations and attempts to provide practical methods and a pragmatic mindset for approaching them. Where differences exist between how pathologists and non-pathologists are recruited, managed, and retained, these will be noted, but often the same kinds of principles and problems are encountered in both groups, only on different pay scales and time frames. Pathologist employment agreements are more completely addressed in Chap. 12.

L. Hassell (✉) · L. McLean
Department of Pathology, University of Oklahoma Health Sciences Center, 940 Stanton L. Young Blvd., BMSB 451, Oklahoma City, OK 73104, USA
e-mail: lewis-hassell@ouhsc.edu

L. McLean
e-mail: linda-mclean@ouhsc.edu

K. Crews
ProPath, 1355 River Bend Drive, Dallas, TX 75247, USA
e-mail: Krista.crews@propath.com

© Springer International Publishing Switzerland 2016
L. A. Hassell et al. (eds.), *Pathology Practice Management*,
DOI 10.1007/978-3-319-22954-6_13

Staffing

Case: Professional Job Description

Dr. Szabo is a veteran pathologist who you believe will fit well with your needs for an additional pathologist to cover the expanding case and medical directorship duties at your 350-bed Mid-Northern hospital and regional practice covering five smaller hospitals. As things have evolved specialty wise in your group, you have a cadre of people to cover the conventional surgical pathology work, with some limited specialization according to interests and specialty training, but that level of specialization is not yet developed on the clinical pathology side, where the two primary pathologists take care of the smear reviews, bone marrow exams, coagulation consults, transfusion management work, and any microbiology-related consults. You are excited to have someone with experience in the clinical lab join your group and help with this burgeoning workload. Dr. Szabo arrives and toward the end of his first week on service, you notice that the stack of bone marrow biopsies is getting taller and ask him about them. He simply replies, "Well, I don't sign-out bone marrows. That was hemepath work where I came from and I'm not suited to it. There wasn't anything about that in my contract and I don't recall anyone mentioning it when we discussed the job duties."

Discussion: This is failure on the part of both the practice and the job applicant. Neither did their due diligence in terms of the job and expectations resulting in a potentially poor (perhaps disastrous) match of skills and needs. A clear job description and detailed listing of expectations could have fleshed out the details of day-to-day work involved. If the job fit is to work, challenges like this are best addressed in advance, rather than after employment has begun.

A characteristic of any successful organization is having the right people in the right jobs at the right time—a noble goal, but very difficult to accomplish. This concept is the essence of the well-known management book, *Good to Great* [1]. In the modern economy, talent (people) increasingly trumps capital in predicting success and survival. In fact, in the tech world, large companies may seek to purchase a smaller company more to potentially capture the personnel rather than add the acquisition's book of business or technology. There are logical steps, however, that can be taken to improve the chances for operational success through optimal staffing. One step toward an effective hire is one of the most overlooked—a well thought out, well written job description. This is important for both pathologists and non-pathologists. Defining the position will provide you a solid concept of the content of the job, the skills and experience required to accomplish that job, and the characteristics and personality traits of the candidate that will complement your organization and its culture. A good job description also provides the candidate with an understanding of the job requirements and your expectations, thereby limiting post-hire surprises such as Dr. Szabo's in the case above. If you find yourself struggling to find the right words or unsure if you have included the major duties, an online search for descriptions of like positions can be helpful, though this may be less valuable for professional positions. Other organizations have been hiring for similar positions for years and well-devised descriptions are often readily available online.

Many times an employee leaves a job early—either by resignation or by termination for "just not cutting it" in the eyes of a manager—due to the parties having differing concepts of the job. This causes disruption in the life of the employee and losses for the practice in the forms of faltering momentum toward reaching goals and the additional time (and money) spent in recruiting, selecting, and training replacements. These kinds of "mis-hires" are expensive to both the practice and the individual and need to be minimized (See *Top-Grading* [2] by Brad Smart).

The temptation to "get a warm body in the job" to alleviate volume pressures or associated overtime costs can be significant, but the right person in the job the first time, even if it takes a little longer, is the better long-term decision. This falls into the mistaken thinking of "not having the time to do it right, but having to make the time to do it over." We have all been there.

In our competitive and resource tight world, look at the job functions being performed by your employees. Assess the level of talent required to efficiently do a job well. For example, a histotechnician or technologist may be needed for competent embedding or cutting of complex specimens, but less expensive skill sets can accession specimens, change solutions in processors, or operate automatic stainers. Matching skill sets to the requirements of the tasks allows for efficient operation of the laboratory and prevents payroll and related costs from being higher than necessary. Occasionally, a position may be designed with a mix of skill sets that would merit a higher salary scale, for example, for a known person such as an existing employee who is ready to move up.

A very good starting point for any employment search is a well-crafted job description.

Case: Cutting Turnover Costs

Middlerock Laboratories had people staffing its accessioning and customer service areas for the primarily anatomic pathology laboratory located in the office building adjacent to their largest customer, Middlerock Memorial Medical Center. Accessioning's clerical functions were seen as essentially high-school graduate, entry-level tasks, while answering the phone calls and giving results or directing calls required a bit more training, but also seemed fairly basic. The manager, however, always seemed to be recruiting and training someone in this department, where the four employees each had an average tenure of less than a year. Employees left for better pay in another department, to return to school or look for better pay elsewhere. Then the accessioning component of the position was redesigned to include doing some simple specimen processing and assisting at the gross bench with the pathology assistant (PA), thereby justifying a higher pay scale, while the customer service component was diverted to a designated billing clerk who found the human interactions on the job added variety to his work. Consequently, quality metrics in both accessioning and customer service improved and employee turnover decreased. Additionally, the quality of the front-end employee candidates seemingly improved.

Sourcing Candidates

Of the many sources for finding candidates for your organization, one of the best for providing longer-term successful employees is the network of people you already know and trust. For example, friends and colleagues of your current staff members are a good source, and your employees will generally want to refer candidates who reflect well on themselves and are a good potential coworker, providing a first-level filter of suitability. Next, do not overlook your own network of colleagues in other organizations, including vendors who have the opportunity to interact with people in targeted positions working for a variety of employers. In this regard, it is important to think of the recruiting/hiring process as being continual, or ongoing, so that you are always on the lookout for good people for future, if not current needs. Likewise, your business should be run in a way that makes others want to work for you.

For more recently trained pathology talent, contact academic program directors in good training programs. They will know the skills and abilities not only of those finishing soon but of graduates from the recent past, many of whom stay in touch and communicate when they are considering job changes. For harder-to-fill positions, whether due to the required skill or experience level, a recruiting agency (although seemingly expensive initially) may be worth the investment in finding the right candidate for your organization. They have a network of sources that generally far exceeds your own.

Keep in mind that depending on the size of your organization, you may be subject to a variety of state and Federal laws requiring steps be taken to ensure employment opportunity is offered to different candidates. Casting a wide net with your recruiting process (advertising in online sources and select print media such as industry periodicals or newsletters) can increase your candidate pool and help meet those employment goals.

For professional and managerial positions, the utility of your network of connections is even greater. While we have all sought candidates and positions using publicly sourced listings such as those in *CAP Today*, Pathology Outlines, and other print or online media sources, the amount of work involved in screening through such options is much less when the lead or opportunity comes through a trusted colleague. This experience has reinforced the mentality that as both a potential employer and potential employee, one needs to be ever vigilant of one's network. The relationship cultivated at a national committee meeting may lead to a job opportunity or a prize candidate next month or a decade from now.

Interview and Selection

Many books have been written on the unacceptable topics for job interview questions. The growing list generally includes such matters as health and physical abilities, religious preferences, gender or lifestyle choices, age, and more recently, questions on genetics.

What you can and should ask are questions that help you assess depth of expertise, honed skills, judgment, attitudes, and the cultural fit of the candidates. This is where that good job description comes in handy. The job duties and required skills and experience written in the description form a framework for developing interview topics. Specific questions should deal with the candidate's experience and technical competence, problem and conflict handling skills, career goals (to ensure the position and company goals align with the candidate's personal goals), and leadership experience when needed—all while assessing attitude and personality characteristics for a cultural fit within your organization.

Ask open-ended questions that require thorough answers, including those that require the candidate to develop solutions to work-related situations or problems. The goal is to ascertain established skills and capabilities, gain comfort with how (and whether) those abilities have been demonstrated in the past, and give the candidate the opportunity to demonstrate their ability to think quickly and articulate succinctly. As you question candidates about their capabilities and accomplishments, delve into *how* they were able to achieve such deeds. This will tell you much about how the candidate interacts with others—from working well with a team and sharing credit with colleagues, or stepping on others to get things done.

Certain positions within the pathology practice or laboratory require specific degrees or certifications. Yet having the right educational pedigree does not always mean the candidate can do the job the way your organization needs or wants it performed. For pathologist positions, do not be fearful of causing offense by administering slide tests, including some form of report dictation. An ill-fitting hire can be avoided by having the candidate actually do the job you are hiring the person to do—for example, diagnose disease and dictate clear, succinct reports. This is perhaps the easiest part of the interview process. Harder to discern is attitude and cultural fit.

If more than one person is interviewing a candidate, consider the wisdom of scripting your responsibilities beforehand, perhaps even developing standard scenarios to use, so that a broader array of skills and perspectives can be seen. All individuals can still assess the degree of fit with the culture and core skills. Experience suggests that multiple interviewers using the more random "sit and chat" approach will more easily miss critical skill or attitude gaps than those using more organized or scripted approaches. Again, the job description can help guide the kind of script used by different parties. The detailed competency-based leadership scripted interviews described in Smart's *Topgrading* [2] may seem onerous in a pathology practice that prides itself as being flexible and easygoing, but their reported success rate in finding "A-players" is difficult to ignore.

When positions are less dependent on specific degrees or certifications, consider the concept of hiring on attitude. Many skills can be taught on the job. A bright, hardworking individual who displays a positive, can-do attitude can add more long-term value to your organization than a highly disruptive genius.

Identify the purposes of your interview process, and verify that all involved know their roles.

Background and Reference Checks

The days of being able to rely solely on the representations of job candidates are well behind us. There are, unfortunately, job seekers who are willing to embellish accomplishments, stretch out tenures to cover gaps, and flat-out invent degrees, certifications, or other pertinent "facts." This is true for professional candidates as well as others and while credentialing bodies will verify graduation and board and licensure status, it is costly to first discover those things at the stage of credentialing. As a prospective employer, you must not only check a variety of sources to validate information relative to experience and education, but your practice may also face increased liability for failing to perform certain checks. Your due diligence in this level of scrutiny will depend in part on which if not all of the potential "downsides" you are aiming to mitigate. You want a fully qualified and competent employee, one who will not be a safety risk to you or your clients, one who is trustworthy for the duties assigned, and who will represent you well to your customers and other employees. Again, taking the time to do things right the first time can save endless headaches down the road.

Work and educational history are verified by most employers these days, although it is getting increasingly difficult to verify much more from previous employers than dates of service and positions held. Legal claims from previous employees for unfavorable references have encouraged some employers to adopt a neutral reference policy negating the value appreciably. It is still worth making the calls, however, as even subtle hints can be picked up in the responses from prior bosses. One useful tool in this regard, particularly if you are conducting the reference check following a phone or other interview with the individual, is to ask the candidate whether the former employer or reference would rate them as an above average or superior performer. Then when speaking to the reference you can honestly state, "this person has said that you would rate their performance as above average/superior in their position. Can you confirm that?"

For jobs requiring advanced degrees or certifications, most of this information can be confirmed through national clearinghouses, websites, or quick calls to institutions. With creative computer packages allowing for preparation of professional-looking documents at home, you can no longer simply accept a copy of a diploma or certificate.

Many pathology practices have employees who work either full- or part-time in the facilities of another company—such as the hospital for which you provide laboratory medical direction and pathology services. Hospitals now require you to affirm that you have performed some level of background verification on the employees you will send onto their premises. These can include checks for criminal background or inclusion on sex offender registries. There will also be requirements to ensure they have had certain vaccinations, medical testing, or drug screening depending on the duties performed. If you practice as part of a large organization such as a university or hospital system, the university will most likely have its own requirements to be met before making a job offer. As an example, for a pathologist to work as a faculty member in a setting we know, a background check and check of the National Practitioner Data Bank are performed before a job offer, the state licensure board carefully verifies training and vets a candidate, the professional liability insurance underwriting committee evaluates the candidate before issuing coverage, the hospital system credentialing committee carefully weighs the evidence, and the potential insurance entities evaluate credentials prior to credentialing. A failure in the first phase would prevent a letter of offer while a failure in the subsequent activities would invalidate the offer.

Within your own organization, you should determine where there is a legitimate business need for background checks. For example, your drivers or couriers should be regularly checked for motor vehicle violations. Even your insurance policies may require certain verifications such as credit checks on employees with accounting, billing, or payroll duties.

All these precautions seem daunting, but take heart; an entire industry of background verification services now exists to help you—for a fee, of course.

Case: The Typo That Was Not

A qualified candidate has applied for an accounts payable job (the position in your practice that pays the bills) and the manager is eager to make an offer of employment. The HR department is assisting with the pre-offer reference checks. During the verification process, which was a combination of using an online service and phone calls to employers, the most recent two positions were verified. The third one back was verified, but two of the last four digits in the social security number were transposed. The assumption was a typographical error. Additionally for that third-back position, the employee's name was shown as Janette, not Janie, which was now being used in the application. As the two names were close, Janie was assumed to be a nickname for the other and the discrepancy was disregarded.

Janie went to work in the accounts payable role and performed competently. After several months on the job, she unexpectedly resigned, refusing to work any post-resignation notice period. The duties were distributed among other employees over the following days and soon irregularities began to appear. Within a few days, it became apparent that Janie had been paying invoices to a fictitious company with a name very similar to other supply vendors for the practice. The false vendor was a front used to steal money from the company.

What happened? What was missed? How could you have seen this coming?

Discussion: Before you express shock in the lack of "internal controls for the protection of company assets," it might be wise, especially if you practice (or will practice) in a smaller pathology organization, to realize how hard it can be to achieve true segregation of critical duties. Most organizations must operate with some level of trust in the employees performing certain functions.

In hindsight, this was a classic case of failure to adequately perform a background check—or to fully explain any discrepancies arising during the check. There is a natural tendency to give the benefit of doubt to another and assume the best, particularly if someone appears sincere. As it turned out, the current social security number (also used at the previous two employers), had been intentionally altered to differ from the real number—but subtly enough that if someone noticed the difference, the discrepancy could be easily explained as an innocent transposition. Three consecutive employers, including the pathology practice, did not find the discrepancy. Although a copy of the social security card had been provided to the practice, no one noticed that the number on the card did not match the one on the application, and the application had been used to perform all verifications. Had the HR department followed up on the "apparent transposition" from the third employer or had they matched the number on the application to that on the card, they would have discovered that this employee had been terminated (three employers ago) for theft and had a corresponding criminal record.

The story does not end there and offers further lessons. Unfortunately, the practice lost a material amount of money and soon became involved in a dispute with its insurance carrier over the expected coverage from its policy regarding employee acts. The insurer took the position that the practice's failure to find the discrepancy was sufficiently negligent to relieve the insurance company from a duty to pay. It refused to pay for an employee's deception due to another employee's error. What a mess!

If you find yourself in a practice with insufficient staffing to segregate duties, a useful "preventive maintenance" step could be to hire an accounting firm to perform a "review" of your functions and processes. A review is much cheaper than a full audit and might just save you much more money in the long run by uncovering weaknesses and potential fixes.

Lessons learned: Do not be deceived by seemingly minor discrepancies in employment data. A small transposition or omission can disguise a much larger issue. Tying up loose ends like pseudo-typographic errors, employment gaps, and reluctant references can prevent substantial loss and heartache. Be just as meticulous in chasing down details about a prospective employee as you are about getting the staging data correct on a complex cancer resection.

For reference checking on prospective pathologist hires, we believe in using multiple references, ideally including references known by members of the practice, if available. While some institutions will require written references to be solicited, we prefer to call as well. Reference checking should be thoughtful and thorough and often will involve multiple members of a practice. Ultimately, in the end, we have found that in cases where reservations remain regarding a candidate, not hiring is most often the best course of action.

Employee versus Contractor

As you make hiring decisions within your organization, there will be times when you wonder whether it would be better to hire an employee or an independent contractor to fill a role. In reality, this decision is more a matter of law than personal opinion or organizational preference. In general, the law says that if the employer can determine what will be done and how it will be done, the person is an employee. In an independent contractor situation, the employer controls only the result of the work, not the "what" and "how." In addition, the Internal Revenue Service considers whether the individual works on a substantially full-time basis or a part-time basis, with a bias toward employment status for substantially full-time work. So if the person is working at your location, using your tools, doing the job your way during the hours you set, he or she likely would be classified as an employee, particularly if working on a substantially full-time basis. If you have doubts or questions, it is always best to check with your HR professional or appropriate attorney who can provide clarity in a given situation. This is a very "facts and circumstances" determination.

Employment Agreements

Once the hurdles are cleared for offering employment, you should then consider the need for an employment agreement. In general, the higher the employee's position within your organization, the greater the need for a written, formal agreement. Again, this is an area where legal counsel can be helpful, especially pertaining to sensitive areas such as noncompete clauses. Once a formal agreement with basic provisions is created, it can fairly easily be adapted for a variety of positions.

The employment agreement for pathologists will be one of the most important for your practice and this is covered in detail in Chap. 12. Quite frankly, once you have an agreement with which you are comfortable and that is fair for the pathologists, usually very little negotiation is required as you add more people. New re-cruits should be encouraged to have an attorney review the offer and employment agreement. After review, some will sign with no (or very few) requests for consider-ation of language changes. When changes are requested, in nearly all circumstances a reply of "this is the agreement signed by all other pathologists" is sufficient to resolve the situation. Every now and then, however, an astute attorney proposes a language change that makes good sense and should be incorporated into your stan-dard agreement for future recruits and for renewals of existing agreements. This is the secondary benefit—it is a good way to continually refresh your forms and to keep them well balanced for both the practice and the pathologists.

The employment agreement should obviously cover the basics of compensation and benefits offered to the employee. Many of the same component areas that you will use in your pathologist employment agreement may be included in agreements for other key employees such as a supervisor, client representative, sales person, billing or accounts manager, etc. We should mention the importance of providing for protection of intellectual assets when devising contracts as well as work policies for this group of employees. While a strict noncompete clause may be difficult to enforce in some settings, an employer is entitled to protect proprietary information such as client lists, fee schedules, and similar materials from inappropriate use by a former employee now under employment by a competitor. Also, in an era when qui tam or "whistleblower" complaints are seen as the way to win the lottery at the expense of a former or even current employer, inclusion of a duty to report potential false claims, or other actionable misbehavior in the workplace is prudent within both employment contracts and company policies.

By now, you realize you need an attorney familiar with the laws of your state who will help you craft a balanced agreement, fair to both parties, but clear on ex-pectations and promises.

One last thought on employment agreements. Your broadest, most pervasive agreement with your employees can be your Employee Handbook. It is a com-prehensive listing of employee-related policies ranging from compensation to paid time off; from general confidentiality to internet usage. It is the place where you can make clear to employees what benefits they have and which rights they do not have (such as "anything that goes through our system is our property without any expectation of privacy"). Each employee should receive a copy (paper or online) and should sign an acknowledgement of receipt (or confirmation of access). The ac-knowledgement should affirm having read the Handbook and include an agreement to abide by all policies therein.

Compensation and Benefits

The goal of your compensation structure and benefit plans are to position your or-ganization to be competitive in your marketplace and allow you to attract and retain good talent. This is critical to remember when you are considering how to structure benefits and which options to include in your plans.

There are several good sources for comparative compensation data—some free and some fee based. On the free side, websites designed to help job seekers know what range of salary is fair for the position they are considering can also be used by employers to ensure they are in the appropriate range. Another free source would be the hospitals or institutions with which you work. They hire people to similar positions in their laboratories and administrative offices and are generally willing to provide you with the pay ranges they use for comparable positions. (But do not, then, use the information to lure their employees away.)

Applicants seeking jobs within your organization will also provide information on what they are currently making in similar positions elsewhere. A word of caution here: the tendency to exaggerate may apply to this data source. Simply asking for a copy of a recent pay stub to "document the file" can help validate this data. If numbers are confirmed you have an additional evidence of the trustworthiness of the candidate, and if not, the candidate will either disappear or struggle to explain the "misprint" on the application. In the latter event, the employer should beware!

More formal survey data is available for purchase from a variety of sources, but that expense may not be necessary if you are able to otherwise gather sufficient data. Keep in mind that the free sources of data may be very applicable to your marketplace, but will generally be limited to a handful of entities. Purchased surveys, on the other hand, may have much wider participation. Each situation is unique.

Employee benefit programs are an important part of the compensation package you offer. Entire degree programs are available for professionals seeking careers in benefit plan design and administration. The important message to take from this overview is to realize that you must offer a competitive benefit package or you will need to pay a much higher salary that allows employees to make their own arrangements for health, retirement, and other needs.

Different benefits are important for employees of different ages and stages of life, but medical, paid time off (including some form of pay continuation for illness or injury), and a contribution toward retirement tend to be the most popular. Additional frequent offerings include dental and vision coverage, long-term disability, life insurance, and tuition reimbursement. Surveying what is offered by your competitors (or the entities with which you compete for employees) can give you a fairly clear picture of what you need to do to compete for good talent. Because of the individual differences and preferences, the ability to offer flexibility in covered benefits may allow you to reduce the cost of actual benefits provided while providing a high level of satisfaction to a broader array of your employees.

In addition to the benefits mentioned above, physician practices may also choose to provide allowance for coverage of various professional expenses such as continuing education, memberships, and licensure fees. Offering additional time for conduct of professional activities such as service on national or regional medical boards, committees, or organizations can be an important benefit. Some practices may choose to cover other professional expenses, such as travel between worksites. Additional liability insurance may also be covered, and provision made for reimbursement for out of pocket health expenses.

When considering benefit plans, realize that the benefits generally cannot be discriminatory in favor of the owners or higher paid employees. There are a few limited situations where benefits can be segregated for owners versus nonowner employees. You can, however, discriminate in favor of the lower paid employees. This consideration may lead to circumstances where the "highly paid" individuals in an organization may have incentive to operate under a different organizational banner, for example, the Professional Corporation, while other personnel involved in an operation, the secretaries, technologists, and so forth, are employed by a different corporate entity. While discussion of the various Employee Retirement Income Security Act (ERISA) tests that determine whether these "related entities" are de facto the same and operating under separate corporate cover for the sole purpose of avoiding taxes or providing equal retirement benefits to lesser paid employees is beyond the scope of this book, consideration of such organization ought to be guided by competent legal counsel with experience in this arena.

Case: The Flexible Benefit Practice

Dr. Cortez-Martinez, a fellowship trained genitourinary (GU) pathologist, had joined the Upper Rockies Pathology group 3 years ago because of their flexible approach to benefits, which allowed her to choose to some degree among several benefit options. She chose to go with family dental coverage over the long-term care coverage option, at no-added cost, figuring that would help cover the projected need for braces for her three children with mal-occlusion. Recently, the practice partners, a status she had just attained, had been discussing how they could accommodate the differences they perceived between one another when it came to valuing time away from the practice. They proposed to "require" individuals to take a minimum of 6 weeks leave (which could include professional activities) and allow individuals to take up to 12 weeks of leave. The year-end practice profits ("bonus pool") would be used to value any excess weeks people worked above their minimum and appropriately reward those who had worked more than others.

Discussion: The proposal was passed enthusiastically with full support from the most senior members of the practice eager to spend more time with their grandkids, and those less senior looking to retire their student loans and build college education funds for their children, like Dr. Cortez-Martinez.

Onboarding and Rounding

So you have hired the right employee, now what? A strong start and positioning the individual for success? We have found, particularly for pathologists, that using an onboarding checklist is key to a fast start. Our checklist is a formal checklist that, for pathologists, is nearly three pages in length. The new hire is assigned an experienced pathologist who oversees completion of the checklist, typically over a few weeks. Checklist items range from access to the laboratory information system to learning how the schedule works. While an experienced pathologist is tasked with overseeing completion of the list, most of the checklist items are achieved using non-pathologist personnel, such as business manager, secretaries, and technologists.

Once an employee has been "onboarded," a process is designed for a supervisory person to regularly visit (round) with the individual. The purpose of these meetings is to help troubleshoot any issues, increase employee engagement, and further facilitate the employee in bonding with the organization. For example, we have hired several recently trained specialists in clinical pathology. Following the onboarding process, our director of clinical pathology meets weekly with each recent hire. They discuss issues in the lab, better ways to interact with the system, and, since we are an academic institution, academic issues. The new pathologists have performed remarkably and have very much appreciated the regular contact with the director of clinical pathology.

Careful onboarding of new pathologists also has financial ramifications. A new pathologist must obtain a medical license, secure malpractice insurance, become privileged by the hospital(s) if hospital based, and become credentialed by the insurance companies including Medicare and Medicaid in order to bill each insurance company. This process can take up to 5–6 months. Additional background checks and querying the National Practitioner Database for any previously reported issues may also be required. For pathologists working at Joint Commission inspected hospitals, there is a required initial practice quality process, Focused Professional Practice Evaluation (FPPE, think initial quality assurance check) that must be performed, with continued quality monitored by Ongoing Professional Practice Evaluation (OPPE).

Goal Setting and Evaluations

Timely, constructive feedback to and from employees at all levels of the organization is helpful for improving performance, building morale, and giving employees personal goals for progressing in their jobs or within the organization.

First, consider the issue of timing and frequency. While most employment situations have followed the practice of having fairly formal annual evaluations, and this periodicity is useful for providing a sufficiently long-term perspective on accomplishments, if this is the only form of and forum for feedback, the pace of organizational progress will be glacial and will likely communicate a message of indifference to the employee. Quarterly, monthly, or even weekly informal or semiformal touch points on performance, and even more frequently if problems are being addressed or specific mentoring provided, can be highly beneficial.

Next consider the setting. An evaluation can be as informal as a hallway conversation to a few handwritten paragraphs or as comprehensive as completion of a several-page form. Consciously choose the setting with a goal to allow meaningful, comfortable interaction, without any risk of embarrassment to either the employee or the organization. This is especially important if you anticipate the need to give corrective or negative feedback. Whichever way you go, here are a few things to keep in mind.

It is good to give employees the opportunity to evaluate their own performance. Ask employees (again, formally or informally) to list their accomplishments for the year, outline their strengths and weaknesses, and list the personal goals they would like to achieve over the next year. This will also give you as reviewer hints and reminders of how the employees have performed. It is easy to be so caught up in putting out today's fires that you forget the progress of the past. In doing this, realize that some employees are much better than others at completing self-reviews. A few weaker performers may have missed their true calling as writers of great fiction, while strong, quiet giants may not be as adept at tooting their own horns. The self-evaluation is a starting point for a review that will affirm, redirect, encourage, and correct.

A basic appraisal will rate employees in characteristics and accomplishments important to their job duties. Most evaluate areas such as job knowledge, quality of work performed, productivity, initiative, communication skills, interaction with others (both inside and outside of the organization), reliability, attendance, compliance with procedures, and problem-solving skills.

Whether for employees or managers, a good evaluation will compare performance (individually and/or departmentally) against goals established in previous reviews. The review process will then modify or replace those goals for the next year or review period. Organizations are dynamic and the health-care world is changing, so it is possible that what is planned for a particular year has little to do with the tasks that are actually accomplished. This tends to be true, however, more for your managers than their employees. Flexibility will be required.

Individual goals should align with practice or departmental goals. Departmental goals should align with company goals. An employee achieving personal goals should not only help that employee's job growth and advancement, but should move the organization toward accomplishment of its goals. Without clear goals, it is easy for employees to gravitate toward duties most enjoyed or more easily accomplished while neglecting more challenging tasks. The organization becomes stagnant, its progress toward goals slows, and it quickly finds itself behind the competition.

Aligned financial incentives are one of the best ways to ensure employees reach goals and the company or practice makes progress toward established goals. Any reward under an incentive compensation plan should be tied to the attainment of individual goals, departmental successes, and the overall performance of the company. One to three clear, measureable goals are sufficient. The more goals, the more complex the plan and the more negotiation will occur on weighting and importance of individual goals. For example, in the histology department, average blocks and slides prepared per hour would serve as good targets—with appropriate modification for errors or mistakes incurred to ensure quality is not sacrificed for speed. For the company, increase in profitability in either absolute value of profits or profit margin (or both) is generally an adequate, singular goal. Without specific performance triggers for incentive pay, employees may perceive payments as arbitrary, based more on managerial opinion or whim than fact. What was intended to be a performance enhancer and reward system quickly becomes a demoralizer.

One additional helpful evaluation is the exit interview or questionnaire. These tools can provide useful information to management in understanding why an employee has chosen to leave and perhaps what can or should be done to improve parts of the work environment. Departing employees tend to be candid about their opinions, so even if negative, the feedback can bring about positive results for the organization.

Performance appraisals for professional employees are also important, yet are probably most often neglected in busy practices, except perhaps as pertains to newly hired pathologists on a partnership track. Even here, however, our observations have been that the most common sense is that "no news (feedback) is good news" and so they continue to do what they do, even when perhaps some fine-tuning or major readjustments are needed. Then, when 1 or 2 years in, it appears they are not measuring up to what is wanted in a partner, the process of salvaging the experience for either the practice or the pathologist is much more difficult. Feedback on cultural issues, client relations, work habits, and interpersonal interactions is often much more important than on how specific cases are handled. For those issues and for more specific norms, such as turn-around time for reporting or overall productivity, feedback should be given early, with regular monitoring or coaching to ensure successful corrective activity and habits are developed.

Given that differing job duties have widely differing reimbursement rates but not widely differing importance to the overall health of the practice, tying incentive payments to clinical reimbursement and/or production is typically done to a lesser extent in pathology practices, as compared with other more "eat what you kill" practice settings such as surgery or gastroenterology. Development of truly reflective productivity indices in a broad pathology practice requires time and complexity in order to achieve the goal of fairness. On the other hand, many academic practices have developed balanced mission-based metrics to rank and more generously reward highly productive members of the practice or department, regardless of their roles.

For more discussion of feedback and specific tools, see Section "Background and Reference Checks".

> Just like in the body, feedback loops are critical in human resource management. Timely, clear and aligned with organizational goals-oriented sessions will go far to enhance organizational performance.

Dealing with the Disruptive Employee

We may need to disrupt the workplace to institute changes in technologies and long-standing practices for revolutionary process improvement that can bring both life and long-term success to an organization. Harboring disruptive individuals, however, can drain energy and reduce morale and productivity for the rest of the team.

Disruptive individuals may exhibit a variety of behaviors including, but not limited to, sarcasm, involvement in numerous conflicts, overall bad attitude, recurring insubordination, crying in response to criticism, sabotaging equipment and/or projects, blaming others for problems, poor relationships with coworkers, inappropriate reactions to criticism, increased tardiness and/or absenteeism, slamming doors, interrupting meetings with side conversations and comments, believing that rules do not apply to them, feeling they have special "rights," persistent complaining, challenging authority, destruction of property, becoming unusually upset over events, intimidation, harassment, physical violence, yelling, verbal abuse, refusing reasonable requests, using profanity, threatening behavior, and inappropriate behavior that interferes with the functioning or flow of the workplace. If these behaviors are not addressed at the outset, they can easily escalate in number and intensity.

A high-performing workplace will have well-established norms such that each worker feels comfortable giving feedback to his/her coworkers. This can work for simple issues such as, "We need to call or finalize all biopsy reports before lunch" or, "As this space is part of the lab, we can't have coffee here." More significant issues will most likely necessitate involving other people, including management.

It is important to create a policy that clearly defines what is acceptable behavior in the workplace and what will not be tolerated. Each employee should sign and date the document agreeing to abide by the standards of conduct. Channels should be set up so that employees are encouraged to report problems/issues and resolution can be attained.

Try to assess and address the causes of the behavior, then address the effect. Speak to the employee in private about the behavior and allow them to respond. Acknowledge their feelings and point out alternative ways to respond to the situations. Emphasize the consequences for repeated behavior. Allow them time to change their behaviors. On occasion, education or training may help them understand that their behavior is and was inappropriate. For issues that extend beyond the simple, documentation of issues and interventions should be maintained.

If the unacceptable behaviors continue or escalate, the disciplinary policy, in place for situations such as these, should be strictly followed. Early involvement of HR and legal is wise since handling these issues can quickly exceed the skills and training of nonexperts.

While in some cases, simple corrections are possible and employees continue to develop, in other cases, progressive disciplinary measures are needed, sometimes leading to termination. While this is time consuming and often difficult in the short term (emotional upset, a gap in the work schedule, etc.), in our experience, the organization is usually stronger and more functional following resolution of these types of issues.

The Importance of Management Structure

Pathology practices and laboratories perform critical, complex functions every day where the possible consequences of error extend to harm and death for a patient. Having clear reporting relationships and lines of communication for decision making are imperative for the operation to function optimally. When structures are unclear and employees receive conflicting assignments and priorities, or face ambiguous accountability structures, the organization risks making errors, missing critical deadlines, interrupting workflow, and affecting efficiency.

The management of a pathology practice can be further complicated by the possibility of having a number of owners routinely working alongside the nonphysician employees. The individual owners may have widely varying preferences and opinions not only on issues of diagnostic import, but also on laboratory processes, procedures, and priorities. The nonphysician employees may regularly be caught in the middle of disagreements on how and when work should be processed.

For example, the laboratory protocol for the number levels cut on a particular biopsy type may be three. Dr. Smith wants six levels and insists that the laboratory prepare the slides on his cases accordingly. The standard location for the comment on slide quality is in the microscopic section of the report. Dr. Smith wants his slide quality comment in the diagnostic comment. The medical director has worked with the laboratory to establish a standard procedure for H&E (hematoxylin and eosin stain) staining. Dr. Smith wants his stains darker and has provided the laboratory with a special staining protocol for his slides. Dr. Smith is also an owner of the practice; a fact of which he regularly reminds the employees when his comments are in the wrong section, his stains are too light, or his slides contain only three levels. Additionally, Dr. Smith has arranged to have Friday afternoons off in exchange for other duties. He therefore insists that his work be prioritized over other work every Friday so he is not delayed in his departure.

The laboratory employees are tasked with preparing slides of high quality and delivering them to the pathologists with maximum efficiency. They perform a wide variety of tasks (often highly skilled tasks) repeatedly every hour of every day. Variability in the workflow (whether to perform certain steps uniquely for Dr. Smith or to stop between cases to determine if the next case is Dr. Smith's) is the enemy of a smooth, accurate, and efficient process. Many a laboratory technician has prematurely neared the entrance to eternity by making wrong decisions on prioritization of cases or by following standard protocol for a pathologist who prefers his work prepared a unique way.

This familiar scenario highlights the need to understand the distinction between ownership and administrative structures, and clearly segregating the ownership/governance processes from the daily operation of the organization.

Whether vested in the medical director or in division heads for subspecialty lines (e.g., GI, hematopathology, dermatopathology, etc.), the employees need to know whom to look to when conflicting messages and priorities arise. The laboratory managers need to be authorized to redirect the Dr. Smiths to the appropriate physician administrative leader for resolution of his individual concerns. Physician administrative leaders must have the recognized authority within the group to direct the laboratory on standardized procedures for their respective areas.

There was a time in the pathology world when higher reimbursement afforded more disparate processes and the staffing to maintain unique protocols for pathologists. But with today's reduced reimbursement (which equates to reduced compensation), even the most particular pathologist-owner is taking note. Errors are minimized and efficiency maximized when workflow is as standardized as possible. When efficiency is maximized, profitability is maximized.

All organizations need effective leadership. Unfortunately, we all did not select our current line of work because we enjoyed continuous interaction with people. Now we find ourselves in roles such as medical directors or division heads with others looking to us for leadership and guidance.

It is much less important for you to be the most intelligent manager ever known than it is for you to be approachable, fair, and trustworthy. Be clear in your expectations. Give feedback when jobs are performed well and when errors occur. Provide "air cover" to your employees when disruptive forces are attempting to give conflicting messages or priorities.

Many of your employees will be bright, intelligent people who may not have had the same opportunities for advanced education or who made different choices for their lives. They may be keen thinkers and observers who very quickly see through manipulation and deception. When trust is lost, there is no reset button. Once lost, some employees will not trust you again; others may, but with reservation. In contrast, hidden benefits accrue when individuals can operate in a "high-trust" environment. Hence, getting there, and staying there are important leadership priorities (see Stephen Covey, *The Speed of Trust* [3]).

Summary

The tools you will need for maneuvering the HR aspects of your practice or laboratory are vast, but a fair, level head and good legal counsel are the starting points. It will be impossible to run a successful organization without employee conflicts, legal challenges, and mistakes being made. An overarching dedication to fairness and doing things right, however, will be your best defense when troubles arise.

Case: The Sudden Departure

Recent growth in specimen volumes has necessitated the addition of a PA to your grossing team. Experienced candidates are hard to find as they have generally landed good positions with organizations that work to keep them. An experienced candidate applies for the position. His resume indicates several years of experience and a solid education, including a PA degree from a good program and progress toward a Master's degree in health-care administration.

In the interview, you ask probing open-ended questions that delve into the candidate's knowledge and skills. The replies confirm substantial experience as a PA and solid understanding of the appropriate handling of complex specimens. He evidences a quiet, positive demeanor that you believe will fit in well with your group. After references are checked, an offer is made and accepted.

The next few months go very well and you are pleased to have a team competently handling the volume of specimens. The team works well together and the operation is running smoothly. After slightly less than a year, and to your complete surprise, the new PA resigns. He gives 2 weeks' notice, which you know is not nearly enough time to fill a position like this. You may be able to fill the gap with temporary help, but that solution is suboptimal as the contractor will not know your systems and the excess burden will fall on the remainder of the staff. This will again leave your PA team struggling to keep up with volumes, tired and demoralized—at least in the interim. *What happened? What did you miss? How could you have seen this coming?*

Discussion: Following good practices, you routinely conduct an exit interview with departing employees. During the exit interview, the departing PA indicates to the HR representative that since he has now finished his degree in health-care administration, he has accepted an entry-level administrative position with a local hospital. He indicates that this had been his objective all along—to work as a PA while finishing the last few hours of his degree and then find an administrative position in a hospital that would set him on the path to his long-term goal of running a hospital.

Here's What Happened Because the position required substantial technical skills, the interviewers' questioning focused almost entirely on the candidate's experience as a PA and knowledge required in performing that particular job. When reviewing the resume, the hours toward the Master's degree were not given much thought as they were somewhat superfluous to the open position. No one picked up any hints from the Masters hours or even considered the possibility that an experienced PA might have plans to become something other than an even more experienced PA. Therefore, no one asked the candidate about career aspirations, long- or short-term goals, whether he enjoyed being a PA, or even why he had pursued the additional education. The candidate did not mislead the interviewers to get the job, as no one ever asked whether this job fit into his longer-term career plans. The candidate, fearing that his short-term interest might reduce the chances of getting the job he needed while finishing school, did not offer that information.

Now you find yourself with an opening—again—for a difficult-to-fill position after having spent several months training the PA on your systems, processes, and technologies.

Lessons learned: There are good reasons for asking the "softer" questions on goals, aspirations, and what a candidate enjoys in a job. It just might save you from hiring a short-term employee who does not have long-term aspirations for the job (or with your organization), and save you the costs of training a short timer. It is also important to pay attention to everything on the resume. The candidate traveled certain roads for reasons. Perhaps the education is a passing interest. But perhaps there is more you need to know.

References

1. Collins J. Good to great: why some companies make the leap…and others don't. New York: HarperCollins Publishers, Inc.; 2001 (Print).
2. Smart BD. Topgrading: the proven hiring and promoting method that turbocharges company performance. 3rd ed. New York: Penguin Group; 2012 (Print).
3. Covey SMR. The SPEED of trust: the one thing that changes everything. New York: Simon and Schuster, Inc.; 2006 (Print).

Part V
Pathology Group Issues

Chapter 14
Group Dynamics

Lewis A. Hassell, Michael L. Talbert and Kimball Fisher

Overview

Case: Dysfunctional Decision-Making

A group of ten pathologists meets monthly for a board of directors meeting. Decisions are by a vote of the eight partners, although consensus is desired and often achieved through pre-meeting discussion. The three youngest partners often speak against issues but vote in favor when the vote is called. However, following the meeting, they undermine decisions and speak against the managing partner. Over time, this leads to group paralysis and a tendency to "second guess" or "revisit" earlier decisions.

Discussion: The inability to make major decisions and move ahead can be crippling. The culture is toxic and the solution is difficult. Perhaps talking out the issues could resolve the situation but this may require an outside mediator who can carefully identify dysfunction as it occurs. Much dysfunction occurs in environments where it is not directly labeled as such, hence, it is allowed to continue and may increase. Enforcing or revisiting employment agreements or corporate bylaws may not be helpful unless the destructive behavior is documented and the offending pathologist(s) is threatened with termination. Perhaps the overall fit is poor for one or more of the junior partners, and they should seek a better practice fit elsewhere.

When highly trained professionals decide to practice together, whether as an independent group, employees, or an academic department, group dynamics become critically important to their success. Basic issues such as work assignments and hire/fire decisions require a good deal of cohesion as do the seemingly simple day-to-day interactions such as call coverage and whose special stains to do first. Group dysfunction can consume immense amounts of time and energy, lead to increased

L. A. Hassell (✉) · M. L. Talbert
Department of Pathology, University of Oklahoma Health Sciences Center, 940 Stanton L. Young Blvd., BMSB 451, Oklahoma City, OK 73104, USA
e-mail: lewis-hassell@ouhsc.edu

M. L. Talbert
e-mail: michael-talbert@ouhsc.edu

K. Fisher
The Fisher Group, PO Box 91452, Portland, OR 97291, USA
e-mail: kimball@thefishergroup.com

© Springer International Publishing Switzerland 2016
L. A. Hassell et al. (eds.), *Pathology Practice Management*,
DOI 10.1007/978-3-319-22954-6_14

turnover, and otherwise render a practice uncompetitive in its environment. In the authors' experience, although some amount of group dysfunction is fairly common, a practice leader who ignores it does so at the peril of the practice. Group dysfunction is often much more of a threat to a practice than external pressures.

Shared values and norms of a practice underpin positive group dynamics. While any individual has wants and needs (e.g., pay off school loans, be active at church, travel and compete in ballroom dancing), each one must interact under a shared contract with the group, a contract which may be in part unwritten. For example, vacation may be part of an employment agreement and decision-making may be enshrined in corporate bylaws, while actual hours at work on a typical weekday may not be explicitly specified. Yet group norms may lead a senior pathologist to quietly counsel a young pathologist who regularly leaves at 3 p.m. that "the pathologists of our practice work until 5 p.m." to help educate as to the norm.

These principles apply to any group of pathologists, whether academic, hospital employed, or an independent private practice. In the first two settings, the existence of a larger structure such as a medical school faculty practice or hospital leadership to which the pathologists are responsible, may lead to more written rules or tighter expectations. This in turn may create the potential for greater dysfunction in a group of relatively equal pathologists.

One key to good group dynamics is communication: communication of norms, expectations, and, when needed, failure to meet expectations. That which is explicit should be made clear, either verbally or in writing (such as contractual language), while regular and transparent communication can facilitate establishment and maintenance of implicit norms. This communication may be written such as behavioral standards or responsibilities while on call or be established through discussion and decision-making via formal and informal meetings.

Monitoring the Mood and Communication

Group dysfunction is often invisible to outsiders but obvious to participants. (We have known situations where the converse is true as well, but this disconnect in perception is more uncommon.) But how does a leader monitor the mood of a practice? One could measure pathologist turnover, but this is a lagging indicator and may be too late to avoid a potentially devastating effect on the practice. A better indicator is the quality of communications. For example, if a group of professionals can talk openly, constructively, and without defensiveness, about how the group will handle breast biopsies and, better yet, whether all individuals actually adhere to established practices or not, that is a clear, positive sign. In contrast, an inability or unwillingness to have these difficult conversations may indicate dysfunctions such as a lack of communication skills, or worse, a lack of commitment to the success of the practice. Avoidance of discussions relating to things such as work styles ("pathologist X doesn't pull his/her weight") or other fairness topics (e.g., money, schedule, and assignments) generally indicates problematic dysfunction requiring the leader to intervene before unresolved issues turn into conflict situations which may negatively affect group morale and productivity.

Note that a lack of communication, however, is not always an indicator of dysfunction. The authors are aware of a stable situation where a senior partner pathologist routinely started work early (sometimes before 5 a.m.), and left for much of the morning to attend to private nonmedical businesses, returned for lunch, and then left work prior to the other pathologists. This pathologist routinely did significantly more than his share of the sign-out but was not always available for frozen sections or the phone calls that would interrupt the other pathologists' sign-out. Yet this arrangement was never discussed by the pathologists, nor was it the subject of sidebar conversations by them because they apparently found the schedule tradeoffs acceptable.

Remember that communication is not always a guarantee of success, either. Contrast the victory above with another situation known by the authors where the partners did discuss alternative work schedules for multiple board meetings and innumerable lunch conversations leading only to the development of "opposing sides" and unmet expectations, and not to any creative alternative scheduling practices. In another similar case of unsuccessful communication about this issue, a pathologist felt forced to retire early rather than scaling back to 75% in an effort to balance work/life or work/health issues, leading to a negative consequence for the practice as a whole. When dealing with professionals who have a wide variety of experiences, concerns, opinions, and expectations, even effective communication practices cannot guarantee effective group functioning, However, ineffective communication almost always results in problems. The role of the leader, therefore, is to ensure that all members of the practice are involved, and that communication is constructive rather than destructive, including during the sometimes emotion-laden discussions associated with giving and receiving performance feedback. Books and training programs on effective communication skills are widely available to help the practice leader learn more specifics on this topic, but as a general guideline consider the following basic communication tips.

Communication and Feedback Tips

- Specific communication is normally better than general communication. Remember to use language that makes sense to the person or persons being communicated with, not just language that makes sense to the communicator. Use examples and data rather than vague or unsupported statements. This is especially important when giving performance feedback. Do not say: "You don't do your fair share." Do say: "You do 30% less sign out than other members of the practice."
- The best communication is highly interactive, not didactic. People tend to zone out or multitask when they are only listening. Ask questions to ensure involvement, interaction, and understanding. In meetings, everyone should speak.

- The best way to demonstrate that communication has been effective is to have the receiver(s) of the communication summarize what they heard. Just because information was "sent" does not mean it was "received."
- When expressing difficult feelings or opinions consider using this general template: "When (this happens), I feel (emotion or mental state)." This helps people express their personal opinions without assigning blame or potentially inappropriate judgments of others. For example, instead of saying, "you don't seem to care about anybody else," or "newer pathologists are treated poorly," say "when you left early yesterday without telling anyone, I had to stay late and cover your calls. I missed my daughter's recital and that made me feel angry." Or, "when the schedule was changed yesterday without asking me, I felt undervalued." The former statements are more likely to cause problems, the latter more likely to open honest and caring discussion.
- Avoid assuming how other people feel. Ask them. Do not speak about people behind their backs. Speak to them directly.
- Silence is not consent.

While as noted above, each group or organization, and even groups within a larger organization, will have its or their own culture, the culture itself may evolve with time as new challenges or circumstances arise. (Remember that organizational culture is defined as the operating "software" for interactions and activity within that organization or group. Norms, expectations, protocols, and policies, along with incentives, rewards and recognition all constitute "culture.") Perhaps thinking of the situation as akin to the variation in day-to-day weather in contrast to the general climatologic setting would be a good analogy. Culture will help you know what the norms are for approaching weather patterns and what the likely range of outcomes are for those, but each individual "weather maker" will have its own nuances and impact.

However, in contrast to atmospheric disturbances that are generally beyond control, a variety of approaches can be useful to mitigate the impacts and duration of the storms of a cultural mood swing within a group or organization. We might not be able to predict how long a hurricane will stall and dump rain on a city or state, but in an organization we might be able to exert some control over how many workers we have trying to pump specimens through an overloaded system. We might be able to determine whether angry employees are assigned to mission-critical tasks, or whether the incentives for performance appropriately match our group goals.

This analogy is further useful in thinking about the tools used to forecast upcoming meteorological events and considering what tools might be useful in predictive planning within the group culture of a laboratory or pathology group. Wind speed, barometric pressures, relative humidity, satellite images, and so forth might enter into the model being used to predict whether we will have sun or storm for tomorrow's picnic. Likewise, in a group, certain sentinels might be placed to monitor workflows, revenues, cultural or administrative stresses, regional or national trends along with awareness of individual variables that all might contribute to either the "perfect storm" or idyllic weather.

Healthy organizational cultures tend to have many similar characteristics. They tend to be quite transparent. With regard to matters of accountability and individual responsibility, they score highly on the accountability end. In contrast, on the axis of risk-averse to risk-taking, they are more centrist, enabling, or even encouraging a reasonable degree of risk taking (freedom) to explore new ideas and opportunities. They also score well on matters of choosing to do things right, to high standards, and without shortcuts.

Other healthy organizational characteristics include a learning approach to mistakes, rather than one of blaming and shaming (which remains consonant with the shared accountability mentioned above), an uncompromising dedication to integrity of word and action, a strong pursuit of collaborative, integrative action, and relentless determination in the face of difficulty. Now it may be evident that these characteristics are not as easy to monitor as atmospheric temperature. There is no "integritometer" that one can post on the break-room wall to show the level of truth-telling today and compare that with yesterday. One cannot just stick a wet finger into the air and tell whether the collaborative winds are from the favorable southwest or forebodingly from the north. Nor can one look at the solid and dotted lines on an organizational chart and ensure that there is a high degree of accountability and individual responsibility. So how does a leader assess the organizational health? Cultural mood-forecasters will use a variety of tools to help them assess the state of the organization, and often develop particular patterns for "taking the pulse" of their group. Patterns of behavior often used to this end include:

Management by walking around (MBWA) is a commonly used method to provide leadership and cultural weather forecasting first popularized by Peters' and Waterman's *In Search of Excellence*, but it can also be misused by creating a feeling of micromanagement. Bidirectional visibility is important for leadership when titrated appropriately. No worker wants to feel like their boss is the equivalent of a helicopter parent, always there hovering. But MBWA does offer the leader the opportunity to communicate and see directly, which can lead to better decisions. And the first hand sense of the demeanor of ones' associates is an exceptional tool in determining the state of the mood in the organization. We have experienced and lived the benefits of this sort of "rounding" activity, used by leaders across our organization, and it is bidirectional, meaning that mid-level leaders are regularly taking stock with both their own reports and their "one-ups" in the hierarchy. The net effect is a greater degree of employee engagement across the board drawn from the sense that "my leaders care about me and my work," which leads to better decisions at all levels, quicker resolution of pain points and so forth.

Case: Management by Walking Around

Bobette, the practice manager for a multisite large pathology group, was hired following some notable group failures, some mis-hires, the separation of a small subgroup at one of the practice's hospitals, and some dissatisfaction expressed by newer members of the practice with the "old guard" who had founded and built the practice. Although the practice spanned several metro areas in more than one state, Bobette began to make monthly visits to each of the practice locations, and to have face-to-face visits with each of the pathologists in the practice, to listen, solicit ideas, report back, and get a better tenor of how things were working. As a result, her efforts during the remainder of the month were better prioritized, problems got solved, and the level of pathologist-to-pathologist conflict decreased. This is an example of the "hub and spoke" model that operates to hold together many extended families as well.

Observational effort—while this is in some ways similar to MBWA, it is really more focused, an effort to see between the trees if you will, perhaps directed toward answering a specific question or issue (Why do we have so many phone calls about accessioning errors? What is happening to slow things down in micro? etc.) A related tool is the use of self-inspections, which may be conducted by a variety of different team members and for a variety of purposes (i.e., not always for accreditation).

Cultural key questions have been used by many groups to track the sentiment of an organization over time, thus helping to monitor the impact of changes, and to assess priorities for future planned interventions. This process can be as simple as informally asking people open-ended questions such as "What gets in the way of you being as effective as possible?" and "How can we work better together as a practice?", or it can be as structured as formal questionnaires. The employee engagement survey is a commonly used means to monitor such factors as relative job satisfaction, quality of management and leadership, and to detect potential irritability issues in advance. However, the utility of such surveys is limited by the frequency with which they can be used (generally not more frequently than once a year) and limited response rates. Customer satisfaction surveys are also a useful insight into organizational mood and such data may be collected on an almost continuous basis. But one should not overlook the general sense of sentiment that can be gathered by just looking around at people during celebratory events, catching the energy in hallway and break room conversations, and looking at what appears on the walls and bulletin boards.

Individual interviews are important for any leader and they may take a variety of forms—accountability sessions, reports, strategy sessions, annual evaluations, exit interviews, "side-bar" conversations, etc. But beyond the direct purpose that may be implicit in each of these varied interactions, some component of energy and engagement assessment should also be occurring that will give a measure of whether that individual, and likely others around him or her, is happy. This can also be the most useful means of determining the nidus of any major discontent that requires intervention. Making some element of the "What do we need to start/stop/continue doing?" assessment a part of these interviews can yield highly useful cultural data to guide action.

Decision process audits or other root cause analyses of adverse or sentinel events can also inform cultural adjustments. Such audits typically evaluate the roles of a host of inputs, including several directly related to culture. The process itself can have a transformative impact on organizational integrity and transparency provided the process is indeed conducted with those motives in mind. They typically include an analysis of decision-making effectiveness by group discussion of examples of both "good" and "bad" decisions in order to determine how to continue the positive attributes of good decision-making and how to strengthen the weaker attributes. It is usually also a good idea to teach practice members a variety of decision-making techniques and learn how and when to use them as illustrated elsewhere in this section and in the following case study.

Case: Bad Decision-Making Leads to a Mis-Hire

Gervais Pathology Partners was clicking along at a high level of productivity and their income statement showed they were doing well. Overhead was low, contracts were secure, and the external environment seemed stable. The six-person group with two mid-sized hospitals had managed to structure and titrate their workload to perfection. Five people did the work and one was off. They loved it. Then the world changed. The most senior pathologist, Dr. Steve Gervais, became ill and was unable to work. The group pleaded hardship with their hospitals to get temporary locum tenens credentialed, but a quality problem with the very first locums pathologist soured the later attempts. They put out ads but were recruiting at the wrong time of year as most recent graduates had already taken jobs and so the options were limited. Desperate to fill the void, three of the partners called a vote (the vote being 3–2) for what they thought was a reasonable choice, or at least a "warm body" (though that was also subject to debate listening to the other two partners later on) to fill at least part of the void left by Steve. The on-boarding process took too long, it seemed, given their anxiety to get back to a "normal" 6 week rotation, and the new pathologist was not particularly adept with hematology or, as they came to discover, client relations. And to make matters worse, he did not know his blind spots. About 6 months following his start, Vick, one of the "minority two," got a call from a hematologist at their larger hospital inquiring about a rather "creative" read he had been given on a bone marrow that had led to his referring the patient to the tertiary referral center he used, only to discover that they could find no support for his referring diagnosis in their evaluation. When Vick had asked the new pathologist about it, the new hire had been glib and seemed not to care, and in fact had called him a quite disrespectful name.

Based on this and some other less well-documented rumors of complaints, Vick called a meeting of the partners to consider a course of action, but could not garner full support to let the new pathologist go. The three partners who had pushed to hire the new pathologist argued compassionately to send him to "charm school" and give him more coaching. A year later, after nearly losing one of their hospital contracts over one of his "issues," they ultimately agreed their efforts had been in vain and terminated the new pathologist, though by now they were obligated by contract to pay a large severance package.

Ultimately, the group did a detailed analysis of this experience and recognized their failure to put all their hidden self-interests on the table at the time of the initial decision to hire and the mistake in using a simple majority vote to decide hiring.

Improving the Mood

Charters are a common way to focus organizational structures, but too often, these documents are created and then not referred to again. If it is to be a useful cultural tool, a charter must be short and clear enough to be memorable, and it should be seen as a living document that guides day-to-day decision-making. In the DMA case (see Appendix A, Case 2), for example, had the Executive Committee charter included a component about ensuring the financial viability of the practice, and the organizational culture been such that referring to the charter was an accepted and expected part of key meetings, any of the members could have asked: "Is there anything else we need to consider relative to our financial viability?" Perhaps this question would have allowed important information to surface that would have accelerated the replacement of Dr. Jones and avoided the subsequent defections of two additional members of the staff. Better yet, had this question been asked prior to Dr. Jones' departure (and the cultural monitoring data concerning his concern about the salary cap been available), perhaps he even could have been retained.

A tool called "*Operating Guidelines*" [1] might prove even more useful in this case. Operating Guidelines are agreements made by all members of an organization that serve as the new or revised cultural norms of that group. They typically include interaction agreements that will help a culture become more functional such as: "We agree to be transparent, open, and honest," or "If we have a concern, we share it directly with that person instead of talking behind their backs to someone else," or "We make medical decisions by consensus," or "We consider facts and data before making decisions," or "We start and stop meetings on time," etc. Importantly, these guidelines must be agreed to—in advance—by everyone affected by them. This creates a sort of positive peer pressure that encourages compliance. To be effective, this must also be a living document that is revised and agreed to whenever there is a change in the culture (e.g., new team members, critical errors, changing businesses, technologies, tools, etc.). If, in the DMA case, there had been an operating guideline that said something such as: "We openly share information about decisions being discussed," or "We don't allow time sensitive issues to go unresolved," and the culture encouraged the application of these guidelines, DMA may have avoided serious problems.

Governance and Decision-Making

Decision-making processes are dependent on the governing structure of a practice/ department. While there is no one absolute right way to structure governance and decision-making, there are typically more choices involved in decision-making compared with governance. In general, decision-making by an individual or subset of the whole group is faster and more efficient in terms of up front time invested while group decision-making is slower but has the potential advantages of broader expertise and consideration of more aspects of an issue with the opportunity for better acceptance and implementation of a decision if all stakeholders have had input. It is helpful to think of decisions as major and minor. Major decisions, such as the sale of the group, would in most instances be discussed and decided by all shareholder pathologists (although this could be a single pathologist), while minor decisions like the purchase of a $100 book, should not be discussed by all of the pathologists. While these are admittedly extreme examples, it is often useful to define who makes what decisions and clearly empower those individuals to act. For example, the managing partner may be able to sign contracts up to a certain amount or purchase items up to a certain dollar limit while situations beyond these limits may be handled by an Executive Committee, a vote of all shareholders, or a decision of all pathologists in a practice regardless of shareholder status. In a like vein, a decision such as reducing vacation rather than hiring another pathologist and taking a pay cut may best be made by engaging all pathologists in the discussion and decision to facilitate buy-in and longer term satisfaction.

On a macroscale, the typical independent private practice is governed by its shareholders (as laid out in the Articles of Incorporation), typically the partners.

They may elect to make decisions by simple vote of shares (may be equal, may be unequal) or consensus. Sometimes, the non-partner/non-shareholders may be allowed to vote on items for which consensus is sought or which do not involve an action involving ownership of the group (such as selling the group or issuing of shares). The authors have found the consensus method to work the best for major decisions in groups in which dysfunction is at a minimum. Consensus decisions, it should be noted, are different from unanimous vote, but rather reflects a decision that will be supported, rather than subverted, by all involved. If consensus cannot be reached following sufficient effort, shares may then be voted. In these situations, leaders should watch for follow-up discussions and efforts to revisit past decisions to evaluate the quality of the decision-making process.

Decision-making for employed pathologists and academic departments can follow several patterns and many decisions may be made outside the department by the parent organization. Typically, decision-making will be by an advisory model or consensus. In the advisory model, the chief/chairman solicits input from stakeholders and decides. A vote may be sought, but a substantially split vote may create factions while a near majority risks creating "losers." A technique for mitigating these risks is additional communications through both individual and group discussions. Additional conversations can at least allow pathologists with ultimately different opinions "to be heard." Consensus is more difficult and may be impossible for some issues but could be reserved for medical decisions (e.g., how does the group handle breast biopsies) or delegated to a subgroup of the department (e.g., the breast "experts" in the department). Once again, communication is critical and discussion should be encouraged with all viewpoints/stakeholders requested to contribute. Decisions should be documented and minutes of decision-making meetings should be distributed as well as saved. While not all decisions are good decisions or perhaps the situation has changed, a leader should monitor for nonconstructive efforts to revisit decisions that are based on initial non-consensus or an inability to accept decisions of the department/leaders.

Recently, Joseph Folkman and Jack Zenger, noted organizational behaviorists, compiled a summary of behavior patterns that led to bad decisions [2]. Their list of nine behaviors or habits may seem self-evident, but in our experience is spot-on when we look at the poor choices we have seen ourselves and other groups of pathologists make. Here is their list:

- Laziness, being unwilling to do complete due diligence, cover all the bases, etc.
- Not anticipating unexpected events (sometimes the worst-case scenario comes about!)
- Indecisiveness, lingering too long over the matter, waiting for one more bit of data, etc.
- Remaining locked in the past, seeing only the status quo, the "way we've always done it"
- Failing to align decisions with strategy
- Overdependence on others, waiting for the other person/group to act, decide, etc.
- Acting in isolation or unilaterally, not getting input or buy-in from other major stakeholders. (Groups generally are smarter than individuals!)

- Lack of technical depth, meaning that when a leader or group relies on the technical expertise of others, without sufficient depth themselves, they may misinterpret the relationships, fail to see critical nonstarters, or other flaws in the decision

There are probably numerous other paths to bad decisions, but analyzing your own personal and group tendencies relative to these high-frequency bad habits may provide insight into how you can develop fail-safe signals that you may be heading toward a terrible one [3–6].

Generational Issues

Recently, much has been written about generational issues in organizations, but it has always been true that pathologists of different ages and at different stages of their careers have different attitudes and needs. For instance, a newly hired, recently trained pathologist may typically be focused on getting a handle on school loans and a mortgage while providing for a growing family, while a more senior pathologist may be more interested in his/her retirement plan and transition out of the practice. Currently, the following major categories have been considered as generations and encompass some general age groups. Clearly, these are just generalities and the age ranges are not absolutes.

Silent generation (1925–1945): Generally characterized as hard working, loyal, and rules based.

Baby boomers (1946–1964): Characterized as believing in hard work to get ahead (currently the generation representing the majority of heads of groups/departments).

Generation X (1965–1981): Characterized as focused on work/life balance.

Generation Y/Millennials (1982–2000): General characteristics of embracing technology and valuing team work and diversity; they seek flexibility and work/life balance; tend to multitask.

For the leader, the critical point is the recognition that each pathologist (and for that matter, person/employee) is an individual with their own needs and attitudes regarding work… and that these differences will partially drive how they interact with others and as part of a group. Furthermore, these differences should be identified and considered by the leader. This also speaks against the idea of fairness through all pathologists having similar jobs and assignments. Rather, the cohesive group/department is composed of a mixed mosaic of needs, desires, and work styles, with the goal of constructing a strong aggregate of skills, attitudes, and work styles. A mixed aggregate may be stronger than an assemblage of nearly identical pieces. Traditionally, senior pathologists have mentored junior pathologists. Particularly today, there is strength in bidirectional mentoring. Where a senior pathologist may share the wisdom gained through years of practice, the junior pathologist may be more familiar with new practices (being recently from a training program), technology, and social networking. By embracing these inherent differences, the leader can work to build the strongest practice by leveraging the synergies inherent in having a range of skill sets, work styles, and attitudes.

Non-partners and Part-Timers

Implicit in the above discussion of generational issues and needs and wants is the importance of a flexible approach to non-partners and part-timers. While employed pathologists and academic pathology groups may not deal with non-partners, other "classes" of pathologists may exist as part-timers or, for academic practices, temporary, "clinical," or other modified titled pathologists. A leader and, more generally, pathology groups, especially since non-partners and part-timers may involve shareholder-type issues, should strive to retain an open mind toward these issues since the alternative may be nonemployment or retirement of a pathologist who seeks an alternate arrangement. On the other hand, the situation should be considered in a structured format rather than as a once in a blue moon unique arrangement, not only for simplicity but also to retain a sense of fairness. For example, a partner may be allowed to reduce to 75 % effort while retaining partner status and a fractional share of bonus while to achieve an effort of less than 75 % level, a partner may need to sell their shares and relinquish their partner status. This could create a structure for subsequent replacement pathologists and inject a greater level of fairness into the situation. Once again, communication and transparency among all the pathologists are critical to achieving a win/win.

Specialization

A similar case exists for specialization as discussed above for non-partners and part-timers. If there is a compelling reason to specialize within a practice (and that is certainly a major trend in pathology), then the leader faces the situation of accommodating a range of individualized "deals" which can build a stronger practice but which can also lead to dissonance through upsetting the sense of fairness in a practice. Specialization may range from relatively simple (e.g., some pathologists focusing predominantly on anatomic pathology (AP) while others do predominantly clinical pathology (CP), but all take AP/CP call) to constructing subspecialty minigroups to deal with each section in CP and every organ system in surgical pathology across a variety of practice sites. In general, specialization is not only better health care by allowing development of greater expertise but, for example, subspecialization in surgical pathology has led to productivity gains of up to 50 % [7–9]

Succession Planning

Succession planning refers to a conscious effort to plan for replacing members of a practice. Succession planning combines strategic planning by being long range and broad reaching and risk management by being an effort to pre-empt or mitigate the loss of certain skills or portion of workload. The skills mitigated may be medical (e.g., we need someone who knows transplant liver pathology), leadership (e.g., who will be our president/chief of service), or other (e.g., Suzanne was our CPT coding expert). Succession planning should be at least an informal activity of a practice leader. More formal approaches include having succession planning as a component of formal strategic planning or striving to have an understudy for each major area of a practice. Succession planning can be as simple as taking an organizational chart and posing the question for each box on the organizational chart, "What if this person were to suddenly leave the practice?"

The "Good" Associate

Thus far, we have mostly considered the "other" pathologists in the practice. But what about you? How can you be a "good" associate/partner? It starts with your fit in practice. Ideally you are doing what you enjoy in a setting/practice site that enhances your professional satisfaction. Recognize that the practice of pathology evolves and that practices change as well. Individuals may change with time in terms of their professional needs and desires. The practice that you joined 10 years ago may no longer be a great fit because of changes in you and/or in the practice itself.

Being a good citizen in the practice is important. Focus on good communication among members of the practice. Listen to others' points of view while being prepared to compromise around yours. Actively support decisions that have been made and live the norms of the practice, both explicit and unspoken. Do your share of the work and a little more. Do your own monitoring of the mood of the group. Seek and listen to feedback, both from peers and subordinates. Even if your group is not doing regular 360-degree feedback, you can elicit useful feedback to help you improve. The health of a practice is every member's responsibility, not just the leader's. And, never lose site of the patients. Simply focusing on doing the right thing for patients can help a practice reset and move ahead.

Engagement

A lot of attention is paid to the topic of engagement in organizations today and health care is no exception. Regular employee engagement surveys are a part of many hospitals and multispecialty physician practices as these entities recognize the value in and need to draw on all the talents of their employees or team members to meet the ever-raising demands of "faster, better, cheaper."

We think that engagement is the natural state for a physician who has entered medicine, and hopefully this applies well to pathologists, with the ideals of using their talents to help others and to make a difference in the lives of patients. But after hours of classroom lectures on the minutiae of an obscure pathway they will never encounter in practice and past-midnight memorization of markers, methods of detection and antidotes or antigens, followed by sometimes abusive training programs where they may be viewed more as "the help" to grind meat and mince the morsels, sacrificing any sense of personal desires in favor of patient or program demands, not a few may enter practice just ready to get their own lives back. And even if they do manifest interest in making more of their situation and the system they have become part of, either the practice itself, or the larger system, sends messages that their engagement is not truly welcomed. Efforts to remove these disincentives to giving their all and to convey the genuine inviting messages for greater engagement can have impact. An article from the October 2014 *Physician Leadership Journal* [10] identified the following 15 traits as helpful to hospitals to enhance physician engagement; we think they can apply on the practice level as well. As you read through this list, you might consider two questions—first, what does my organization do to communicate this? And second, in what ways is that message diluted or undercut by what my organization actually does?

1. Respect for competence and skills
2. Feeling that their opinions and ideas are valued and sought
3. Good relationships with their physician colleagues
4. Good work–life balance
5. A voice (control) in how their time is structured and used
6. Fair compensation for their work
7. Good relationships with their non-physician clinical staff
8. A broader sense of meaning (mission) over and above day-to-day duties
9. A voice in clinical operations and processes
10. Opportunities (and funding) to expand their clinical skills and learn new skills
11. Opportunities for professional development and career advancement
12. Good relationships with administrators
13. Alignment with the organization's mission and goals
14. Working in an organization that is a leader and innovator in patient-centered health care
15. Substantive participation in setting broader organizational goals and strategies

Key differences between employees (their employee status, specialty, generational origin, leadership role in the practice, etc.) may lead to challenges in generating cohesion and group synergy.

Case: The Prima Donna

Dr. Mason believes he is the best diagnostician in his six pathologist group and belittles his associates when talking with clinicians. Dr. Mason's associates are aware of this and sarcastically refer to him as "the gifted one." To avoid feeding Dr. Mason's ego, Dr. Perry did not show him a frozen section she was unsure about, and some unwarranted additional surgery was performed.

Discussion: This is an example of major dysfunction that led to unnecessary surgery. The norms of the group are poor and the issue needs addressing. A highly functioning group will have ongoing quality assurance (OPPE). If there are true quality issues, they should be addressed. Beyond this, it is never appropriate to talk down your fellow pathologists and this issue must be talked through by the pathologists. Additional case studies that may provoke thought or discussion on these topics are presented in Appendix A.

References

1. Fisher K. Leading self-directed work teams. New York: McGraw-Hill; 2000.
2. Zenger J, Folkman J. Nine habits that lead to terrible decisions, Harvard Business Review, Sept 1, 2014. https://hbr.org/2014/09/9-habits-that-lead-to-terrible-decisions/. Accessed 7 April 2015.
3. Weisbord MR, Productive workplaces. San Francisco: Jossey Bass; 2012.
4. Peters TJ, Robert H, Waterman Jr. In search of excellence: lessons from American's best-run companies. 1982. New York: Harper Business Essentials (2004. Print).
5. HBR's 10 must reads on making smart decisions. Boston: Harvard Business Review Press; 2013.
6. Levi D. Group dynamics for teams. 4th ed. Washington DC: SAGE; 2014.
7. Black-Shaffer WS, Young RH, Harris NL. Subspecialization of surgical pathology at the MGH. Am J Clin Pathol. 1996;106:33–42.
8. Louis DN, Colvin RB. The later years, in keen minds explore the dark continents of disease: a history of the Massachusetts general hospital. http://www.massgeneral.org/pathology/assets/book/pathology_chap25.pdf. p 366. Accessed 2 Feb 2015.
9. Groppi DE, Alexis CE, Sugrue CF, et al. Consolidation of the north shore-LIJ health system anatomic pathology services: the challenge of subspecialization, operations, quality management, staffing and education. Am J Clin Pathol 2013;140:20–30.
10. Whitlock DJ, Stark R. Understanding physician engagement—and How to Increase it. Physician Leadersh J.2014;1(1)8–12.

Part VI
Better Practice Management

Chapter 15
Skills and Tools for Better Practice Management

Michael L. Talbert and Lewis A. Hassell

Case: The Big Plan

On-Cyte Pathology Group has just finished a grueling weekend retreat with an extensive review of their marketplace, new technologies and shifts in health care, and their own strengths, weaknesses, and history, and have come out of the gate with a new and ambitious strategic plan to move forward in a big way. They plan to take their practice virtual, emphasizing their expertise in the interpretation of the new images acquired through in vivo microscopy methods. They will continue to extend their mobile-van-based service to select regional surgery centers and dermatology practices, while expanding into a truly national market with IVM GI services. Their retreat was facilitated by a business consultant they retained for the purpose, and one of their next calls was to a well-known legal firm specializing in multistate practices as they foresee their clinical duties will become more national in scope and their corporate bylaws may need to be revised if not totally restructured. They have also begun plans to investigate various funding options, ranging from self-funding the expansion to seeking venture capital to a novel approach like one of the crowdsourcing funding services. They also recognize they will need to properly structure and staff their marketing campaign, but have not solved that problem yet. They have tremendous internal information technology (IT) expertise, but anticipate a greater demand for IT personnel to complete development of their apps and keep the portals secure and functional 24/7. They will likely move their in-house billing operation to a larger firm with more national experience as they begin to accrue work in more diverse settings. Discussions with various large gastroenterology (GI) practices and consideration of hiring their own interventionists are also planned.

Discussion: On-Cyte's pathologists, while obviously skilled and ambitious, also recognize the wisdom in the team-based approach to their business. They recognize their limitations as well and have sought competent, skilled help in key areas of their practice beyond their individual prowess.

M. L. Talbert (✉) · L. A. Hassell
Department of Pathology, University of Oklahoma Health Sciences Center,
940 Stanton L. Young Blvd., BMSB 451, Oklahoma City, OK 73104, USA
e-mail: michael-talbert@ouhsc.edu

L. A. Hassell
e-mail: lewis-hassell@ouhsc.edu

© Springer International Publishing Switzerland 2016
L. A. Hassell et al. (eds.), *Pathology Practice Management*,
DOI 10.1007/978-3-319-22954-6_15

Overview

In a rapidly changing health-care environment, every practice must continually improve, adapt, or otherwise change to thrive or, at the least, survive. Since the authors first outlined this project, Medicare payments for immunohistochemical stains, both technical and particularly professional components, have been slashed; reference-based pricing seems to have grown; on-the-fly modifications to the Affordable Care Act have been made; the healthcare.gov website fiasco has occurred; and while the sustainable growth rate threat has been repealed, Congress has set the framework for Medicare payment schemes to drive changes in how physicians work through the Merit-based Incentive Payment System. So what has been the effect on practices, how should practices respond, and, perhaps more importantly, what is coming next and how should practices prepare? In this chapter, we explore "tools of the trade" in practice management.

Scanning the Horizon

So what is happening and what is coming next? A key component of practice management is monitoring the external practice environment as well as following developing health-care and pathology-specific news. These are active processes and should involve all members of a practice in every facet of the environment from changes in local primary care groups to national legislation. The successful practice must be "plugged into" the local health-care environment through interactions with physicians from other specialties, service on hospital, health plan and national pathology medical society committees, and ties to the local business community. Also useful are the day-to-day gleanings of couriers, office staff, and social contacts to keep abreast of developments in your immediate environment. As you assemble this data stream, consider the broader implications of changes and any drivers such as money, market share, or positioning. Many changes will not immediately make sense as the environment evolves; much information will prove incomplete or even incorrect with additional time. The key will be those developments which provide an immediate or long-term opportunity or threat to your practice. For example, a courier report that, "Our Town Urologists, Inc. didn't have any specimens today and the receptionist thought they were being sent out of state," could be the first indication that a major source of outpatient diagnostic material may be at risk. An immediate response such as confirmation and discussions with the head of that group is probably in order. Further assessment would also be in order: Did you miss earlier clues this might happen? Does this signal a wider risk that other clients might seek other out-of-state solutions unfavorable to you? Does this development signal a problem with your service, diagnostic accuracy, or pricing? In short, is there a better value equation than what you offer? For pathology groups with significant outpatient markets, we have many times seen abrupt changes in referral patterns leading to reduced incomes and/or downsizing of groups. This is a facet of practice management you need to get right.

Changes in the local environment also often create opportunities. Hearing that a fellow pathologist from a small hospital is thinking about retirement may create the opportunity to transition that hospital into your practice's sphere. Learning that a local dermatologist has been dissatisfied with the attention to service issues she receives from a national laboratory creates an opportunity to offer your group's services. Talking to a state's academic practice leader and discovering you have complementary subspecialty pain points and excess staffing may lead to a way to share cases or coverage in selected areas to the benefit of both practices. Larger structural changes such as hospital- or large-group mergers may offer an opening for the new entity to reconsider pathology service providers. Monitoring the larger environment is necessary to understand pending legislation or rule-making and its potential effect on your practice, to monitor regional/national trends that may become increasingly powerful in your practice region, and to identify potential mechanisms to improve your own practice. National payment schemes, particularly for Medicare, are often discussed in the national media and are closely followed by national medical organizations. You should belong to multiple pathology organizations and will receive periodic communications regarding proposals under consideration, pending legislation, and results of legislation and rule-making. From time to time, you will be solicited to lobby your congresspersons regarding pending legislation. Recognize, though, that much of what is discussed does not come to pass and some things that are legislated may be modified through rule-making or delayed. Even if a debated proposal does not become law, thinking through its effect on your practice and potential responses can be a good exercise.

As health-care delivery changes, it changes in an uncontrolled manner and effects typically play out differently and at different times and rates depending on the locale. Given this, it is very useful to monitor developments in other areas as well as responses of pathology practices to the changes. For example, some pathologists are part of newly formed accountable care organizations (ACOs) while most are not. Those without experience of working in an ACO can learn from those who have and perhaps be better positioned when ACO formation is explored in their service area.

Monitoring the national environment is also important to identify, evaluate, and monitor new tools, techniques, and services. There has been much discussion regarding molecular testing, next-generation sequencing, Big Data, digital pathology, patient-centered care, population health, and ultrasound-guided fine needle aspiration among other topics. What are the legal, practical, and billing statuses of each of these new areas? How do they or would they fit into your practice? What are the benefits of waiting? What are the risks? What possible scenarios exist 2–3 years in the future? Are you or someone in your practice closely monitoring each of these areas (and many others)? It can be useful to follow the science and technology of these new areas through the literature and meetings of national organizations, but for the practical implementation and billing aspects, a network of leaders of practices similar to your own can be invaluable. These can be developed through national organizations such as Association of Pathology Chairs, American Pathology Foundation, College of American Pathologists and American Society for Clinical Pathology, among others, or through random connections over time. It is also a not uncommon experience to just call pathologists featured in an article or who gave a talk at a meeting or whom you can identify through Internet search and just "pick their brains" regarding what they are thinking and planning. Many pathologists are very open and perhaps through the sharing of ideas, both pathologists and their groups can benefit. Social media should not be overlooked in this matter either. A variety of such services have pertinent discussion groups where useful (but not infrequently, irrelevant) information is exchanged. And you can also create your own page or topic groups to attract like-minded individuals from around the world who may have valuable perspective on a topic.

Professionals for the Practice

Pathologists are acknowledged experts at what they do. Years of medical school, residency, fellowship, and, perhaps the best training of all, actual practice, take most pathologists to a level of specialization at which scope of practice issues with other physicians only infrequently become an issue. Pathologists do not, however, typically develop a similar level of expertise in some areas vital to the operation of the practice such as legal, human resources (HR), accounting, billing, marketing, and IT. These are infrequently available in training programs or available to only a very limited extent and given little weight in credentialing or certifying hurdles that trainees traverse, and hence get very little early attention. Depending on the setting and a practice's size and sophistication, such expertise can and should be obtained, then maintained, and developed as the practice develops. For the hospital-employed pathologist and some academic practices, many of these functions will be provided by the hospital or other parent organization. Accounting, legal, billing, marketing, management, and IT services will be provided by in-house or contracted services. If a specialized consultant is desired, such as a consultant engaged to evaluate expanding molecular pathology services, that person will most likely be contracted by the hospital.

For the independent practice, however, many of these services will be selected, contracted, and paid for by the practice. As such, the advantage of practice size to allow for greater professional expertise in its pathologist ranks can also allow for increased expertise in business assistance. This desire or mandate for greater access to IT and business expertise that can be allocated over more people's income is one key driver in the movement to larger groups over the past decades. Depending on the size of a practice, in-house accounting and billing may be considered. Professional management of the business aspects such as contracting can often be more efficiently managed by a non-pathologist professional, freeing the higher dollar pathologist to practice in their area of greatest expertise. Legal expertise can also be improved as a practice is able to devote more resources to support functions. Transitioning from a local general attorney who helped you incorporate a practice and who reviews contracts to a firm with more specialized attorneys even extending to attorneys with deep knowledge of pathology can be a major step ahead for a practice. Marketing is another area in which many practices can effectively invest.

Developing and marketing a practice's brand is often best managed by professionals. Marketing can also be used to build business and service clients with some larger groups electing to hire full-time client service and marketing personnel. IT can be a huge expense for practices today that will continue to increase as information management becomes more central to a pathologist's role in clinical care. Wise investment in both systems and personnel with the right match for the practice's needs can be critical to success in the long term.

Another area for investment can be consultants. Whether a consultant is used to advise on a specific project such as taking over histology services from the hospital or is engaged to do a general consultation of some aspect of a practice, many times the combination of new thinking and a new viewpoint can be a valuable investment. Selection of consultants can be by word-of-mouth recommendation, by a Google or LinkedIn search, or may result from hearing a consultant present at a national meeting. Contracting for such specialized services should be done carefully and with a clear idea of the desired outcomes ("deliverables").

The decision to hire such talent versus contracting with another entity will hinge on the scope and intensity of the desired service. Most practices would not hire full-time legal counsel but rather would use legal help as needed with the flexibility to engage specialized legal counsel if indicated. The volume of services simply would not merit full-time counsel. On the other hand, many pathology practices do the entire billing process in-house. With billing, a moderate-size practice can generate enough work to employ a small cadre of billing personnel. For this situation, a practice must evaluate the cost of in-house billing (including overhead, HR, etc.) versus using a billing company. In this scenario, as well, one must evaluate the efficiency and effectiveness of the actual billing operation (see "Revenue Cycle Management," Chap. 4).

Case: A Consultant Finds Money

Barry Bowen is a nationally known Current Procedural Terminology (CPT) coding consultant. Big University Pathology engaged Barry for a 1-day consult to review the billing practices, perform a CPT and International Classification of Diseases (ICD) billing audit, and lecture the faculty, residents, and billing staff on CPT coding. The visit was something of an eye opener. Not only did Barry find that 5–10% of CPT codes were simply never assigned to cases, but during the lecture there also were several instances where individual faculty piped up "Well, I don't code that." Dr. Chase Smith was so fascinated by the nuances of coding, he carefully reviewed the provided handouts, obtained a CPT coding manual, and subscribed to a well-regarded CPT newsletter. Within a month, Dr. Smith was regarded as the local CPT coding expert and quickly devised a process whereby he checked all surgical pathology coding at the end of each work day. Six months later, Perry Johnson, the departmental business administrator, was happy to report that collections were running some $200,000 annualized ahead of last year's pace and that most of the positive variance was due to Dr. Smith's coding efforts. Dr. Smith was a hero.

Discussion: Sometimes an outside expert's eyes (i.e., a consultant) can make a large difference. CPT coding is something you need to get right. Over-code and risk fines or worse. Under-code and leave money you have earned on the table. As the health-care finance environment continues to tighten, money cannot be left on the table. Where once there may have been excess resources, complete and correct coding now relates to meeting payroll. You should periodically review your entire coding and billing process with more frequent focused audits similar to quality control (QC) in the laboratory. Ideally, an outside expert can be periodically utilized to conduct a review. Judicious use of consultants can be very beneficial for a practice.

Tools for Improving the Practice

Pathologists become adept at using certain tools in their training. The microscope, decision support database, information system, and other resources become as much second nature as driving a car or tying ones shoelaces. Many of the elements we have illustrated above—coding, financial statements, and such—also fall into the category of tools that should be familiar to leaders in the practice. We strongly recommend that pathologists and practice leaders become facile with several additional management tools.

Process improvement using Lean and Six Sigma has become more than a business fad since these management tools bridged the gap from the manufacturing sector to health care over a decade ago. Yet despite that long history, it is still common to find practices cementing over the cow-path processes of the past rather than finding the shortest ways to add value or accomplish the quality improvements they need. *Value stream mapping* is one tool that can provide a useful overview of operations and identify where the wasted effort, time, or other resources are, and thus the targets for improvements. *Spaghetti diagrams* likewise can be useful to track movement of people or product along the path to production. Identifying the various kinds of waste in a system and empowering the organization with a culture that drives out waste is part of the toolkit as well. Even seemingly simple disciplines such as *Five 'S'* (Sort, Set in order, Shine, Standardize and Simplify, Sustain) can have remarkable impacts when rigorously applied. Likewise, the use of visual cues for process status, dummy-proofing processes, single-piece flow, and other Lean tools accelerates the generation of quality services and products, and improves financial and patient-care quality performance. In-depth study and practice to learn and master the use of these tools is worthwhile for every practice.

Active cultivation of a healthy organizational culture is critical and can be one of the outcomes of application of Lean and Six Sigma. But the ingredients for many of the soft skills that contribute to healthy or unhealthy organizational culture are not always exclusively found in quality or financial improvement tools such as these. Sports teams with top talent and high payrolls in lucrative markets often underachieve because of the "locker room" effect of a misbehaving player, or a poor manager or coach. Understanding the emotional individuality of one's team can be a starting point in the quality improvement effort here as well. Use of formal testing tools such as the Myers–Briggs type indicator is not common in pathology practices though some do and report favorable impact. Other tools to foster healthy communication and bridge various cultural barriers, such as Erin Meyer's eight axes of cultural expectations or approaches, can also be useful to defuse misunderstanding or misbehaviors stemming from differing expectations or assumptions [1]; see Fig. 15.1.

Team-building exercises, or use of organizational consultants and facilitators have also been productive in our experience, particularly when the leadership of a practice or organization is part of the conflict that may be holding an organization back from higher performance. Attention to cultural dynamics and proactive discus-

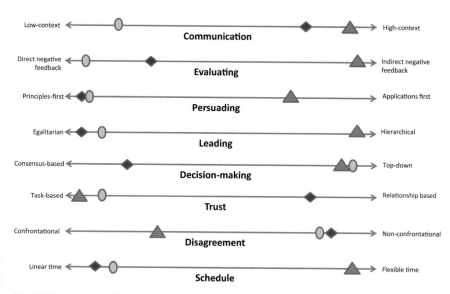

Fig. 15.1 Eight axes of cultural contexts that may be sources of organizational conflicts (adapted from E. Meyer, Cultural Map, HBR, 2014). Different *colored shapes* represent individual or group culturally favored operational points on the different domains. By identifying which axes have the widest divergence of individual profiles within an organization, one can devise coping strategies to ensure that decision-making and communication, or other processes, do not falter

sion or training in cultural issues may be particularly important when practices are consolidating or merging, or when other significant shifts are afoot.

Case: Succession Challenges

Cougar and Lugar Pathology had been doing well since its founding over 20 years ago by Kit Cougar and Bill Lugar. They had solidified their geographic reach by bringing in all the hospitals within a 100-mile radius using their model of top-tier lab services and consultative "always available" mantra. Things had gone well as they had brought in new associates to support the model. Lugar was gone now, having retired to Arizona near his grandchildren, but Kit still seemed engaged, though he had always had a penchant for diverse interests, everything from high-altitude mountain-bike racing to classic cars. You joined the practice 2 years ago when Lugar retired with ambitions to bring your molecular training to bear on the next generation of growth for the group of ten pathologists and a lone PhD. But while organized as a professional corporation, the group really ran pretty much as a sole-proprietorship under Kit's benevolent wisdom and ample energy. Even when Lugar was around, he mostly did the job of picking up any loose ends that Kit might have missed as he pursued the grand design.

Lately, some of the newer hires have been voicing concern over commiting significant resources to seeming tangential ventures. At an inopportune time, this low-level grumbling came unexpectedly to Kit's knowledge through a nonphysician employee of one of their client hospitals. The very next morning, Kit delivered a letter of resignation specifying that in 3 months he would be out the door. In the interim, he would cooperate to train and orient whomever they chose to lead the organization.

This earthquake-like announcement immediately provoked a call by two of the senior partners to the group's legal counsel to establish what their corporate bylaws stated about governance. Not much. They called a meeting of the group to map a plan to transition to a new governance model. After a rather acrimonious meeting in which all sorts of finger-pointing took place ("Well, if you hadn't gone blabbing to Nancy, we wouldn't be in this mess…" etc.), the senior leaders recognized that reorganization was going to be a challenge on many fronts. While recounting the boardroom drama to your wife afterwards, she says, "It sounds like the group could use a therapist, or at least a good consultant. Have you ever talked with the Ponds, you know, that pleasant older pair we sometimes see at church? I think they have some sort of organizational behavior background."

After a phone call to satisfy your own curiosity and assess suitability, you arrange for the two senior partners to meet Jane and Jerome Pond. The Placid Pond Group, who have done quite a bit of organizational counseling and facilitation through comparable crises in the past, listen and take notes, getting much more of an earful on the various dysfunctions in the group than perhaps they expected right off the bat. They define the initial "deliverables" to be an independent assessment of stakeholder interests, development of a new governance structure supported by the group, and definitions of new decision-making methods to promote a healthier organization and prepare future leaders. The proposal is ratified by the partners and the Ponds go to work with them. Over the next 3 months and beyond, the group is coached into a participatory model of decision-making. The "big issues" that require consensus are defined, and new officers are installed and trained to become conversant with the organization's processes, client relationships, and fiscal details. The sentiment following the first group meeting following Cougar's severance is that they are going to do well. There is a new energy, a great sense of empowerment, and vigor to tackle the challenges they face together.

Discussion questions:

What kinds of problems in a practice group are the most vexing in terms of being able to independently resolve them?

What are the risks and benefits of using an independent consultant to help resolve "dirty laundry" kinds of organizational issues?

How should a potential consultant or practice resource be assessed for value? What if the two parties cannot agree on "deliverables?"

Case: Strategic Advance at Mountain Valley Partners

One of the long-term habits that had always helped to unite the Mountain Valley pathologists was their summer weekend get-together at the camp (really a family vacation lodge) owned by one of the partners, an hour drive from their main base of operations. It began as a "by invitation only" event that was as much recreational as operational. But the conversations in the evenings, when they were not on the lake fishing or hiking one of the surrounding peaks, inevitably turned to the state of their mutual practice affairs. And just as inevitably, they would have ideas surface that could be totally crazy or wildly profitable. As the reality of the business value of this annual foray into the wilderness became clearer, they began to consider ways to exploit it for the business value, rather than just as a time away from work together where they could strengthen bonds of friendship.

The group was growing, but the property would easily accommodate the numbers they had for the first few years of inviting everyone. They tried calling it their "escape" or a "retreat" but somehow those words did not fit particularly well. What they often ended up with was more like a strategic plan for the coming year or so. They ultimately settled on the term "advance" as sufficiently capturing the image of a forward-looking event. People began looking forward to the opportunity to have more extended periods of time to discuss matters of importance that could not always be adequately handled in a routine business update or group meeting when people had to rush off for a morning frozen section or got called away with a massive transfusion situation. So some topics began preparation a few months in advance, and the schedule got harder to balance between the "renewal and team-building" ends of things and the strategic thinking and planning side. Also, as the group diversified culturally, they noted that it got harder to bring everyone into the discussions and see buy-in or commitment afterwards. So they began to engage a facilitator to guide the discussion and take responsibility for capturing the ideas that would pour out, often at rapid-fire pace. Sometimes, smaller section groups or task forces would meet in advance or even in the woods somewhere during the advance, to hammer out an aspect of their plans or proposals.

On occasion, Mountain Valley partners would invite various advisors (legal, financial, etc.) to join them for a portion of the weekend, particularly if there was a known issue or project for which a particular perspective could be invaluable. But sometimes, it was just to assuage members of the group whose risk tolerance might differ from others.

Now the group has evolved into a multistate operation, approaching 50 pathologists. The annual advance has been a key method in reaching that level of success, and remains one of the "don't miss" dates on the calendar. Though it has long-since outgrown the camp on the lake, the ways in which it has been used to the group's advantage—everything from replicating Lean training in a nutshell to giving time to "listen to the customer" in the form of key clients, to highlighting and celebrating new services being developed, continues to serve the group well. You might say the advance is one of the most valued practices (MVPs).

Discussion questions:

What sorts of celebratory events are useful for a practice group?

In what ways can strategic planning and thinking be facilitated so that they do not become passé or even irritating?

Organizational traditions help to perpetuate the culture for new members of the tribe. What did MVP do that improved their culture and avoided the pitfall of factionalism?

Reference

1. Meyer E. The culture map: breaking through the invisible boundaries of global business. New York, NY: Public Affairs Press; 2014.

Part VII
Managing Risks and Opportunities

Overview

Case: Is It Opportunity or Risk?

The partners at Community Pathology, P.C. were chatting at lunch with some of their colleagues about new changes ahead in medical practice and how they would like to get out of the bind where their incomes were so subject to the next CMS ruling about payment rates and rules. Bob, an OB, suggested that they should form a self-insurance consortium for their malpractice insurance. Tim, a gastroenterologist, suggested that they could easily collaborate to build an outpatient surgery center and capture the technical fees that were now going to the hospital. Tom, the general practitioner, said that with the range of incomes in their relatively closed community, they could consider a concierge-type integrated practice model to offer quality services to paying customers, allowing them to cut out the various insurers who kept coming back to them with progressively more stringent contracts each year. The youngest of the pathologists, Frieda, listened with eager ears, but the anxiety inside her grew, as she interpreted the body language of her colleagues and senior partners who seemed ready to commit their income stream (and hers!) to fund almost all of the suggestions.

Discussion: Different individuals have differing degrees of risk-tolerance and differing perceptions of what constitutes risk itself. Some of this is generational, or age-related, but a variety of other factors enter in as well. Awareness of this fact and a willingness to deal respectfully with this are important to group dynamics and the success of a group. Management of risks can also lead to shifts in understanding and tolerance of risk, much as a practiced gymnast feels confident in attempting new moves on the balance beam as she gains confidence in herself and her spotter while performing more routine tasks.

Every business deals with risks in some manner. Paired with those responses are the ways in which businesses deal with opportunities. Often the choices around

L. Hassell (✉) · M. L. Talbert
Department of Pathology, University of Oklahoma Health Sciences Center, 940 Stanton
L. Young Blvd., BMSB 451, Oklahoma City, OK 73104, USA
e-mail: lewis-hassell@ouhsc.edu

M. L. Talbert
e-mail: michael-talbert@ouhsc.edu

J. P. Wood
McDonald Hopkins, LLC, 956 Main St., Dennis, MA 02638, USA
e-mail: jwood@mcdonaldhopkins.com

these two issues are intimately intertwined and delicately balanced. And since the perception of one or the other is critically important as well, in a group setting using some form of healthy or unhealthy decision-making, the culture of the organization affects the ways risks and opportunities are managed. In this section, we will examine the different types of risk usually encountered and the ways in which practices may cope with those risks. We will conclude with a discussion of opportunities and entrepreneurialism.

> Risk, general or professional, needs to be managed. Doing so requires consideration of what the risks are, the likelihood of their occurrence, the potential cost, and steps to mitigate the damage to the persons and businesses involved. Prevention is the most cost-effective means of mitigation.

Chapter 16
Professional Liability Risk

Lewis A. Hassell, Michael L. Talbert and Jane Pine Wood

Case: Am I Covered?

Fresh from training, Dr. Petermann joins Consulting Pathologists, PC at a modest starting salary. Anxious to repay his student loans as soon as possible, he willingly agrees to provide weekend call coverage for Jim Journe, a solo pathologist who is nearing retirement, who serves a hospital not within the contracts of Consulting Pathologists. Dr. Petermann only read his contract cursorily and believes his activities on his own time are his, so he is not infringing on Consulting Pathologists. He also assumes that his activities on the weekend will fall under Jim's liability policy. On his very first weekend, he is asked to review a blood smear he believes shows a leukemoid reaction. However, he misses the diagnosis of acute promyelocytic leukemia, and the patient dies from profound coagulopathy without being referred. When the legal papers for wrongful death are filed, neither Jim's nor Consulting Pathologist's liability insurer is willing to accept responsibility.

Discussion: Liability insurance policies define what acts are potentially covered. Knowledge of one's coverage is paramount. Dr. Petermann should have fully investigated liability coverage regarding his weekend call activities.

Professional Liability

It has not always been the case that a practitioner of medicine could face economic impoverishment at the hands of the legal system, but it certainly has been recognized at least as far back as Hippocrates that a physician held the potential to inflict harm on their patients. Despite the oath to "do no harm" in these caring

L. A. Hassell (✉) · M. L. Talbert
Department of Pathology, University of Oklahoma Health Sciences Center,
940 Stanton L. Young Blvd., BMSB 451, Oklahoma City, OK 73104, USA
e-mail: lewis-hassell@ouhsc.edu

M. L. Talbert
e-mail: michael-talbert@ouhsc.edu

J. P. Wood
McDonald Hopkins, LLC, 956 Main St., Dennis, MA 02638, USA
e-mail: jwood@mcdonaldhopkins.com

© Springer International Publishing Switzerland 2016
L. A. Hassell et al. (eds.), *Pathology Practice Management*,
DOI 10.1007/978-3-319-22954-6_16

relationships, physicians are human and make mistakes, whether intentional or not. Even the best and defensible efforts may produce bad outcomes, which in the hands of skillful plaintiff lawyers may result in a sympathetic jury awarding in favor of the injured party.

As the "doctor's doctor," pathologists were often shielded from the patient's view in the past, and thus in large part, free from the emotional context that governs the filing of most malpractice suits. But pathologists are not immune, and while not as frequently sued as many other specialties, several notable areas of professional risk are present. The majority of these generally center on failure to diagnose a malignancy or premalignancy such as a melanoma, breast cancer, or cervical cancer. Data published by Troxel [1] and a major pathology malpractice carrier illustrated these areas of risk from a historical standpoint. Another study from the New England Journal of Medicine [2] indicated that although the frequency of suits against pathologists were in the lowest third of physician specialties, the mean settlement in pathologist cases was second only to pediatrics in dollar value payments to plaintiffs.

These data also illustrate the magnitude of the awards to plaintiffs in cases involving pathologists and thus can provide guidance about levels of liability insurance that should be considered. Of course, these may vary by region and practice setting, due both to the legal and cultural climate, as well as the nature of the patients being served and under what auspices.

While managing professional liability may appear to be simply a matter of determining the level of liability coverage needed, selecting the particular terms of coverage, and completing the appropriate paperwork to enroll, there are a variety of significant factors that impact liability risk generally and specifically. For example, the hiring decision itself is one of the key times to influence the overall liability risk of the organization. Certain personality types and behaviors are known to be more prone to incur suits (brusque, poor listeners), whereas other types of behaviors and personality types prone to avoid them (empathetic, good listener.) While liability risk managers have seen progress in risk prevention through educational efforts aimed at a host of activities and attitudes, starting with the best mix of personal attitudes and traits is clearly helpful.

The choice of policy terms and nature of covered actions will determine in large part the policy premium to be paid. Generally, policies are written with two dollar amounts, one referring to the maximal amount that can be paid under the policy and a second number, usually about half the first number, indicating the amount that can be paid for a single claim. So, for example, a $3,000,000/$1,000,000 policy (the numbers may be presented in either order) has a maximal annual payout of $3 million dollars, but only 1 million for any one claim. With the trajectory of claims settled and dollar amounts steadily increasing at around the rate of inflation, policy values and premiums will likely also continue to inflate, although some evidence indicates that many of the quality and educational initiatives have reduced risks, and thus helped maintain lower premiums.

A second key variable to consider when choosing a policy type is whether the policy covers activities conducted during a specified period of time (covered period) ("occurrence" policy) or claims filed in a given period ("claims made" policy). While the former type generally seems more appropriate in terms of simplicity in covering the various sorts of professional activities one may be engaged in during a career, the second type has certain advantages, such as a somewhat lower cost, particularly for someone entering practice, that may make it more desirable as a choice. On the other end of these claims-filed policies is the matter of claims that may arise out of activity performed while employed and insured but which are not filed until after employment has ended or shifted to another employer. This "tail" of potential liability is lower than the liability one has while actively practicing but potentially just as devastating personally and financially. So, the matter of ensuring that "tail coverage" is provided should be a part of the discussion of benefits and employment arrangements. The following summarizes the differences between these two policy types:

Occurrence Policy

An occurrence policy protects you from any incident occurring while the policy is in force. The policy then covers those incidents forever. For example, you buy a policy in 2009, treat Client X in 2010, and terminate the policy in 2011. In 2014, Client X sues you for an incident that occurred in 2010. You are covered because you were insured when you treated Client X. With an occurrence policy, it does not matter if you are covered when the suit is brought.

2009	2010	2011	2012	2013	2014
Start policy	Treat client X	End policy			Client X sues

Claims-Made Policy

A claims-made policy covers you for any covered claim provided it meets two criteria:

- You are insured when the claim is made. If you no longer need coverage, you can purchase a "tail" to protect you for the past (see below).
- You have continually renewed the policy from the time the incident occurred until the time the claim is made.

In this example, you buy a claims-made policy in 2009 and renew it every year. You treat Client X in 2010. In 2013, Client X decides to sue for the services you provided in 2010. You are covered because: (1) you were continuously insured up to when the claim was made and (2) the treatment was provided after the policy started in 2009.

2009	2010	2011	2012	2013	2014
Start policy	Treat client X			Client X sues	

Adapted from *The Trust* http://www.apait.org/apait/products/professionalliability/faq/claimsmade.aspx

Most employer-provided liability insurance is explicitly for activities conducted under the terms of the employment agreement, so practitioners who may be inclined to "moonlight" in another setting or offer volunteer services domestically or internationally may find their actions unprotected by specific professional liability. Relying on an umbrella-type general personal liability policy is one option in this setting, if the policy specifically covers professional medical liability, but there are many others. It is critical to consult with a knowledgeable agent, providing him or her with a complete description of all of your activities and copies of all policies, so that he or she can assist in determining whether you are adequately covered.

Careful scrutiny of the extent of different activities being covered under the policy is also an important way to limit the cost of liability coverages. While some policy underwriters may not distinguish between activities solely devoted to the clinical laboratory and those involving cytology or surgical pathology, these activities all have rather different liability risk profiles, and savvy consumers and underwriters may wish to negotiate on these more explicit terms. In this arena then, it may make sense to deal with a policy provider who has more experience with pathology-specific underwriting to take advantage of potentially lower areas of risk for certain providers in the practice.

It is also important to determine whether the policy(ies) extends to the practice entity (the professional corporation, limited liability corporation, or other legal entity) as well as the individual pathologists. Because the practice entity has assets, even if a hospital-based practice (the accounts receivable are a significant asset), it is important that the practice entity also be covered by insurance.

Case: Risk Management

Southeast Pathology had the philosophy of giving back to the communities they served and derived their successes from. Hardly ever turning down a request for advertising support, their names, either as a group or just the practice, had appeared in playbills, on YMCA kids' athletic teams, and other community venues. Over the years, board members of the local ballet company had acknowledged their particular support and invited members of the group to various gala events for donors and supporters. Then came the misadventure that started simply enough with a biopsy of a pigmented lesion on the thigh of a ballet board member's young daughter. The sample encountered a processing glitch in the laboratory, resulting in poor-quality sections that were unreadable. The specimen was reprocessed and sectioned with little improvement, but eventually diagnosed after significant delay as a variant of melanoma. Unfortunately, the processing and sectioning mishap used all the lesional tissue, making it unavailable for molecular testing that might have qualified the girl for a promising clinical trial. Dr. Madoff, leader of Southeast Pathology, following the protocol for event management in their quality management plan, called the mother to express his apology for the mishap and less than optimal outcome and to explain what they had done to prevent such things from happening again to others. It was only then that he recognized the connection between the patient and his acquaintance on the ballet board. Because of their friendship and the group's status as community contributors, established before the adverse event, and because of his apology, she chose not to file a complaint with the medical practice board or a negligence suit, even though it appeared her daughter might not do well as a consequence.

Mitigating risk is something best done before the risk event arises. That is what we have been talking about in disaster preparedness, employee screening, and liability insurance. Once the water is rising or the suit is filed, it is too late to build the levee or buy the policy. This section will discuss the role that certain good practices play in doing that, even though they may not be strictly seen as "risk management" in the traditional sense.

A healthy quality management plan prospectively identifies activities or areas in the laboratory that are high risk and determines means to monitor and reduce these risks. For example, mislabeled specimen trends may reveal opportunities for education of specific personnel or adjustments in technologies or methods to reduce the chance for "wrong blood in tube" or other potential disasters. Likewise, a proper quality management plan also includes processes, as noted in the case above, for follow-up on sentinel events, near misses, and patient/clinician complaints. This can include various tools from Lean and Six Sigma, such as root cause analysis (RCA) or failure modes and effects analysis (FMEA), to fully characterize the milieu in which an event occurred and how a process or situation might be improved. The more robust these plans are, the easier it will be for a practice or laboratory to weed out areas of risk and drive the level of risk downward.

Since much and typically most pathologist professional liability occurs in surgical pathology and cytopathology, very robust quality systems, plans, and risk mitigation efforts should be in place in those areas. Well-designed patient identification processes can mitigate the risk that a diagnosis is mistakenly assigned to the wrong patient. A carefully designed reporting system can ensure that a complete and understandable report will be reliably delivered to the appropriate health-care provider. Good practices will also focus on the accuracy of diagnosis with judicious use of second pathologist review (particularly of high-risk cases) and outside consultation. A robust quality assurance (QA) plan can help identify the rare instance of a misdiagnosis to allow for group education and mitigation of any systemic issues in process or diagnosis. Further examination of anatomic pathology (AP) QA programs and risk management are beyond the scope of this book but excellent resources exist, and the authors know of multiple practices that have engaged consultants to review their procedures [3–5]. A high-performing practice will have a well-designed system to reduce errors with a practice-wide culture that is proactive and open. The authors would personally avoid practicing in an environment that was not well designed to minimize error.

One area that has been the topic of considerable debate is the issue of error disclosure and apology [6, 7]. Increasingly, more states have medical apology laws on the books that generally preclude the use of a medical apology as evidence of wrongdoing or negligence in malpractice suits. While some have argued that these practices may manipulate and are tainted with insincerity, in other settings, the process can be part of the quality improvement effort and offer significant emotional closure for both victims of such errors and those responsible. One should be familiar with the legal treatment in one's state and recognize that error disclosure is an activity distinct from apology.

Case: Tail Coverage or Not?

Dr. Kane has been a shareholder in his small group practice for 8 years but is now retiring. When he joined the practice, his employment agreement specified that he would be provided malpractice insurance, but did not specify which type of coverage would be provided. His three other partners are feeling the financial pinch and have always gone with the cheapest option, which was a claims-made policy. Since the group is relatively new, they have never faced the issue of "tail" coverage. They are also a bit peeved at losing someone they were relying on for another decade or so and dismayed at having to recruit a replacement in the time frame of the 3 months' notice Dr. Kane has given them (much as they like Dr. Kane and wish him well). The three other shareholders are inclined to model their approach on what they have heard others do, that is, only cover the tail for partners who have been with the group for 15 years or longer. Dr. Kane has been signing out all their gynecologic (GYN) cytology cases and directing the blood bank and transfusion service in the clinical laboratory. Given that they live in a rural area where the ratio of lawyers to farmers is considerably less than 1:1, Dr. Kane is inclined to take the risk of "going bare" on his tail of liability.

What should Dr. Kane do?

Is the partners' position defensible under legal terms?

What should they do to avoid this painful position again?

What if instead of leaving for another career, Dr. Kane were joining another practice or had died unexpectedly?

Discussion: Clearly, these are issues that should have been carefully questioned and resolved at the time the employment contract was written and negotiated. Attempting to negotiate or rectify the gap later, particularly when one of the parties is aware of specific or potential plans that might affect the decision, is much more difficult. As noted earlier in this book, some policies are transferrable to a new employment setting, and tail coverage may be waived upon death of the practitioner.

Case: QA and Risk Management in Surgical Pathology

Dr. Michael Armstrong, director of surgical pathology at Coastal Medical Center, gazed with interest at the pretty lobules of cartilaginous tissue well demarcated from the surrounding pulmonary parenchyma. "Well, they certainly got it all," thought Dr. Armstrong. Then, he realized, "this is a lobectomy specimen; I wonder why they did this?" Glancing back at the paperwork, he stopped on the preoperative diagnosis: "Adenocarcinoma of the lung. Please do genetic studies." Dr. Armstrong's pulse quickened as part of a generalized sympathetic response as he realized that some type of error had been made. He quickly flipped to the patient's previous pathology specimens. There it was: "Lung: adenocarcinoma." Thirty minutes later, as Dr. Armstrong reviewed the previous cytology specimen, he realized that while the specimen was cellular, typical features of chondroma were not present, and the cells were predominantly bronchial epithelial cells complete with cilia and clearly benign. This triggered a focused review on a new pathologist with two fellowships, who had been hired 6 months before. The focused review revealed more issues and was followed by a complete review of every case diagnosed by the new pathologist. Despite a rigorous on-boarding review of cases as part of focused professional practice evaluation (FPPE), the practice had allowed the new pathologist to sign out independently for some 3 months. The new pathologist was let go. Fortunately, except for the index case, no significant harm was done to any patients.

Questions for discussion:

Could this happen in your practice?

What systems does your practice have in place to prevent this type of occurrence?

When was the last time your group reviewed your quality plan for surgical pathology? And cytopathology?

Does your practice have a method to identify high-risk specimens? Is this policy/procedure followed by all pathologists?

Do you collect quality data by pathologists to look for gaps or trends?

Are any/all "misses" reviewed with the individual? Are these "problem" cases seen by all sign-out pathologists?

References

1. http://www.thedoctors.com/KnowledgeCenter/PatientSafety/articles/CON_ID_000295. Accessed 24 Apr. 2015.
2. Jena AB, Seabury S, Lakdawalla D, Chandra A. Malpractice risk according to physician specialty. N Engl J Med. 2011; 365:629–36.
3. Nakhleh RE, editor. Error reduction and prevention in surgical pathology. New York: Springer; 2015.
4. Nakhleh RE, Fitzgibbons PL, editors. Quality management in anatomic pathology: Promoting patient safety through systems improvement and error reduction. Chicago: CAP Press; 2005.
5. Valenstein P, ed. Quality management in the clinical laboratories: promoting patient safety through risk reduction and continuous improvement. Chicago: CAP Press; 2005.
6. Dintzis SM, Rendi MH. CAP Foundation Keitges program on medical ethics: disclosing harmful pathology errors to colleagues, treating clinicians, and patients. CAP'14 Chicago, Il. http://www.cap.org/apps/docs/annual_meeting/2014/pdf/S1366_Course_Presentation.pdf. Accessed 19 Jan. 2015.
7. Carmack HJ. A cycle of redemption in a medical error disclosure and apology program. Qual Health Res. 2014;24(6):860–9.

Chapter 17
Corporate and General Liability

Lewis A. Hassell, Michael L. Talbert and Jane Pine Wood

Case: Organizational Risk

Dr. Roberts is the only neuropathologist in his group that serves three neurosurgeons, one of whom occasionally operates on tumor cases. When Dr. Roberts travels for meetings, he makes himself available to do remote consultation on frozen sections using scanned whole-slide images of the frozen section viewed on a mobile device and a cell phone for verbal reporting of his opinion. While traveling in Asia, he is asked to consult on a case when he is in the waiting area of a busy airport. People on both sides of him can readily view the images of the slide and the information on the label of the slide.

Is this a reportable Health Information Privacy and Accountability Act (HIPAA) violation that subjects the practice to risk?

What kinds of policies might be put in place to manage that risk while not restricting Dr. Roberts' ability to view the images wherever he is?

Discussion: There are issues here that could place the organization at risk and create a need to have policies about using mobile devices and accessing patient data in public places, on phones, tablets, or other tools.

Storage of personal health data on such devices has proven a very costly risk for several high-profile institutions as well as individual medical practices when such devices were lost or stolen and a security breach needed reporting. The HIPAA imposes rather stiff penalties for even inadvertent release of patient medical information to unauthorized persons, a liability that is not covered by most general business insurance. Prevention in the form of good practices, solid policies, training, and awareness is critical to escaping the potentially large fines for release of protected health information (PHI). A number of notable large institutions have received

L. A. Hassell (✉) · M. L. Talbert
Department of Pathology, University of Oklahoma Health Sciences Center, 940 Stanton L. Young Blvd., BMSB 451, Oklahoma City, OK 73104, USA
e-mail: lewis-hassell@ouhsc.edu

M. L. Talbert
e-mail: michael-talbert@ouhsc.edu

J. P. Wood
McDonald Hopkins, LLC, 956 Main St., Dennis, MA 02638, USA
e-mail: jwood@mcdonaldhopkins.com

© Springer International Publishing Switzerland 2016
L. A. Hassell et al. (eds.), *Pathology Practice Management*,
DOI 10.1007/978-3-319-22954-6_17

negative press and faced liability following the loss of electronic media such as hard drives, laptops, or other media containing even seemingly innocuous patient-identifiable data such as admission dates, accession numbers, zip codes, etc. Federal law requires practices to have HIPAA policies in place, as do quite a few states. Every practice should have an HIPAA privacy and security officer who is responsible for ensuring that appropriate practices and policies have been implemented, and who can assist in coordinating a response in the event of a possible privacy breach.

Besides the harm resulting from professional neglect or malpractice, a host of general potential liabilities exist for pathology practices. The degree to which these are or may be covered by other entities (the hospital, e.g., for hospital-based physicians) varies but should be examined and discussed with legal or other advisors. For a practice employing any nonphysicians to perform services, some level of additional risk is present which should be covered under general liability insurance. For a practice operating as a corporate entity with some form of officers and possibly a governing board, consideration should also be given to officers and directors insurance to cope with the potential for everything from financial malfeasance to sexual harassment allegations. These kinds of risks can be as costly and destructive, not to mention disruptive, as professional malpractice suits.

Key to managing risks in these arenas are healthy practices and solid policies governing employee behavior, adherence to policies, management of grievances, and attention to relationships within the workplace. Equitable pay and benefits may also help keep employees engaged and disinclined to seek financial windfall through a legal claim. Again, this is an area where hiring scrutiny and painstaking review of references and personality are critical prior to a hiring decision. Care in maintaining an employee handbook with regular review of same, as well as thorough training and orientation to both initial and any additional tasks, is important.

Financial mischief afflicts small and large practices far more often than it should simply because the officers and managers running the practice have not developed and incorporated practices that both protect the practice and the individual from reproach. Dual witness handling of receivables and deposits, appropriate and timely audits, documentation trails, and dual signature requirements for disbursements are important measures, but are beyond the scope of this book. Designing systems and controls that make it impossible to misappropriate funds to private advantage should prevail over trust of long-standing or new employees or partners. Malfeasance happens because people are human and because the opportunity exists. One cannot change the nature of humans, but one can manage the situations and the opportunities that are offered. It is very difficult to recover resources lost to embezzlement occurring over even short periods, much less decades.

Case: Love in the Lab

Dr. Petrole has been with your practice since finishing his training and is developing nicely in terms of his expertise. He directs your chemistry lab and handles the growing volume of the molecular testing you have brought in house. The chief technologist you have hired to perform the molecular testing is young and seems to work well with Dr. Petrole. She and her husband become well acquainted with Dr. Petrole and his wife, and often engage together socially. As the years progress, you note that the good doctor and your chief molecular technologist regularly attend the same professional meetings. Eventually, their behaviors lead to suspicion that their relationship has passed beyond a purely professional one.

Is this a situation that poses risk to the practice?

What sorts of protections might be put in place to prevent harm?

Discussion: Certainly policies cannot prevent people from falling out of love or in love with the wrong people. But given the environment where the least suspicion or allegation of inappropriate relationships, favoritism, or sexual harassment can lead to disastrous consequences, organizations are wise to scrutinize accepted practices to avoid situations that might leave them vulnerable in the event of such accusations.

Another risk that falls into this general category is loss of proprietary information. While patents can offer some protection for certain kinds of intellectual property, a host of other keys to business success lie in the form of business process information, client lists, provider contracts, supplier pricing, and other data that are also subject to walking away in the brain or electronic media carried by a current or former employee. Often practices have not taken a careful inventory of these assets or considered them the assets worth protecting in some form. While it is common to have some sort of noncompete clause in an employment agreement to protect from talent defections that could harm the business, these are often difficult to enforce and may not cover all information that one desires to protect. Prudent management should ask the question of themselves as to what a departing employee is or could be taking with them and whether that has detriment to the business. Clear policies about accessing or maintaining such information outside of the workplace, however defined, may offer some protection, but careful hiring practices are probably the best insurance against such potential losses.

Case: The Missing Money

The branch manager of the local bank your practice uses calls one morning to say that the deposit left in the depository the previous evening is short $500 from what was listed on the deposit slip, and he wanted to alert you to the possibility that one of your employees had taken some of the money. You are of course dismayed at this allegation, not because of the amount of money, but because you have trusted your clerk and secretary to handle the deposits each day. You recall that yesterday there was a patient who came to pay the bill with cash, rather than the usual credit card or checks. As you think through your processes, you assume they cannot be so dumb as to have shorted the deposit that way. So you query them each independently about what happened yesterday with the deposit. Did you count the money or tally the paid bills in the computer? Were there cash payments? Others? Was the money ever left alone? Did you seal the deposit bag? Did you both drop at the bank? After closely reviewing their answers and your policies, you can see no gaps when the money could have left the company in someone's private possession. There were no unwitnessed gaps. In passing, one of them mentions how crisp and new the bills were and that they had clipped them all together in the bag, while the checks were left loose with the deposit slip.

With that knowledge in mind, you go to the branch bank and ask to see the manager about the discrepancy. You describe the company protocol of dual management of the funds, and the fact that both stories from the prior day lined up precisely. "So you think the $500 made it to the bank?" intones the manager in disbelief. "I've seen a lot more lying employees than bank errors, if that's where you're going." You ask to see the room where the deposits from the night depository are opened and where the teller sits as they open the bags. You note that they use a knife to open the plastic sealed bags. "Is the teller left-handed or right handed?" you ask. "Well, I believe she is left handed" the manager states. The wall and the table where the envelopes are opened has a small gap, just big enough to hide a few bills. Leaning over, and nudging the table slightly, you see something lodged in the space just a ways down the narrow canyon. Reaching in and moving the desk further from the wall, you retrieve five crisp Ben Franklins neatly clipped together where they had lodged when the teller slit open the practice deposit envelope while looking the other way such that she did not notice she was flinging the neatly clipped cash to her left.

What would you have done if there had been just one employee handling the deposit and such an allegation had come from the bank?

What other systems could be put into place?

Chapter 18
Disaster Risks and Preparedness Planning

Lewis A. Hassell and Michael L. Talbert

Case: Hurricane Katrina

It is May 2005, and a monstrous slow-moving hurricane Katrina is bearing down on the Gulf Coast of the USA, with the lives and livelihoods of millions squarely in her sights. The ensuing disaster is of a scale far beyond the preparations of individuals and communities whipped by her winds or flooded by her rains and sea surge. Holed up in his office equipped with sleeping bag, bags of Chex Mix, and Gatorade, Dr. Johnson bravely attempts to help care for the patients remaining in the hospital, but the laboratory ultimately succumbs to the darkness following loss of power and failure of flooded generators. His multihospital practice group with their simple condo-style first floor office is likewise ruined and the practice records are totally destroyed by the storm. The duration and extent of devastation mean that they will not have any income beyond whatever receivables are electronically deposited for a very long time ahead. Once the moral demands of the acute situation are attended to and they are able to regroup in some form, Dr. Johnson and his fellow pathologists determine that their best choice is to close the practice and reestablish their lives elsewhere. However, they soon discover that the gap in records and the inability of many of their former credentialing hospitals to respond that they were in good standing have placed them in a very unenviable position of waiting for exceptions to policy, response from nonexistent medical staff offices, and the like.

Discussion: The example illustrates that although one may have a disaster plan in place, at times the magnitude and extent of the disaster can overwhelm one's preparations.

While it is possible to spend one's life thinking through extreme "Katrina-like" disasters that might threaten the practice and attempting to prepare contingency plans, we believe there are probably better uses of time, provided that one has attended to certain principles and priorities. This is particularly true since no amount of simulation, drill, or other planning and preparation can enable an organization

L. A. Hassell (✉) · M. L. Talbert
Department of Pathology, University of Oklahoma Health Sciences Center, 940 Stanton
L. Young Blvd., BMSB 451, Oklahoma City, OK 73104, USA
e-mail: lewis-hassell@ouhsc.edu

M. L. Talbert
e-mail: michael-talbert@ouhsc.edu

© Springer International Publishing Switzerland 2016   221
L. A. Hassell et al. (eds.), *Pathology Practice Management*,
DOI 10.1007/978-3-319-22954-6_18

to be perpetually completely prepared for all possible overwhelming disasters. We suggest that six principles be followed:

1. Make disaster preparation a part of normal activities and conversations by regularly asking the question "What if......?" and filling the blank with the most commonplace kinds of disasters, both natural and human, seen in a given area. It would be imprudent, for example, for a Northern California practice to not have an idea of how they would manage things in the event of a destructive earthquake, or of a Kansas practice to not take into account the potential impact of a tornado. On a lesser scale and perhaps more likely, consider loss of your computer system for various time frames, tissue processor and other equipment failures, and loss of key employees among other challenges.
2. Drill regularly, with attention to the communication elements of the disaster plan since this element above all impacts outcome.
3. Cultivate a culture of empowerment in everyday situations. Evidence shows that when conditions are stressful, independent action by empowered team members can make the difference between success and failure. Individuals fearful of stepping beyond the scope of their job description in a disaster situation can be a risk rather than a benefit.
4. Encourage learning within the organization via debriefs following drills, and open discussion of decision-making in other settings resulting in less-than-optimal outcomes. Enhancing the collective wisdom will make individual choices by empowered employees more effective than relying on hierarchical leaders' choices.

   Think outside the box of conventional disasters. Consider the extreme weather event, sudden death of a key employee, utility failure (including such things as IT infrastructure and security), employee malice, or localized fire or flood that, if it came to pass, could sink or significantly impair your practice's ability to continue to survive.

   Prioritize your preventive actions and preparations, but do not let the "important but not (yet) urgent" nature of disaster preparation allow you to perpetually procrastinate.

Disaster preparedness depends much more on the preparation and empowerment of capable employees than on policies or safeguards.

Case: The Bolt from the Heavens

Pine tree pathology was a ten-pathologist practice centered in a small city with a regional hospital and a second smaller hospital but serving over a dozen small hospitals in a 150-mile radius. Histology services to the outlying hospitals were centralized in a pathologist-owned laboratory on the grounds of the smaller hospital in the central city. Surgical cases were signed out at both hospitals in the central city with the outreach hospital cases and physician office cases handled at that smaller hospital histology site as well. Pathologists drove to the outside hospitals for specific meetings, to provide laboratory medical direction, and to perform frozen sections. Billing was done in an old building at a third site in the central small city. Pine tree pathology owned its own information system and used high-speed dedicated lines to connect the two surgical pathology sites in the central city with the billing system using a triangular configuration for its architecture with "mirroring" of information between sites such that cutting one leg of the network would not isolate any one site.

One night, the building that housed the billing operation was struck by lightning and despite the typical protective gear designed for voltage surges, every electrical device in the building was "fried." While the fix ultimately required a major purchase of desktops and memory, due to the mirrored configuration, no data were lost and the billing operation was quickly brought back online.

Discussion: There are many hazards and many, if not most, strike with limited warning. Thinking through the key elements to remaining up and running through various disaster scenarios can pay great dividends.

Chapter 19
Market and Valuation Risks

Lewis Hassell and Michael L. Talbert

Case: Market and Payment Risk

UroGiants, Inc., a regional urology practice, has decided to consolidate the management of their specialized pathology needs and enhance their shrinking profit margin by retaining their biopsy samples and processing them in their own histology lab. They have offered your group the chance to continue providing diagnostic reports on their patients and the samples produced in their histology lab. Basing their projections on the technical component reimbursement rates in 2010, they calculate they can add about US$200K in profit to their practice of seven urologists each year if they do this, and they have offered your group the opportunity to provide the professional component as well as direct the histology lab at an attractive monthly rate. Having heard the stories of great profits from histology at national meetings, UroGiants gets the lab equipped, hires away one of your histotechs, and starts the operation in October of 2011.

The Centers for Medicare and Medicaid Services (CMS) then announces a 50% reduction in the technical component reimbursement for 88305 and the business manager for UroGiants comes to you to say they will no longer pay you the current medical director fee. She proposes that you can continue providing both services, but UroGiants needs to cut your medical director payment by 75% to "maintain profitability."

Discussion: This case illustrates both market risk and "regulatory risk" in a very dramatic way and points out that they can affect not only your own operations, but also how you interact with other clients or partners. Up-front due diligence in establishing relationships might expose settings where such risks are more likely to suddenly occur if a particular client or relationship is dependent upon a single contract, payer, reimbursement rate, or similar circumstance vulnerable to change. Continued monitoring of the practice, regulatory, and payment environments may also help mitigate potential negative impacts.

L. Hassell (✉) · M. L. Talbert
Department of Pathology, University of Oklahoma Health Sciences Center, 940 Stanton
L. Young Blvd., BMSB 451, Oklahoma City, OK 73104, USA
e-mail: lewis-hassell@ouhsc.edu

M. L. Talbert
e-mail: michael-talbert@ouhsc.edu

© Springer International Publishing Switzerland 2016
L. A. Hassell et al. (eds.), *Pathology Practice Management*,
DOI 10.1007/978-3-319-22954-6_19

Market Risks

Pathology is not practiced in a vacuum or a single market. Even those working in the smallest clinical settings are influenced in part by the flutter of butterfly wings in China, which is to say that the globalization shift that has happened in other economic sectors is underway in pathology practice as well. Assuming that the economic moat that surrounds a practice because of geographic isolation, captive referral sources and solid long-term contracts cannot be breached is like assuming that the borders of a modern country can be secured by Maginot Line-like physical barriers alone.

Of course markets can expand as well as contract or shift, and we will have more to say about this in the entrepreneurial segment later on, but the important thing to recognize is that the health-care market is becoming a much bigger and more fluid market than it has been in the past.

Simultaneously, one of the biggest risks in the market is that a single large customer, such as CMS (Medicare), can, with a single regulatory shift, change drastically how profitable or unprofitable your segment of the market is (or if a type of specimen or procedure is even covered). This is a major reason why organized medicine and organized pathology have taken such an active advocacy role through the various national organizations. The vested interests of the profession and individual practices are sufficiently great that it is prudent to monitor and actively participate in the educational and relationship-building activities to ensure that regulators and legislators properly consider a correct and broad view of the market and profession. This is one key to managing the market risks associated with regulatory and legislative action. Become engaged in and monitor what is happening on the national stage that can affect your practice and learn to become an effective advocate. One of the lessons that should be emphasized here above all is that when the need to exert influence arises, the time for building an effective relationship is usually long past. These relationships with both local leaders and national representatives are based on history and political currency, principally money in the form of contributions, and organization, the kind of organization that gets additional contributions and mobilizes voters and public opinion. These are activities that are best carried out in advance of the acute needs. Build individual relationships based on contact and communication, such as through hosting laboratory visits for legislative leaders, while engaging in the political "game."

Beyond the advocacy on the national level, proactively interacting with insurance providers and other payers, public groups (including patient advocacy groups), and major clients such as hospital administration and health system leadership is also wise. Multiple surveys of the general public, policy-makers, and even fellow physicians have shown a surprising lack of awareness of what pathologists are and do. While this should not be surprising to those keenly aware of the stereotype of the pathologist prowling the basement of a hospital or hidden behind the proverbial "paraffin curtain," it has undoubtedly contributed to the market vulnerability of the profession and many pathology practices as medicine and health-care finance undergo momentous upheavals.

Conversations with private insurers can be beneficial, allowing pathologists to make the case for any value-added services they provide. These conversations can set the stage for contact when an issue arises in the future as well as potentially result in preservation of current payments or even enhanced payment rates when the circumstances and practices warrant. While practice managers can fill this liaison role in many instances, it also helps to have practice leaders in the discussion at times.

Some of the most dangerous market risks are those in your local market. The two most significant areas of risk are market share loss and structural changes. While there is growing consolidation and larger numbers of employed physicians which tends to define outpatient referral patterns, meaningful fractions of most markets still have some flexibility to referral patterns. For instance, a primary care practice may choose a new reference laboratory based on the laboratory's ability to report results into the practice's electronic health record. This may mean the biopsies will follow the lab work away from your practice and toward pathologists at the reference lab. Similarly, a group of urologists or gastroenterologists may wish to either capture the technical component for their biopsies by starting a histology lab (perhaps they will invite you to be the medical director) or the professional component by hiring their own part-time pathologist. While these arrangements are somewhat less attractive than several years ago for a number of reasons, continued downward pressure on health-care expenditures could lead to increased marginal moves in the market. Mitigation of this type of market risk involves developing as strong a position in the market as possible using a combination of market-leading quality/service and market domination that, in itself, creates barriers and raises cost to entry. This should be coupled with strong client relations (make them love you) and active market surveillance. You should always be aware of changes in your market as well as identifying potential new clients.

The structural risks in the local market are more difficult to defend against. There is little you may be able to do if a small hospital that you serve joins a competing large network that employs its own pathologists. Similarly, previously independent groups of physicians that your practice serves may be employed by a hospital that directs their specimens to the hospital's lab and employed pathologists. Often your group will have little say in such matters. However, structural changes in the local market may also be beneficial. Your group may be adding business as the system you serve expands its footprint in the market.

Case: Market Risk Comes to Roost

Coastal Pathology, a 15-pathologist group covering three hospitals with a six-county outreach, was considered a powerhouse and a very desirable practice to be part of. It had defined the pathology market in the eastern half of their state for over 20 years. Then one day, incredible news was brought by the courier. Skin Consultants, PC had no specimens to pick up. In fact, the courier was told that Skin Consultants had hired their own dermatopathologist who was also the medical director of a new histology lab. A phone call to one of the Skin Consultants senior dermatologists confirmed the bad news and established that arrangements had been made with the nearby university to provide immunohistochemistry and immunofluorescence studies as needed. Within an hour, the damage had been tallied. Six hundred thousand dollars in annual professional revenues gone and no work for one of the group's two dermatopathologists. For the pathologist-owned histology lab, the damage was similar: US$500,000 in annual revenues now gone; a loss which would necessitate loss of personnel. The initial shock was great, personnel would need to be RIF'ed (reduction in force) and pathologists' income would take a hit.

Questions for discussion:
  Could something like this happen to your practice?
  How could a practice mitigate this risk?
  How would your practice handle a sudden decline in revenue? How would decisions be made?

Valuation Risk

Another type of "market risk" worth mentioning is the valuation of the independent practice and its assets, which can change with the changing environment but which can also provide challenges within the practice. The foundation for understanding this has been laid in the earlier chapter on mergers and acquisitions (Chap. 9: Practice Sales and Mergers). There are generally two types of practice situations that are quite common today: those with virtually no physical capital assets and those who have invested in a range of tangible assets such as support structures, real estate, and laboratory equipment. These have been discussed in detail elsewhere in this book. Here we will primarily deal with the issue of valuation of these assets and attitudes toward them.

The model of practices with virtually no tangible assets has been pursued to easily provide essentially a flow-through mechanism for a pathologist's professional services income and to simplify the matters of joining and departing the practice. The nominal "buy-in" cost in these settings makes them attractive to recently trained candidates seeking to retire student loans and such. This approach also appeals to those who want to maintain simplicity in their partnership agreements and at the same time maximize their income. But a problem arises when a different valuation structure is imposed and senior shareholders are faced with the potential of reaping a windfall. This alternate valuation is based not on a tangible asset basis but on an income stream model, which then may cast the total value as a four- to six-time (or more) multiple of the adjusted net revenue, typically resulting in a much higher value than just assets. This multiple of adjusted net revenue varies according to the strength and market position of a practice as well as current interest rates and the potential rate of return in the broader financial market for a revenue stream. The "risk" here is twofold; on the one hand, majority shareholders may "sell out" control of the practice for a windfall, and on the other, capital availability and marketability of the practice may fluctuate due to market, regulatory, structural, or even technical factors. More is discussed on this matter, particularly as it pertains to potential practice mergers or sales, in Chap. 9.

Case: Promises, Expectations, and Risk Mitigation

Dr. Armstrong had found the ideal practice, a 15-pathologist, regionally dominant group only 4-h drive from his family. He could apply his breast subspecialty skills while continuing to develop his broader diagnostic abilities. The salary and benefits exceeded his expectations. Dr. Armstrong was told, "Nothing in, nothing out," by the president of the group, which was explained to mean no buy-in for new pathologists and no buyout for retiring pathologists.

Three years after he joined the practice and made partner with no buy-in, several of the senior partners began looking toward retirement. Citing the group's market strength, reputation, and great financial results, four senior partners proposed adding a buyout to reflect the value of the group. Much animosity arose around the desire to change "nothing in, nothing out." Two years of painful negotiations did yield a program that would provide a significant buyout, but this also created abundant ill will between the younger and senior pathologists. Over the ensuing few years, the ill will dissipated, helped by having the most senior pathologists indeed retire (also referred to as "take the money and run").

Within a few more years, Dr. Armstrong was president of the group and learned that similar groups were being purchased by national companies for millions of dollars, a share of which would greatly exceed any buyout that a departing pathologist had yet received. Dr. Armstrong perceived a valuation type risk and that failing to consider selling the group at a high valuation could lead to issues in subsequent years if the option no longer existed in our ever-changing world of health care. So the group engaged well-known consultants to both value the group and educate the group. In the end, Dr. Armstrong held a formal vote of the shareholder partners. For a number of reasons, some personal, the partners voted overwhelmingly not to seek a sale of the group.

Discussion: Pathology practices do have value which can and will fluctuate. How that value is handled is a key to the long-term success of that practice.

Chapter 20
Technologic and Regulatory Risks

Lewis A. Hassell, Michael L. Talbert and Jane Pine Wood

The core tools of histopathology—seventeenth-century optical microscopy and nineteenth-century aniline dye chemistry—continue to undergird the practice of pathology. However, the rapid strides in science and technology over the last several decades imperil the traditional methods and models of diagnosing disease. The threat of a "disruptive technology" that will change forever the means by which the job of diagnosis is performed (and often who does it and where it is done) seems greater today than even 5 years ago. Examples of this are easy to find and seem to appear almost daily. For example, a recent publication summarized some research with a surgical tool termed "rapid evaporative ionization mass spectroscopy" believed to be capable of detecting and differentiating tumor versus non-tumor based on the computer-analyzed signatures of gases captured from the surgical field during the course of electrocautery [1]. If validated and suitably cost-effective, the technique would appear poised to eliminate the need for intraoperative (and potentially postoperative) margin analysis by frozen section methods. Another method with similar ability to erode or supplant a significant portion of routine pathology (although it could also be directed to augment pathology practice) is in vivo microscopy using confocal microscopy or optical coherence tomography. Some within gastroenterology have advocated that use of these tools during endoscopy could eliminate the need for pathologic evaluation of upwards of 80 % of colon polyps, currently a significant component of many pathologists' workloads [2]. Similar concerns related to shifts in who does the

L. A. Hassell (✉) · M. L. Talbert
Department of Pathology, University of Oklahoma Health Sciences Center,
940 Stanton L. Young Blvd., BMSB 451, Oklahoma City, OK 73104, USA
e-mail: lewis-hassell@ouhsc.edu

M. L. Talbert
e-mail: michael-talbert@ouhsc.edu

J. P. Wood
McDonald Hopkins, LLC, 956 Main St., Dennis, MA 02638, USA
e-mail: jwood@mcdonaldhopkins.com

© Springer International Publishing Switzerland 2016
L. A. Hassell et al. (eds.), *Pathology Practice Management*,
DOI 10.1007/978-3-319-22954-6_20

work or where the diagnostic work is done could be raised with expanded low-cost testing methods such as those offered by Theranos, a company promising inexpensive laboratory tests on small blood volumes, or the high-tech deoxyribonucleic acid (DNA)-sequencing-based "liquid biopsies" able to detect circulating tumor DNA long before clinical signs appear.

But this "death of the profession" risk may be less an issue than two other technology-related risks. These are the risks of being too soon (and hence on the bleeding edge) to a new technology or being too late to the technology (nothing left in the punch bowl). Both of these mistakes can be costly for a practice, opening the door for shifts in market share, erosion of margin, and even poor medical decision-making due to skewed incentives for utilization. Best practices to avoid these pitfalls require careful scrutiny and due diligence of the technology and the reimbursement/value to be added. It also requires a bit of the entrepreneurial spirit and organizational culture that understands the risk and the means of coping with uncertainty for the future. More about this is said below.

Case: Early Adoption of New Technology

In the early days of flow cytometry, a moderate-sized pathology practice providing services to several hospitals in a region decided to bring a new fluorescence-activated cell sorter (FACS) flow cytometer to their community, in keeping with providing "university quality" services to all within their service region (the practice's overall mission). They recognized that this might lose money for a season, so it was organized within the structure of a nonprofit organization with the purpose of attracting research grants and allowing operating expense "grants" from the practice to be deductible for tax purposes. There were no trained operators within their catchment area, so a worldwide search was conducted to locate someone with sufficient training and experience to operate the new device. The bright young pathologists of the group were excited by the foresight and largesse of the other group members in taking on this venture, and it set the group apart when it came to attracting new talent as well.

While they performed routine analyses on certain tumor types, the reimbursements for these were slow to come. A number of times hematolymphoid neoplasm evaluation was shown to have significantly affected the accuracy of their diagnoses, but the numbers of these cases were fairly small and did not alone cover the costs of operation. Revenues never reached the level of covering operations, and although some professional component revenue did accrue, it also did not cover the costs of ongoing grants to the nonprofit institute for at least the first 10 years of operations. Eventually, the medical landscape changed, and flow cytometric evaluation demand and reimbursement increased on the hematolymphoid side of things as instrument cost and operational complexity diminished. In addition, the institute had developed a strong reputation for quality, service, and fast turnaround times, thereby attracting cases from a wide region. "That was one of the smartest things we did, about 10 years too soon" remarked one of the partners of the whole saga of the institute and flow cytometry.

When is being on the "bleeding edge" justified?

What might happen to an organizational culture if a venture becomes a cash sink rather than the exciting, but "break even" operation they had been led to believe?

What factors prevent "pulling the plug" when the losses are continuing?

What other structures or avenues might there be to mitigate the pain of losses in such a setting besides the one chosen by this group?

Regulatory matters also pose a significant risk (in the sense of sudden change to the playing field) to operating successfully in the laboratory and pathology practice

Table 20.1 Regulatory entities and their domains

Regulatory entity	Primary domain	Examples of lab regulations
Centers for Medicare/Medicaid Services (CMS)	What gets paid for	CLIA regulations regarding lab medical directors and accreditation requirements; payment or coding policies
Occupational Safety and Health Administration (OSHA)	General safety issues in workplace	Chemical use and storage; exposure limits
Food and Drug Administration (FDA)	Broad oversight of food products, drugs, and medical devices	Blood product preparation and administration; laboratory-developed tests as in vitro devices
Department of Health and Human Services (DHHS) and the Centers for Disease Control (CDC)	Disease reporting and safe handling of communicable diseases	Lab safety with infectious agents
State Health Departments	Health and testing issues for laboratories serving state residents	NYDOH accreditation requirements
Nuclear Regulatory Commission (NRC)	Oversight of radioactive products or devices	Use and storage of radioactive reagents or devices
Department of Homeland Security (DHS)	Use and availability of items of potential public safety threat	Blood irradiation equipment; storage of biological agents

CLIA Clinical Laboratory Improvement Amendments, *NYDOH* New York State Department of Health

arena. Table 20.1 lists some of the regulatory bodies holding differing degrees of leverage over the operations in US laboratories. In Canadian and European labs, some degree of comparable regulatory oversight is also found.

The announcement in 2012 by the Food and Drug Administration (FDA) that they were concerned about the safety of laboratory-developed tests (LDTs) and intended to exercise regulatory authority created a great degree of uncertainty in the various Clinical Laboratory Improvement Amendments (CLIA)-certified labs, which in some cases were deriving the bulk of their income from such testing. This was followed in 2014 with a proposed framework for regulation of these tests and the entities offering them to patients. While this issue is still in the comment phase at the time of this writing, it seems certain based on the nature of comments received so far that stricter regulation of LDTs poses a potential for significant cost to many laboratories offering these tests.

This scenario also illustrates the need to be engaged in the advocacy process and to adroitly choose partnerships in the process to be effective. The various alliances in the health-care world in this debate may include various patient safety groups, the drug and pharmaceutical companies with FDA-approved or in the pipeline companion diagnostic tests (CDTs), the digital pathology companies and other novel device companies whose equipment has been operating under the LDT framework for various purposes, the large reference labs serving multiple institutions as well as smaller labs primarily serving single institutions, and the physicians operating the labs and receiving results therefrom. Also in the picture is the entity that has previously been the sole regulatory gate in the LDT process—Centers for Medicare/Medicaid Services (CMS) with CLIA certification.

Case: Dr. Jim and Advocacy Mitigates Pap Risk (James Navin, Personal Communication to Lewis Hassell, January 2015)

A large lab doing a variety of forms of testing decided to charge a very low rate per Papanicolaou (Pap) smear to the gynecologists who were sending them smears, in hopes of capturing the "pull-through" business for the rest of their test menu. Their success quickly became the model for other labs seeking to exploit the expanding payment opportunities under both government and nongovernmental payers. Soon Medicare noticed the pricing discrepancies and naturally moved to reprice their payments in line with the lower charges from the labs using the Pap test as a "loss leader." As Medicare imposed further reductions on other areas of testing, the pull-through business became less profitable, and labs began to look for ways to cut their losses, leading in some cases to quality compromises that harmed patients. Private payers followed Medicare, and over a few years the (global) reimbursement for a Pap test in Dr. Jim's state went from US$16.45 to 11, leaving labs offering the test inadequate payments for a test that cost US$14–16 to perform.

After many attempts, Dr. Jim met with the local carrier and persuaded them that a professional fee (for those Paps reviewed by a pathologist) was appropriate, but they continued to hold their routine reimbursement under the cost thresholds. Together with other lab leaders in his state, he attempted to bring the cause to other insurers, but got only refusals. Over the ensuing year, Dr. Jim arranged speaking engagements to women's groups and TV and radio audiences, making the case for fair reimbursement, and copied the publicity to the insurers. One responded, "It is inappropriate to discuss reimbursement issues with women," which gave him more fuel for his battle. Meanwhile, Dr. Jim took his case to his legislative delegation and managed to get a favorable response from one of the senators, who in turn wrote to the insurance carrier. After another meeting with the insurer outlining the rationale for a payment increase, and his lab's choices if none were offered, he scheduled a visit to his legislators in Washington, DC.

Turning from the local insurer to Medicare, Dr. Jim proceeded to contact his legislators and other leaders and their staff on Capitol Hill. He sought and obtained support for increased reimbursement from one of the gynecologist's national organizations. As support began to materialize among the legislature, data regarding the actual costs of preparing and interpreting a Pap test were collected. This was surprisingly difficult to obtain, so Dr. Jim sought the help of several national pathology organizations to secure reliable data. In the interim, he also solicited support from the American Cancer Society, which in turn sought letters of support from their regional offices. Dr. Jim continued to engage support from concerned legislators, who eventually met with the director of the Health Care Finance Authority (HCFA), precursor to CMS. She was stunned at the problem and asked, "Why hasn't anyone complained about this before?" But HCFA still did not act.

Dr. Jim continued his almost one-man battle, reaching out to other common interest groups and leadership, ranging from AARP to the White House, with no response. He engaged his network to support sympathetic legislators and hosted lab tours and fund-raising events for those up for reelection. At times he was literally in daily contact with their staff or regional offices. One of these introduced legislation in the US House to increase the Pap payment under Medicare to US$14.60, representing the average cost data from a survey he had done with the American Pathology Foundation. Comparable legislation was also introduced by his senator in the Senate.

Further meetings with HCFA led to requests for more data, more stalling, and no action. Ultimately, they were able to obtain reliable cost data from 20 additional labs and supply that as part of their case. Interestingly, the new data raised the average cost to US$15.60. An officer from HCFA on seeing the data told the Office of Management and Budget (OMB) on Capitol Hill that the data supported the request in the legislation. The response was reported as "derogatory expletive, we aren't going to give it to them." After contact with his representative again, the legislation was reintroduced with more cosponsors in both chambers. Ultimately, the provisions were incorporated into a "must pass" act and signed into law.

Discussion questions:

Does one person have a voice in the advocacy process? What is needed to make one's voice heard?

What excuses could Dr. Jim have offered for acquiescing to the status quo along the course of his battle?

Where do national medical organizations fit in the advocacy process on issues of professional duty, patient care, and quality/reimbursement issues?

What are the unforeseen consequences of a single test pricing policy by one lab?

References

1. Shafer KC, Denes J, Albrecht K, et al. In vivo, in situ tissue analysis using rapid evaporative ionization mass spectrometry. Angew Chem Int Ed Engl. 2009;48:8240–2.
2. Sanduleanu S, Driessen A, Gomez-Garcia E, et al. In vivo diagnosis and classification of colorectal neoplasia by chromoendoscopy-guided confocal laser endomicroscopy. Clin Gastroenterol Hepatol. 2010;8(4):371–8.

Chapter 21
Opportunities and Entrepreneurism

Lewis A. Hassell and Michael L. Talbert

Case: Taking Out and Centralizing Histology

The Regional Pathology Group not only contracts with eight hospitals to provide pathology services but also serves much of the region's physician office outpatient market. While the eight hospitals comprise two hospital systems and two independent hospitals, all are amenable to allowing the pathologists to create a regional histology and cytology lab as a means of controlling histology costs and sending out immunohistochemistry tests. The pathologists' consultant showed convincingly that the pathologists could achieve economies of scale, greatly increase the available immunohistochemistry menu, and create a positive margin while charging back to the eight hospitals total annual amounts that would essentially equal the current cost of operation of each of the smaller histology and cytology operations. The consultant also believed that the pathologists and hospitals would further benefit from the increasing expertise of the pathologists and faster turnaround time for difficult cases requiring additional studies.

How might this histology lab be achieved?
How could the shares be valued?
How could buy-ins and buyouts be structured?

Discussion: Obviously this not only represents an opportunity but also a challenge that the group must assess from financial, operational, and structural standpoints. Acquiring equipment and staff from existing operations would be a natural first proposal, but even before that can be done, some sort of operating entity must be created. Doing this within the structure of the practice might be possible, but would likely change the nature of their corporation or partnership. So, a new structure would need to be capitalized before space and equipment, much less employees, could be brought in. If the pathologists become the owners, as they are likely the source for the capital and operating experience in this case, they need to identify and think through possible future events, such as the addition of new partners and the departure of existing owners very carefully, and preferably with wise counsel. For small closely held companies such as the lab described here, valuation is difficult and can be costly to ascertain. Book, or liquidation, value usually underestimates

L. A. Hassell (✉) · M. L. Talbert
Department of Pathology, University of Oklahoma Health Sciences Center, 940 Stanton
L. Young Blvd., BMSB 451, Oklahoma City, OK 73104, USA
e-mail: lewis-hassell@ouhsc.edu

M. L. Talbert
e-mail: michael-talbert@ouhsc.edu

© Springer International Publishing Switzerland 2016
L. A. Hassell et al. (eds.), *Pathology Practice Management*,
DOI 10.1007/978-3-319-22954-6_21

the value, while revenue-based valuations may mistakenly overestimate the value by failing to consider various forms of market risk.

The Entrepreneurial Pathologist

Pathologists are inherently problem-solvers. They look at a patient's biopsy or surgical specimen and relish the challenge of providing the answer to the puzzle. They consider aberrant coagulation results and devote their understanding of pathways, genetics, chemistry, testing platforms, and kinetics to making a diagnosis and predicting future consequences and potential treatment. The reward is in finding the solution and solving the clinician's dilemma. But another common trait is a reluctance to expose themselves or the patients they serve to risk, primarily the risk of a misdiagnosis, since they are keenly aware of how small features, such as lymphovascular invasion or extension to a serosal surface, can alter perceived prognosis and chosen therapy for a patient.

Both of these characteristics need to be appropriately balanced for a pathologist or group to engage in entrepreneurial ventures. There are certain other key characteristics that may help practices successfully use their talents in new endeavors. One of these is the ability to "see" differently. An entrepreneur sees opportunities where others may see only obstacles or hardship. Entrepreneurs see their resources differently as well, often both in themselves and in others around them. This optimism can be a temptation to get out ahead of the group tolerance and capabilities, so would-be entrepreneurs are wise to temper their enthusiasm with the balance of more risk-averse colleagues, without always being totally shot down by expressions of risk aversion or fears of failure.

> Another key competency often present within a group of pathologists is leadership and management experience. David Frishberg [Personal communication, APF Bootcamp in Practice Management, Redondo Beach, CA, Nov 15, 2012] said that "leadership density needs to be higher among pathologists than most other physician specialties" due to the number of settings where they must exert leadership, oversight, or management skills in their daily life. The process of evaluating and bringing on a new instrument, immunohistochemical stain or other new technology is a fairly common experience for most pathologists, and is not entirely dissimilar to the process of incubating a new venture to launch.

While an in-depth discussion of the generative process for successful entrepreneurial ventures is beyond our scope, the following stages might be considered as critical to ultimate success.

1. See the problem, catch the idea, the dream
2. Construct a mental image of the solution
3. Examine the available resources to realize the solution

   1. Structural, organizational (infrastructure)
   2. Technology, existing or new
   3. Market factors, moat (intellectual property)

4. Finances, venture, operational
5. Human resources
6. Legal, regulatory, licensing (and exit strategy)

4. Conduct gap analysis of each of the above
5. Implement business plan
6. Check nurturing to maturity (profitability) vs. knowing when to fold

With attention to each of these phases of the process and engagement of a healthy balance between the risk-takers and risk-avoiders in a group, success can be achieved [1–4]. We have witnessed a number of successful entrepreneurial ventures over the years, some within practices and some structured outside a practice to limit risk. We have seen large practices dragged down by and ultimately submerged into failure by major ventures that proved unsuccessful or that could not be optimally operationalized in time.

> Successful entrepreneurs balance opportunity and risk, but may have more failures than successes.

Case: Molecular 1: Private Practice Fears

By the midpoint of the first decade of this century, molecular testing was creating quite a buzz in pathology and laboratory medicine. Single nucleotide polymorphism testing, infectious organism including human papillomavirus (HPV) identification, and neoplastic alteration testing for classification, treatment, and prognosis were expanding rapidly. The Association for Molecular Pathology meetings reflected great energy, and testing platforms and methodologies seemed to evolve at three times the rate of other areas of the clinical laboratory. Clinical testing, however, required specialized personnel and was primarily performed at university laboratories and specialized or large commercial laboratories. Many tests were laboratory developed and payment for testing was haphazard and difficult to pursue except for the most established tests. In fact, we know of one mid-sized university molecular pathology laboratory that operated at an annual loss of greater than $100,000, which was seen as a necessary evil to continue developing expertise, fulfill the educational mission, and support research on its campus.

Against this background, many private practices became worried, and pathologists and business thinkers in the molecular world were regularly consulted about what to do. Private practices were concerned that (1) they might be missing a bus that they needed to be on, such that if they did not get into molecular testing, they would never be able to catch up and (2) with the rise of molecular testing of tissue specimens (cytology and surgical pathology), the risk would increase that the private groups would lose control of the specimens which would either be sent directly for molecular testing or that the significant value added of molecular testing would relegate their role to that of triage pathologists. This represented a classic playoff between (too soon) technological risk with attendant resource loss or consumption and downstream market risk. This frenzy of worry ran for some 5 years as reflected by educational courses, change in demographics of attendees at Association for Molecular Pathology meetings, and numerous commercial webinars and meetings devoted to examining the challenges. A few of the largest private practices began to develop expertise and bring on well-established testing such as HPV, Her2, and certain single nucleotide polymorphisms while other practices took a wait-and-see approach. With the rapid advances in platforms and technology with its attendant diminution in the need for assay troubleshooting expertise and design and validation of laboratory developed tests, coupled with a slow rise in the U.S. Food and Drug Administration (FDA)-approved tests, the "leading edge" of the technology curve moved quickly ahead, such that the very early adopters spent relatively little time at the "bleeding edge." As of this writing, many private groups have modest and growing menus of molecular testing and increasing expertise in this area.

Case: Molecular 2: The Case for Next-Generation Sequencing

As we assemble this book, there is an incredible dilemma for medium and large commercial laboratories, academic medical centers, and even large private practices—a dilemma that even challenges the role of pathologists in prognosis and therapy driving diagnostic decisions. While deoxyribonucleic acid (DNA) sequencing has been possible for some years, in just the past few years, large-scale sequencing has become practical (cost and turnaround time) for clinical use and information regarding potential clinical uses is exploding. Identification of driver mutations with targetable therapies (so-called precision medicine) is now not only feasible, but in some clinical scenarios, a standard of practice or part of clinical trials. Even the president of the USA has weighed in on precision medicine. But what to do from test design and case selection is being hotly debated across our profession. There are multiple possible platforms ranging up to $1 million just for purchase, and the technology continues to rapidly develop towards faster and cheaper alternatives (cost per base identified). It is not inconceivable that an entirely new technology that would render existing platforms essentially obsolete might be introduced in the relatively near future. And the initial platform expense may be the cheapest component. Whether one deploys a small panel, say 15–40 known important or actionable hot spots, or a larger panel, the personnel, time, and effort to validate the panel can dwarf the cost of the platform. Beyond this, and perhaps most vexing, the bioinformatics support required to turn the sequencing data into an actionable report is significant, if you can obtain it. And, all of this with the attendant risk that exome sequencing or even whole-genome sequencing (currently too slow and expensive for limited additional clinical utility) may supplant panels or that epigenomic factors, ribonucleic acid (RNA) expression, or even proteomics could be identified as necessary keys to the prognosis and treatment puzzle.

So how does the practice leader approach this challenge? This is a difficult balancing act involving missions and market positioning interacting with costs and resources. There is attendant regulatory risk in that FDA oversight regulations have not been finalized and could eliminate smaller or weaker players. There is also a payment risk; it is not clear how and if these tests will be covered and how much payments might be. That leaves collecting from patients, which, especially for high dollar tests and tests that do not count towards deductibles in patients with rapidly growing health costs, is problematic. Finally, there is a risk that typical practicing pathologists will not be involved in this key area at all—the testing, bioinformatics, and ultimate interpretation of this testing may prove to simply be beyond the typical pathologist and our key roles will be initial diagnosis and selection of an appropriate specimen for testing; a negative development in such an important area. In fact, some postulate that tumor classification may one day be on the basis of driver mutations, pathways, and actual targets rather than organ-based morphologic features.

Questions for discussion:

What is the role of next-generation sequencing in your patient population?

How is your practice involved in next-generation sequencing testing?

How does your mission (or missions) relate to next-generation sequencing testing?

What strategy for next-generation sequencing would make sense for your practice?

How do you see next-generation sequencing testing developing in your patient population in the next 2–5 years?

Given these postulated developments, how should your practice position itself?

If your practice lacks the resources or has no strategy for next-generation sequencing, what risks can you identify?

References

1. Anthony SD. The first mile: a launch manual for getting great ideas into the market. Boston: Harvard Business School Publishing; 2014 (Print).
2. Bush J, Baker S. Where does it hurt? An entrepreneur's guide to fixing health care. New York: Penguin Group (USA) LLC; 2014 (Print).

3. Osterwalder A, Pigneur Y. Business model generation: a handbook for visionaries, game changers, and challengers. Hoboken: Wiley; 2010 (Print).
4. Osterwalder A, Pigneur Y, Bernarda G, Smith A. Value proposition design. Hoboken: Wiley; 2014 (Print).

Chapter 22
Identifying and Capitalizing on Opportunities

Lewis Hassell, Michael L. Talbert and Jane Pine Wood

One of the most satisfying moments in practice management comes when there is a significant positive change in a practice. In general, opportunities may be internal, such as reducing expenses or improving practice efficiency, or external, such as adding to the revenue stream through more work or better contracts, improving your competitive situation, or having novel arrangements that make your practice a more attractive place to work.

Identifying and capitalizing on opportunities requires two basic underlying competencies: scanning and understanding your environment and understanding your practice metrics and capabilities. But identifying opportunities extends beyond understanding the unique "lay of the land" of your practice environment. Many opportunities for new business come from networking contacts; a courier may report hearing that Medical Associates' office practice is unhappy with their reference laboratory or a surgeon at the state medical society meeting might mention that his hospital is looking to change pathology providers. These are obvious examples but many other opportunities may be recognized using a more active approach: for example, the solo pathologist across town is nearing retirement age and perhaps your practice can back him/her up and support a transition into retirement after which your group would grow by adding a small hospital and its attendant work … and, maybe there would also be an opportunity to grow your practice's presence in that part of town by using your practice's advantages in, say, courier and outpatient result reporting.

L. Hassell (✉) · M. L. Talbert
Department of Pathology, University of Oklahoma Health Sciences Center,
940 Stanton L. Young Blvd., BMSB 451, Oklahoma City, OK 73104, USA
e-mail: lewis-hassell@ouhsc.edu

M. L. Talbert
e-mail: michael-talbert@ouhsc.edu

J. P. Wood
McDonald Hopkins, LLC, 956 Main St., Dennis, MA 02638, USA
e-mail: jwood@mcdonaldhopkins.com

© Springer International Publishing Switzerland 2016
L. A. Hassell et al. (eds.), *Pathology Practice Management*,
DOI 10.1007/978-3-319-22954-6_22

So what are your practice's advantages? And how do you identify internal opportunities? This requires a solid understanding of your practice's metrics, capacities, strengths, and, unfortunately, weaknesses. For internal opportunities, you will want to know and follow measures of efficiency such as productivity, cost per unit volume, and turnaround time. You will also want a good idea of your operational processes and limiting factors of each major process (e.g., our turnaround time for histology suffers when we have more than 500 blocks because the histotechs are overloaded). The authors have found the concept of a dashboard very useful in following metrics. Much like a car will have speedometer, odometer, and gas gauge, a practice dashboard can be used to regularly (typically monthly, although specific monitors may make more sense daily, weekly or, for less time critical measures, even quarterly or annually) monitor the key metrics of a practice. Metrics can be compared to nationally available data such as nationally available relative value units (RVU) productivity by pathologist data. Generally, however, the authors have found that self-comparison with your own practice experience in earlier time periods such as month-to-month or, to smooth out variations, prior year-to-date with current year-to-date, to be perhaps the most useful. When doing so, one must account for known changes in the practice to achieve an "apples-to-apples" comparison. A practice must strive to steadily improve, an imperative in a time of declining or stagnant payments. This kind of line-by-line scrutiny of your existing data may not sound very much like entrepreneurialism; certainly it is not flashy or sexy. But it forms a foundational experience that better equips you to launch into external opportunities. By seeing and plugging the holes in your bucket before you try to pour in ever greater amounts on top, you position yourself to offer better solutions and inspire greater trust among the more risk-averse members of the group.

For external opportunities, one must understand capacities and capabilities of a practice. For example, could our practice cover a small hospital across town 8 a.m.–2 p.m. 5 days a week without hiring a new pathologist (an expensive, multimonth process but if this hire allows you to expand specialty expertise or position your practice to go after other opportunities, the calculation may change), or can our practice do an additional 1000 diagnostic biopsies without having turnaround time suffer? And, as important, is the recognition of what is beyond capabilities or sufficiently outside the strengths of a practice as to be impractical. For example, looking to expand a hospital-based practice to include a broad range of physician office work would be difficult for a practice with no couriers and no experience in the outpatient arena in a metro area where there is a highly capable regional laboratory with excellent courier service and IT capabilities allowing a wide variety of result reporting options. Just as athletic teams attempt to control the pace and scale of the game to exploit their strengths (or protect their weaknesses), practices must be keenly aware of these and avoid encounters on turf or terms that are not to their advantage.

Internal Opportunities

While external opportunities often present the most exciting opportunities, internal opportunities can be a reliable source for significant practice improvements through improved efficiencies and/or reduced expenses. The knowledge of your practice is again the key. How much is being spent to send out test X, or in contrast, how much is being spent to keep service Y in house, which when coupled with careful consideration of outsourcing or in-sourcing options and costs can yield significant improvements. A keen understanding of the fixed and variable costs in the practice and the stretch capacities is important when making these kinds of analyses and decisions.

Sometimes, however, the purely economic considerations might drive bad choices. For example, at one point a practice we know had developed a cadre of locum tenens candidates who could work successfully to run large portions of the practice at a lower-marginal cost than a practice partner. This eventually led to jocular comments about farming out the majority of their work to such lower cost, itinerant personnel and just pocketing the difference. Such a decision of course would have eventually been as disastrous to the group as similar decisions by various technical companies that find their outsourcing of manufacturing, engineering, accounting, and eventually even marketing leaving them only a hollow shell that may eventually be disrupted or consumed entirely by their outside sources.

In the authors' experience, there is no absolute limit to improvements in process, efficiency, and expenses although so-called low-hanging fruit can become increasingly difficult to identify.

Pure expense reduction is usually the least effective internal improvement, but should be an ongoing process. It is both a culture and a process. Each member of the team from courier to billing person to technologist to pathologist should be looking for cheaper alternatives. Whether renegotiating a significant reagent contract, eliminating unused phone lines, or restructuring a benefit package to better reflect the needs of the participants while reducing expenditures, the employees closest to any particular part of the practice often generate the best ideas. To complement this, a rolling systematic review can be used to great effect by sequentially targeting areas or line items of expense on the income statement. For example, while targeting sequential lines in the expense area on a monthly basis, if communication devices are targeted, one can review the need for and cost of all landline phones, cell phones, pagers, data plans, and broadband accounts. Unused capacity can be eliminated, services can be bundled, and contracts can be negotiated or renegotiated. In our academic practice, our multitalented business administrator has an annual target for savings such as these. Savings are celebrated, and best of all, resources can be repurposed for more valuable uses.

In most practice settings, people represent the greatest expense. In an independent pathology practice, up to 85 or 90% of all expenses may be for the pathologists' salaries and benefits with the remainder being allocated for basic functions such as billing, marketing, and legal. Given the high cost of personnel, the greatest gains for a practice are often through process improvements and improved efficiency. Happily, such gains also typically produce better service and higher quality, thus yielding a better product and gains in market prowess. Even more than cost savings, process improvement should be a way of thinking and a part of the culture practiced by all participants. Lean and Six Sigma are excellent tools for process improvement, and identifying areas ripe for improvement may be as simple as attacking a regular bottleneck (e.g., three times a week, the pathologists are waiting for slides to sign out), responding to a service complaint (e.g., the mammographers want at least a preliminary diagnosis by 2 p.m.), or creating capacity to service a new client (e.g., can we reliably have all cases out of histology by 10 a.m.?). Beyond this, productivity enhancement of the most expensive personnel (i.e., the pathologists) should also be considered. Tools such as voice recognition, enhanced information technology, or office redesign can increase pathologist efficiency. Similarly, eliminating unneeded slides, decreasing distractions, and standardizing reporting can directly reduce nonproductive time. It may also make sense to relatively overstaff lower-paid personnel functions such as secretarial and histotechnology to further smooth workload fluctuations and more productively use pathologists. Of course, this decision may be a difficult negotiation if different entities' interests (e.g., the hospital/laboratory vs. the practice) are aligned differently on an issue. Improvements such as these are often synergistic: A series of small changes sum to a much larger improvement than a simple addition may suggest. Also, eliminating the final 10 % of a difficult day, when multiple histotechs are out sick and workload is higher than average, can avoid needless stressing and tiring of personnel, which may have its own attendant drop in productivity and quality.

External Opportunities

Conventional wisdom has always been that by simply sticking to your core competencies, you could come out ahead … or at least you could be saved from being on the bleeding edge of a new opportunity. However, given the flat or downward trending reimbursement curves of the past decades, opportunistic practices have often been rewarded when they have embraced new opportunities outside their four walls or their conventional markets. Identifying, evaluating, and capitalizing on external opportunities can be one of the most interesting and varied aspects of practice management. External opportunities may be classified as additional business similar to one's current business, margin improvement, building barriers, and novel (dissimilar) business arrangements. We will examine each area in turn, but successful opportunity evaluation and exploitation first requires a solid understanding of one's current practice dynamics and metrics.

How can you judge an opportunity without clearly understanding how (and if) your practice can successfully manage the opportunity and what an opportunity's impact might be on your practice? A simple example: Your courier reports that GI Partners is adding two new gastroenterologists to its practice and, since they are generally happy with your diagnoses and service (how do you know this?), you assume you will receive the additional specimens. Can you handle the volume? Grossing? Histotechnology? Pathology coverage? Will this affect turnaround time of your general workload? Presumably, your couriers are already picking up the specimens and you have worked out reporting for GI Partners. What if GI Partners wants an interface to their electronic medical record (EMR) or a new correlation conference? And what does this additional business mean to your practice financially? Technical component? Professional component? What would be the expected incremental case volume? Specimen type and payor mix? Can it really benefit your practice? What is the rough upside over, say, 1 year? What are the down sides? Are there any bigger practice risks? Is GI Partners now large enough to now consider its own histology laboratory and/or its own part-time pathologist? Is your relationship with the gastroenterologists at GI Partners such that you can pick up the phone just to congratulate them on their new hires? Or better, are your services so good that your practice and/or particular members of your practice who specialize in gastroenterology (GI) pathology were part of the recruitment and enticed these new hires to join GI Partners ("We have excellent pathology support—we set you up to meet with Dr. Kolin; he's outstanding"). And those would be just some of the considerations surrounding a simple addition to specimen volume.

So our first question centered on our practice's ability to handle volume while maintaining the desired turnaround time for results. This would suggest that workload and turnaround time would be measured through the process (e.g., grossing, histotechnology, microscopic, secretarial) and that any choke points where work could slow down would be understood (and resolved).

Judging the financial impact requires having an understanding (i.e., being able to manipulate) of the data set regarding case mixes, typically by the Current Procedural Terminology (CPT) code, submitting practitioner, payor, and collections. Additional business from insured patients can have a very different financial profile as compared with additional specimens from an uninsured population.

Building on the financial knowledge around the impact of additional specimens is the idea of an improving margin to receive additional payment for the work performed. The most straightforward approach would be to renegotiate the contract covering the work. For example, it is time to renegotiate your group's Blue Health Insurance contract. Is it possible to negotiate for better payment rates? Can you convince their contracting person that your pathology group adds more value or has better outcomes? Can you convince their contracting person that your group has aggressively reduced utilization of blood products and frozen sections and will continue to do so? Do you know about developments in your practice environment that make your group's participation critical? Another way to improve revenue per case through external means would be shifting your payor mix toward a more favorable mix. This is difficult in many if not most practice settings since we typically process and read the work we are sent. Payor mix can shift through obtaining a new hospital client that has a better mix or geographically expanding into a new outpatient market.

Another area of opportunity would be improving your practice's position in its market by directly elevating the practice's visibility and/or market dominance or through creating barriers which would tend to protect your practice's current position. Identification of high-visibility marketing opportunities such as a unique sponsorship or co-branding effort, development of a member of your practice group as a local expert in a particular disease type as a recognized consultant, as a media expert, or through intellectual property and research can be fruitful ways to elevate your practice. While many, if not all, group hospital contracts will be exclusive arrangements, a degree of market preference could be obtained through contracting as a preferred provider with payors. Perhaps the most straightforward opportunity to elevate a practice in a geographic area and create a nearly unassailable market position is through an unrelenting focus on the service and quality aspects. A high-performing diagnostic organization that is easy to use and provides high-quality and outstandingly reliable service with a palpable focus on all types of customers (patients, providers, hospitals, payors) is not only difficult to do but also very difficult to challenge. So a continued focus on customer needs, service aspects, quality, and overall costs (perceived value is a function of service, quality, and cost) is something every practice group should have and something every practice leader must stress.

Healthcare, and hence pathology, is in a period of increased pressure and accelerated change. As such, the development of novel arrangements has transitioned from an opportunity to an imperative. For many years, pathology practices have undergone an evolution toward more specialization and greater sophistication (such as professional marketing and business management). Practices have also developed their own technical operations such as histology and cytology not only to better control the processes but also to capture the technical component revenue. Some groups have developed in-house billing operations and couriers. Many of these actions have been facilitated by group growth or mergers of groups. Some groups have been forced to merge as their hospitals have combined into systems, while other practices have simply failed. We have even seen venture capital deployed to create new models.

In this time of change, identification of new/novel arrangements is critical. Simple evolution of our current practices may not be enough and, for those practices that are part of large hospital systems or large practice groups, much of your success may be tied to the success of the larger organization. For example, if you are part of a hospital system that is struggling to break even but which also provides the technical component support that allows your practice group to provide services, you may find capital to be scarce and struggle to update equipment and maintain appropriate staffing in your laboratory. In this situation, pathologist productivity may suffer and morale may be a challenge.

The range of possible opportunities is limited primarily by the capabilities of your practice and the flexibility the practice may have to pursue arrangements. We have seen development of a wide variety of arrangements and the only practical limits are defined by your practice and situation. An obvious area of possible exploitation is leveraging your practice's current expertise or strengths. For example, a practice with the only fellowship-trained, board-certified hematopathologist in the metro area could leverage consultative expertise in support of testing such as flow cytometry. Similarly, a practice with a dedicated courier (typically a money-losing proposition) could present a better service option to local office practices through coordination of specimen pickups and improved turnaround times as compared to other local pathology practices or even national laboratories.

The opportunities are almost limitless but subject to antitrust, antikickback, and billing laws and regulations among other challenges. Involvement of appropriate legal assistance and consultants may be needed. Among arrangements, we have seen (not an exhaustive list but intended to give the reader a sense of the diversity):

- Independent practice takes over histology/cytology technical operation and bills services to patients, insurance companies, and hospital. Hospital saves money and does not worry about a noncore function (core function is taking care of acutely ill patients and supporting inpatient surgery).
- Practice provides professional component services to a GI group that owns its own histology laboratory that is in turn directed by the pathology group (depending on technical component payment levels, volumes, and efficiency, a histology laboratory can be profitable and certainly was until Medicare technical component payments for histology were slashed on January 1, 2013).
- Regional pathology practice in-sources courier and contracts for courier services with other providers (e.g., radiologists) as well as local banks to defray the cost of courier operation.
- Practice partners with a regional clinical laboratory to bid on pathology and laboratory services for a large multispecialty group. The combination allows for "one-stop shopping" in which the pathology group provides anatomic pathology (AP) services and the regional laboratory provides clinical laboratory services.
- Private practice provides support for research. This can take many forms: biorepository and tissue banking, diagnostic support for grant-funded research, and provision of histology service. We have even seen a nonprofit flow cytometry operation setup that solicited (and received) philanthropic support.
- Legal consultative services and/or expert witness work.
- Pathology group creates gain-sharing arrangement with hospital. This is quite challenging and should be done with legal support to avoid construction of a "kickback." With increasing focus on saving money, improving outcomes, and demonstrating value, pathology groups can look to share in the savings through use of savings or performance targets. This approach may portend how pathologists are increasingly paid in the future.
- Pathology group partners with a diagnostic radiology practice to develop a comprehensive diagnostic center with a full array of modalities and a high focus on patient-centered care and convenience.
- Pathology group seizes an opportunity to invest in a new technology to become an exclusive provider within a region that merges both diagnosis and treatment

for selective disorders, and engages clinical colleagues to assist, essentially forming a small multispecialty group for the purpose.

- Seizing on a particular market segment's interest in patient-directed testing, a practice opens a mall kiosk for delivery of selected point-of-care testing with virtual consultation backup by a clinical pathologist available.
- A multicultural, polyglot pathology group capitalizes on its international character by exploiting relationships the pathologists have with foreign-based colleagues and institutions to begin offering international digital consultations on whole-slide images.
- Seeing an opportunity to offer better service to outpatient surgical centers and in-office procedures, the pathology group capitalizes the purchase of a mobile Clinical Laboratory Improvement Amendments (CLIA)-certified frozen section and rapid cytology van to provide on-site services in these disciplines at a lower-cost point to the clients.

So with a good understanding of your group's strengths, capacities, and finances, there are many potential opportunities to grow and/or strengthen your practice (with appropriate legal and regulatory cautions). In addition, many arrangements can make for a more interesting and diverse practice, a practice that is more rewarding to practice in, and one that is attractive to future recruits.

> Opportunities to improve the financial performance of your practice by solving current problems or doing new things are found both within the practice and in the broad world outside the practice.

Case: An Opportunity or a Hammer?

Arborview Medical Center was struggling with its bottom line in an increasingly competitive market. Although they had been successful in launching some new programs to meet the community needs, declining reimbursements and some high-profile time above the fold in the local news had been crimping profitability as well as patient and doctor loyalty. The newly hired CEO had a mission to clean things up, clear out the dead wood, and get the system on a growth path again. His VP of Ancillary Services also had his marching orders and decided to start with laboratory and pathology services. He informed you, his laboratory medical director, that although there are no specific problems he is aware of, they are going to develop and distribute a "request for proposal" (RFP) for laboratory and pathology services at the hospital and its affiliates. He anticipates that it will take the executive team a month to define the parameters in the RFP but wanted to give you the first word so you can prepare. They have not yet determined who else will be invited to submit proposals, but expect other local groups as well as some regional players, and potentially a national group as well, to be there since they are considering outsourcing the entire laboratory operation.

How should you respond? Should you collaborate in the development of the RFP?

Discussion: Business entities use a variety of processes to select new systems, partners, and providers when their internal or existing resources are not meeting or able to meet their needs, be those real or perceived. The RFP process is one of the more common of these and typically is used when there is more detail involved than simply a price or specification quote. The request itself may have value internally if done properly, since it facilitates synthesis of key strategic issues, including technical, fiscal, and personnel issues. Ideally, the RFP process alerts suppliers that an organization is looking and encourages them to make their best effort in the form of a response. It alerts suppliers that the selection process is competitive and allows for wide distribution and significant responses. It should also "level the playing field" by insuring that suppliers respond

Table 22.1 Nonmonetary value to practice of responding to a request for proposal for pathology services

Perceived value or cost to organization of responding to RFP	Percentage identifying value or cost
Improved group culture, communication, identity, or unity	68
Development of new leadership	32
Better marketplace positioning, more able to compete successfully	47
Greater understanding of group strategy, strengths, and weaknesses	68
More efficient operations	16
Lost opportunities of potentially greater value while working on RFP	0
Better prepared for next RFP	74
More understanding of key personnel abilities	58
Other	28

factually to the identified requirements and encourage requesters to follow a structured evaluation and selection procedure, so that they can demonstrate impartiality in the decision-making process.

In the realm of pathology services contracting, except in the cases where new hospitals or services come into being, the preparation and presentation of an RFP often means that there is a level of dissatisfaction with the existing providers that has prompted the contracting entity, usually a hospital or hospital system, to put the service "out to bid" with an RFP. While in many cases this is for clearly identified and understood reasons and comes as no surprise to the existing provider(s), it can also come seemingly out of the blue. Because of the presence of an existing provider in so many situations, those pathology providers receiving an RFP from an organization with an existing service provider often face a significant dilemma in deciding to respond or not. They may very reasonably ask themselves, "Is it going to be worth the significant effort, or are we just being asked to respond as a means of creating leverage in the negotiations between the organization and the existing provider?"

An informal survey we conducted several years ago of individuals who had been party to an RFP showed that the time involved to prepare a response could easily top several hundred hours, depending on the complexity and nature of the request. But interestingly, even though the odds of success in obtaining new business through this process were only about 50%, the majority of respondents found great value in the work of preparing a response. A sample of the relative proportion of our respondents who found nonmonetary value in this work, and what those values are, is presented in Table 22.1.

Summary

There is a lot to be gained by adopting an "entrepreneurial" spirit or approach to your practice. This section has used a very broad definition of the term in hopes of opening your eyes and mind to some of the myriad possibilities within and beyond your current practice and processes that might be ripe for harvest, if you have eyes to see them. As a means of extending this perspective to others, we suggest you consider working through more of the cases and discussion questions in Appendix B (You and Your Environment).

Case: Defense Wins the Day

The landscape of Newtown was as pockmarked as a World War I battlefield. There were hulks of old medical juggernauts littered around, burned out practices, physician alliances, and such scattered beneath the thin veneer of public appearances and placid goodwill that the two competing health-care titans of Newtown (Eastern New Hope Healthcare and St. Everywhere General) hoped would lead to their ultimate dominance and triumph. The various boundary lines seemed to shift with each skirmish and the physicians in the community generally tried to play the neutrality flag while simultaneously holding the trump card of relocating their services to a competitor.

The pathology group served both masters, and occasionally labored under the delusion that they could somehow broker a peace deal, at least in their technology-intensive domain. Most recently, they have tried to craft a joint venture reference laboratory to serve all three entities' interests. The latest sessions at the peace table had ended fairly brusquely with New Hope walking away with the intent to launch their own regional outreach reference laboratory unilaterally without participation of St. Everywhere, and only nominal medical director support from the pathology practice. The head of the pathology group, Dr. Algan, had recently been in a bit of a tiff with the New Hope CEO, and found no love for the manager of the new entity, United Consolidated Reference (UCR), considering him totally untrustworthy at worst, and fundamentally manipulative at best. The problem, however, was that both entities would need to derive their lifeblood, their specimen stream, from essentially the same marketplace of smaller regional hospitals scattered about the serviceable circumference of 150 miles. The pathology group was already receiving AP samples from these locations and UCR had their eyes squarely on the reference testing from these locations as well. Who would control the movement of this work loomed as the next likely battle in this repetitive cycle. But that was probably a ways off.

Then the call came. The director of marketing for UCR called the medical director to say they had the reference contract for Lower Falls Hospital 50 miles away and there were specimens at the hospital that would need to be picked up that afternoon along with the surgical specimens. Up to that time, these specimens had generally ridden along with miscellaneous patient transports or other exchanges between sites on a catch-as-catch-can basis. Suddenly the stakes had changed. Dr. Algan and the medical director, Dr. Witt, saw the future of their livelihood flash before them: UCR picks up specimens including surgical cases from client hospitals and delivers them to the pathology group for a while, then someone gets testy and they put the cases into play for others to bid on, or hire their own service to do the work at UCR's behest and whim. The current pathology group is then crippled and limps off the battlefield like so many injured entities before them.

Thus, the Done Right Delivery Service (DRDS) was born and began making daily runs. At first it was the practice business manager and selected support personnel driving the miles of roads that linked the small hospitals in their network, but eventually, regular drivers were hired, usually cheerful semiretired individuals looking to cover the gaps and extend their Social Security income. A small fleet of DRDS vehicles was acquired and a dispatcher/manager was hired to coordinate them. It was immediately evident to Dr. Algan that the enterprise, while effective at thwarting their "congenial" colleagues at UCR from stealing their lunch, would lose significant amounts of money so he cast about for ways to minimize the losses. One day in casual conversation with his banker, the topic came up and he learned that the regional savings bank had a host of nonmonetary documents that they moved around between branches, with little time-specific demand, that might be easily added to the collection of pap smears, biopsies, and small surgical samples that were on the list already. Other nonmedical delivery items were also soon added, and within the first year, the operation was no longer losing money, but in fact, turning a small profit. Again, Dr. Algan's partners thought he had proven his golden touch.

What is the role for courage and nimbleness in bringing an entrepreneurial concept to market? What must precede the launch in such "seat of your pants" endeavors?

What if UCR had launched a competing courier service despite the presence of DRDS? In that competitive environment, what would determine success or failure?

How long should Dr. Algan's partners in the venture tolerate losses before they close the books on the operation?

Case: Rosco to the Rescue!

Dr. Rosco and his three partners have been successful in their sophisticated practice setting in meeting the needs for the physicians of their small regional hospital. Although small, the area seems poised to grow significantly as it is somewhat of a hub for development in a new oil- and gas-rich region. One of their colleagues on the medical staff, Dr. Chase, is an endocrinologist who is keenly interested in managing his patients according to the much more accurate and physiologic data available from a newly developed test methodology. He has approached Dr. Rosco about getting the new technology added to the test menu of the hospital. Talking with his administrator about the opportunity to acquire such an instrument outside the normal budget cycle, Dr. Rosco realizes that the proposal will sit silent for another 10 months, as the budget is already set and has so many big ticket radiology and surgery instruments on it that there is no room for this analyzer. Dr. Rosco approaches his two partners who reluctantly agree to invest the money to start a specialty laboratory to do endocrinology testing for Dr. Chase and the few other people who may order it, provided they have clearance from the hospital that they will not interfere or compete for a couple of years.

Dr. Rosco goes back to the hospital for their blessing. The administrator assures him that they have bigger fish to fry than to worry about a small reference laboratory testing menu. Dr. Rosco finds a small vacant storefront for the laboratory, orders the analyzer and reagents, and hires two individuals to run the testing part time.

One of their part time employees has some business background in addition to testing credentials and is asked to market their reference menu to a few of the smaller hospitals in the region, who also have not yet developed the capability in house. They readily agree to send any requests they receive to the Rosco BioAnalytics Lab, LLC, as it is now called. Within the first year, they are running testing 5 days a week and have hired a courier to service their clients. Net cash flow has turned positive in the range of $1000/month. Dr. Rosco's partners are thinking they may have misjudged their partner, since they had indicated privately that they both thought the $20,000 they put in was money wasted, only put up to keep Rosco (and Chase) satisfied and uninterested in going elsewhere.

By the time the laboratory is 10 years old, the service line has diversified considerably, and they are doing a host of esoteric tests on several different platforms. The pathologists spend about two afternoons a week in the laboratory, now employing 20 full time equivalent (FTE) technologists, and another four clerical/administrative types and one courier. They use contract couriers for other work coming from further afield and have begun to test the use of a national "overnight" delivery service to serve distant clients. Their testing volumes have grown commensurately with the personnel, and cash flow continues to be strongly positive, with revenue of almost $3 million annually.

One of the national reference laboratories approaches Dr. Rosco to explore the possibility of purchasing the business. After some deliberations, they settle on a purchase price that is a healthy multiple of the net earnings averaged over the past 2 years. At the last minute, Dr. Rosco's partners, mostly AP types, persuade him to ask to hold back the small AP component of the business. (They had been drawing in a few thousand biopsy samples from various outpatient settings that they had processed initially on a contract basis with the hospital, and then later onsite in their own histology facility.) The reference laboratory purchaser is fine with that decision, since they had planned to just send that work back to the pathologists anyway and they back out the net revenues attributable to the AP work. They also agree to have the pathologists continue to serve as medical directors for the laboratory at a contracted rate. Rosco BioAnalytics ceases to exist, transferring its assets to National Lab and HistoTech, the new AP only venture. The checks clear and everybody is happy.

What risks were taken by the pathologists? What did they see that the hospital didn't see? Why didn't the hospital see the opportunity as they did?

What skill set is needed to bring a venture to scale as they did? How are those skills different from the skills needed to conceive and launch?

What factors determine when it is right to exit a venture? Would there have been value in having the discussion regarding exit strategy in advance of the initial launch?

Part VIII
Looking Ahead

Chapter 23
The High-Performing Practice into the Future

Lewis Hassell and Michael L. Talbert

We recognize that the topics and case studies up to this point have been largely based on past experience, which in some settings might not be predictive of future success given the pace of changes happening in medicine today. However, we do believe that it is not just one principle that will define a practice as successful and that regardless of the changes in the global environment of medical practice and health-care delivery, the principle of being able to effect a synergy of the various aspects covered in previous chapters will be essential to both effective health care and rewarding work as a practitioner of pathology. That said, we recognize that it can be difficult to see how these pieces come together into a cohesive solution for all the various iterations of medical practice that do or will exist. With that in mind, we have asked a number of individuals from a wide variety of backgrounds and practice settings to give us their take on what the high-performing pathology practice will look like in the future. Herewith are some of their responses.

For years, the practice of pathology has enjoyed the enviable status of "well-kept secret" in medicine: Excellent case mix, superb lifestyle, and above average (to spectacular) income levels. However, with increased competition for health-care dollars, keeping what we do and how we do it secret from other colleagues and the public at large is not going to play to our advantage anymore, not that we had anything to hide in the first place: Our expert contribution to direct patients care accounts for 70 % of all subsequent medical decisions; this secret most definitely needs to get out!

L. Hassell (✉) · M. L. Talbert
Department of Pathology, University of Oklahoma Health Sciences Center, 940 Stanton L. Young Blvd., BMSB 451, Oklahoma City, OK 73104, USA
e-mail: lewis-hassell@ouhsc.edu

M. L. Talbert
e-mail: michael-talbert@ouhsc.edu

© Springer International Publishing Switzerland 2016
L. A. Hassell et al. (eds.), *Pathology Practice Management*,
DOI 10.1007/978-3-319-22954-6_23

To do so, a series of structural and organizational changes need to happen in order to (re)position pathology in the sweet spot of medical practice:

- Integrate pathology into the broader and more visible world of diagnostic medicine:
  - (Re)design internal floor plans and workflows, within hospital institutions and outpatient settings, to provide patients with a one-stop shop for all diagnostic services, including radiology and pathology.
  - Urgently transition pathology diagnostic practice to the digital platform.
  - Smoothly integrate pathology, radiology, and endoscopy digital portals.
  - Build user-friendly bidirectional reporting and test ordering platforms for clinicians and their patients.
  - Associate all diagnoses to social media and web pages linked to relevant critical sites.

- Bring pathologists to the forefront of direct communication with patients:
  - Make it known that we welcome direct communication with patients.
  - Assign pathology resources for extemporaneous and/or live (in person and electronic) communication with patients and other stakeholders in their care.
  - Coordinate with clinicians and create pathways that include pathologists in the communication of critical results to the patient.

- Broaden the pathology department membership tent:
  - In tertiary-care facilities and other complex settings, we will need the expertise of "nontraditional professionals" in order to get invited to the table of accountable care organizations (ACOs) and other new health-care delivery models. Pathology departments and businesses will need to demonstrate added value (and subtracted waste) at all levels of the diagnostics value chain. Experts who understand population health analysis, and know how to tease relevant statistics from big data, will need to be included in our departments' rosters, irrespective of their clinical or professional affiliation.

- Become the standard bearer of enhanced connectivity at all levels of health-care delivery:
  - Lobby hard to have state and federal laws and regulations eliminate IT firewalls between institutions and mandate smooth interface between the various pathology, radiology, and electronic medical record (EMR) digital standards. We generate the information that leads to 70% of subsequent care in medicine, and yet, we accept the fact that most of this information is "boxed" within the narrow confines of a single institutional IT system.
  - In the absence of such regulations, find ways to provide patients with a complete electronic record of their diagnostic tests (including digital images).

Although I am a strong proponent of merging the business interests of related diagnostic specialties (radiology and pathology, in particular), I also realize that such business and organizational merging will not always be possible. However, bringing these specialties and services together from a logistical and workflow point of view is feasible and should be the minimum goal desired. Radiology and pathology benefit more than any other specialty from fast-developing progress in technology, including the explosive field of molecular and personalized medicine. A walk through a modern laboratory and radiology department is akin to a walk into the future of medical science. I am confident that bringing these two giants together will exponentially enhance their individual visibility in the eyes of the patients and unequivocally assert their central relevance in the mind of all critical health-care stakeholders.

Karim E. Sirgi, MD
CEO, LambdaX3 International
Denver, CO

One must make certain assumptions when attempting to predict the future. Plus, one should not attempt to predict too far in the future, because with each passing year, the predictive accuracy steadily diminishes. Or, as Winston Churchill put it: "I always avoid prophesying beforehand, because it is a much better policy to prophesy after the event has already taken place." With those caveats in mind, I provide one possible picture of pathology practice through the rest of this decade (through 2020) and, in particular, the nature of the successful "Pathologist of the Future" (POTF). It is predicated on the following assumptions: (1) there will be a steady decline in fee-for-service compensation arrangements, with increased payment bundling and risk/reward sharing, (2) hospital and physician group consolidations, including hospital ownership of physician practices, will increase, (3) technology, particularly in the "-omics" domain, will continue to develop and its clinical utility will expand, and (4) the number of practicing pathologists will grow at a rate that lags the increasing demand for pathology services, resulting in a net deficit in pathologist supply.

The POTF in a high-performing practice will avoid marginalization from clinical health care by being fully engaged with clinician colleagues and their patients. The goal of that engagement is high-valued (high quality, lower cost) patient outcomes. The POTF will be a master diagnostician and clinical knowledge-generating consultant, driving diagnostic accuracy in anatomic and clinical pathology services. He/she will develop, validate, and provide access to appropriate new technology for optimal patient care. The POTF will be a steward of patient data sets that drive patient outcomes management, quality of care improvement, and population health management through early predisposition prediction and disease prevention or mitigation interventions. He/she will be an effective and appropriate steward of limited health-care resources, serving as a critical source of appropriate utilization management information for clinicians and patients. This includes improving test selection, improving test accuracy, improving the knowledge derived from these tests, improving the timely and informative communication of results, and improving the follow-up and management of clinical information. This means becoming integral and indispensable members of patient-care coordination teams in the evolving new delivery systems. He/she will cultivate effective interpersonal communication skills and be "good citizens" of their health-care institutions. The POTF will understand their environment—particularly the culture of the clinical care settings—in their health-care institution, their community, and the greater health-care delivery systems at large.

This future "sweet spot" has a number of implications. Organizationally, pathology practices/departments will demand effective leadership, including a meaningful place at the institutional leadership table/organizational chart (e.g., C-suite, medical board/staff leadership). Pathologists must be willing to participate in key institutional committees, including as chairs. They must be effective at interpersonal communication and team play. The financial infrastructure of the practice must understand risk/reward-sharing arrangements, and must have a voice in payer contract negotiations and billing systems. New group members should be recruited from forward-thinking residency training programs that engage trainees in the competencies necessary for success in the future. Recruiting for attitude and effective behavior is as important as recruiting based upon academic achievement. This will be particularly important, because these future high-value practice settings will be collegial and collaborative, with high performance, high expectation and accountability, and open and transparent working environments. The values' threshold will be set high, and incentives will be aligned accordingly. Recalling Winston Churchill, remember that "A pessimist sees the difficulty in every opportunity; an optimist sees the opportunity in every difficulty."

Ronald Weiss, MD, MBA
Department of Pathology, University of Utah,
Salt Lake City, UT

Wayne Gretzky said that to be successful in hockey you have to "skate to where the puck is going to be, not where it has been." It is tempting to try and lay out a vision of where pathology is "going to be" in a few years and offer that as the secret to the "high-performing" practice. But Gretzky's success was determined in large part by "playing by the rules" in a context in which the rules were relatively static, as determined by the National Hockey League (NHL) and physics (of puck and player speed and trajectory, that is, rules governing gravity, friction, and conservation of energy). Pathologists (and all physicians as well as other stakeholders in health care) are now playing in an arena in which the rules are changing and to a large degree being rewritten as we go along.

One cannot even say that rational "market forces" can be relied upon, as we are now engaged in a grand experiment to replace one set of nonmarket-driven incentives, with another that (as was the first set) is deemed by some authorities as more likely to produce optimal health for individuals and society. A high-performing pathology practice in the past might rationally have built its success upon a strategy of highly efficient, quality production based upon the reimbursement of an 88305, coupled with the ability to market to physician clients who had the independence to choose a pathology lab based on quality and service. Of course, there were other forces acting too, such as local politics and referral patterns, and even (let it be said) legal and nonlegal kickbacks and inducements. But all of this, for better or worse, made up a more predictable context in which decisions could be made about how to organize one's practice of pathology. At some point (likely only in the distant future), there will perhaps be another relatively stable and predictable context that determines the rules of play within which a pathology practice could rationally lay out such criteria and strategies for success. However, for the foreseeable future, pathologists will be in an environment of high unpredictability that makes the approaches of the past (which *were* successful for many pathologists) hard to replicate.

So I will take a different track and answer the question not of what the "high-performing" pathology practice will look like, but instead: What are the characteristics of the "high-performing" *pathologist* likely to be? That is in essence answering the question: What are the personal qualities or guiding principles that can help an individual pathologist thrive in a time of great uncertainty and unpredictable and often negative change for our profession and society?

- Be adaptable—Darwin demonstrated not survival of the fittest but of the most adaptable. Our morphology skills, most valued in the past, may become commoditized, and the skills that might be most valuable in the future, such as leadership, knowledge of informatics, health-care economics, molecular medicine, or direct engagement with patients (!), may not be the ones we learned in school or residency.
- Focus on quality and integrity in your work—These make life worthwhile, which is the gift given to all who do meaningful work—by doing it better, we can also do more good.
- Be "patient centered"—This is the *cliché du jour* in health care, but there is a useful application for pathologists: Make sure (as much as possible within the context of what you are required to do) that what you do *actually* matters to the patient that it adds value and passes the "common sense" test—that it is not done mindlessly in the *false* pursuit of "quality" or "value." We can all fall victim to this. For example, while templates, synoptics, and checklists are useful tools to assure better care, they can be overused in a slavish fashion and result in nothing more than a longer, less efficiently produced pathology report that contains meaningless information and pseudo-quantitative measurements of characteristics beyond the mathematical significance of the measurement itself or any enduring usefulness to the patient. It is easy to create complexity where simplicity will do.

- Follow the money—Not in the crass sense of self-interest but with the enlightened realization of two facts: (1) As a society, we can no longer afford the health care we buy (or more properly borrow from our children's future), (2) No pathology practice can survive standing alone or as part of a business entity that spends more than it makes.
- Be willing to innovate and try something new—When the outside world is changing, defending the status quo (the principle activity of most medical professional organizations) may not be the best strategy: Wayne Gretzky also said, "You miss 100% of the shots you don't take."

Luke Perkocha, MD, MBA
Kaiser Permanente
San Francisco, CA

I looked around my office for my trusty crystal ball, but could not find it. Either it was stolen, confiscated as a hazardous material, or considered outdated along with my adding machine. Without that assistance, I will try to summarize my thoughts, while remembering that health care as an industry continues to be driven by providers at the local and regional setting. There is much discussion about the impact of the Affordable Care Act on the execution of health care as though standardization at the national level is inevitable and just around the corner. In my experience, ACO models, hospital systems, physician practices, and managed care contracting remain local. Even large multistate organizations are forced to adapt to the local level in order to provide care in that setting.

We find ourselves in a challenging and ever-changing environment. Health care has always been the realm of change. However, it is the rate of change that causes concern for so many. There are a few common threads that tomorrow's pathology group will embrace as essential for success

Size Only large groups will survive. According to the College of American Pathologists (CAP), it has long been held that the average pathology group size was 5–7 members. Technology and economics will change this long-held statistic. I predict that metropolitan areas will probably be served by a single pathology partnership that might encompass 70–80 pathologists under a single tax identification number (TIN). There will be a greater need for fellowship-trained or organ-specific experienced pathologists in community settings where there is (currently) insufficient volume to support such talent in a small group. This diagnostic need will bring pathology groups together in the interest of mutual survival. Technology will improve to the point that digital pathology will become a reality, allowing cases to be matched with those most capable of rendering diagnoses, while allowing pathologists to reside miles apart from one another. Some might speculate that such technology will cause pathology to be outsourced overseas. I do not believe this will be the case as medicine will still require communication between pathologists and specialists in order to maximize diagnostic accuracy and efficient health care. Medical staffs will never accept the loss of pathology relationships from their health-care teams.

Infrastructure With larger groups comes the need for more infrastructure to support practices that are spread over larger distances and not represented in a single hospital setting. When a group's service lines include multiple health systems, the complexity of the group will require much more support. The need for contracting, management coordination, billing, coding, accounting, and compliance will place burdens on the group that a single managing partner would never be able to keep up with. Instead, formal administrative structures will be the norm.

Sources of Revenue In the future, pathology will lose the battle to sustain component billing. Managed care entities will go directly to the health systems, requiring data mining and regulatory compliance. They will defer the cost of laboratory medical direction and quality control to the health systems. Sources of revenue will derive from three key sources.

Anatomic pathology will remain a significant portion of a pathologist's income. However, many battles will be fought to protect this aspect of reimbursement. Managed care entities will attempt to roll these reimbursements into diagnosis-related group (DRG) bundled payments where many specialists will be forced to fight over pieces of the reimbursement pie.

Part A Another source of income will be that which we traditionally refer to as Part A. These are the services typically related to laboratory medical direction. This will be another battle hard fought to retain. However, the emphasis to control laboratory testing, as well as the cost of molecular and genetic testing will open opportunities for the pathologists. These arenas may find increased needs for clinical pathologists to work full time with health systems in controlling these expenditures.

Clinical Diagnostician The future is certainly an information age. However, it is the management of information into concise blocks that can be used for effective treatment that will be most valuable. The pathologist's role as a diagnostician and coordinator of information will create new opportunities. Pathologists will manage more algorithms and data sets to reveal individualized diagnostic conclusions that are used to create custom treatments. Consultations will be requested that draw upon the pathologist's knowledge of pathology and data mining to create an invaluable health-care asset.

Over time, we find that many things change but remain the same. Pathologists will need to be flexible and resourceful but also cunning in their positioning in the future. They will need to band together to build groups that can provide the best of all pathology specialties. They will need to market their trade to best effectiveness in settings they may not have considered before.

Robert De La Torre
Manager, Pathology Specialists of Arizona, LLP
Phoenix, AZ

The following section comes from a colleague who began his career in a large academic center but left academia to pursue a variety of successful private laboratory ventures primarily in the anatomic pathology (AP) arena, with an array of partners, including hospitals, physicians and other labs, until his last venture was sold to one of the large national labs.

My last years in practice were different from my earlier professional life. I was based entirely in the outpatient sector, primarily in clinical lab medicine. As a dyed-in-the-wool anatomic pathologist, I nevertheless came to believe that much of what we will be doing in the future requires us to move back in the direction of clinical lab medicine. I founded ConVerge (a full-service lab serving patients, physicians, and some hospitals in New England) based on our volume and experience in womens' pathology in my old lab and expanded from there into general clinical lab services, chipping away rather successfully at the block of medicine controlled by the national labs.

We worked with local-area pathologists, but interestingly, I found myself looking from the outside in and wondering what the hospital-based practice would look like in the future. One of the groups we worked with was Spectrum Medical Group. This is a multispecialty group with surgical specialties, rehabilitation, radiation oncology, radiology, anesthesiology, and pathology all together. Their size and diversity meant they had some very experienced administrators. Perhaps that is one of the options for the future practice of pathology. Structure and size may become much more important. It is the smaller and medium-size hospital-based groups I wonder about. I really doubt that there is much justification for their financial or business independence once fee-for-service disappears. And that leads me to the question of the future practice of pathology in general.

Basing my thoughts on the Massachusetts experience with Romney/Obamacare, it was clear that Massachusetts considered the "health insurance for all" mandate only the beginning. They knew it would cost more than they were willing to tell the voters. They immediately appointed a commission to look at how to really cut cost. After a long and careful deliberation, the commission declared a crisis unless meaningful reforms were made in how the country pays for health care. Among the many recommendations there was one that stood out: Fee-for-service reimbursement had to go. In fact, they blamed it for most of what is wrong and why health-care costs have spiraled out of control.

In Massachusetts, the legislature has already passed the first laws overhauling the system.

In the commercial sector it appears that some major players have accepted that we must change in the direction of the "Affordable Care Act" model. Hospitals and physicians are going to regroup in order to deliver care under a new model.

I may be retired, but I am an ardent observer and cannot wait to see how this all turns out. But if it goes the way I think it likely will, we must rethink what constitutes the optimally organized pathology practice. If I were to bet, I would say that the best pathology practices will be those that are dedicated first and foremost to the quality of their professional services and can leave much of the administration to business professionals. It is almost inevitable that pathologists will be practicing in larger aggregates. The lucky ones may be those that are part of a large medical (multispecialty) group or a medical center type of practice.

I wonder if there will be many entrepreneurial lab opportunities. I wonder if I am one of the last of that breed. On the other hand, I suspect there will always be restless innovators and, thanks to them, I may not be the last dinosaur.

Karl Proppe, MD
Retired
MA and ME

As the alarm band on my wrist wakes me with a gentle vibration, I lie in bed for an extra 5 min and get up. The sensor on the wrist band communicates with my bathroom light and shower. The water heats on demand, and after I finish shaving, the shower comes on, with a preset water temperature and flow. The shower runs for exactly 7 min and then shuts off. I leave the shower, and the heat lamp in the bathroom comes on, helping dry me faster. I brush my teeth with the help of an electronic brush, preset to my individual dentition. Flossing is accomplished with an automatic flosser.

Once dressed, I move to the kitchen where the flat-screen monitor delivers the important news/weather of the day. Once I pour my coffee that began brewing as I left my bedroom, I am on my way to the hospital lab. My future car is customized to adjust to my fingerprint as I touch the door handle. The engine starts, the seat is positioned, and the high-definition (HD) radio tuned to Entertainment and Sports Programming Network (ESPN). I review overnight messages and appointments and work for the day as the car navigates itself to my parking spot.

Five minutes prior to arriving at the office, the thermostat adjusts the room temperature. My computer/workstation starts, and the log-on process is initiated. Once I enter the office, the sensors identify me and the password sequence is finalized. One screen lightens up and reminds me of the day's appointments/meetings/conference calls. The other two screens also boot up—one with a virtual log of the cases I need to sign out and the other with the first digital image of the first case.

My office phone rings and the caller's info is displayed on one of my screens. I answer with a movement of my right hand, and the speakerphone is activated. The caller is one of the general surgeons wondering when I will review one of her cases; I can see the case on the log and call it up with a voice command. I let her know I will get back to her within 15–20 min. After the surgeon hangs up, I can append the caller's number and pager to the case as I review it. Magnifications of the digital image are adjusted by voice command; movement of the slide is accomplished by touching the screen or by voice prompt. Once I have determined that the breast lumpectomy is malignant, I complete the diagnostic template on the report by voice prompts. If I miss an important part of the template, I am prompted by a voice from the workstation.

After the report has been proofread by the virtual intelligence built into the program, I sign it out and it is transmitted to the surgeon electronically (smartphone/office/desktop). The sign-out routine is repeated for the 50 cases on my log; I am finished with the log by 1:00 p.m. Any special stains needed or deeper levels are also ordered by voice prompts customized to my own needs.

Specimen processing is performed rapidly, with biopsies ready to be examined in less than 1 h. Larger specimens require at least 2 h for proper fixation. The fixative of the future is nontoxic and used routinely by all histology labs.

Clinical pathology consultation for providers and patients is reimbursed (real time) by all carriers and Centers for Medicare and Medicaid Services (CMS). Real-time virtual discussions with the patient and their provider are supported, as are individual outpatient consults. As a phone call comes in for a patient-requested consult, I am able to retrieve the important clinical history by voice command. If I need to search the Internet, this is also accomplished by voice command. There is no longer any manual typing involved.

As the end of the day approaches, I have signed out 50 surgical pathology cases, communicated with 10+ providers and patients, and participated on three conference calls. I have sent out five cases for digital consultation to colleagues in Nebraska and Oklahoma and received their consultation reports within 2 h.

Bone marrow aspiration specimens are no longer examined microscopically; all are done by imaging cytometry and molecular markers. In fact, most hematologic disorders can now be diagnosed from peripheral blood specimens, with rare intervention to obtain bone marrow samples.

Also during the workday, I have been able to participate in virtual continuing medical education (CME) exercises when I have the time available.

Genomic studies have become commonplace in community hospital labs, and all pathologists have received training on the interpretation of these studies.

Apps are available for me to review anything I have signed out during the day, should a provider or patient call me after I have left the hospital.

As I return home, my heater/air conditioner has sensed that my car is within 5 min of arrival. The climate in my home has been stabilized, and the video screen reporting the day's events is ready to come on as I enter from the garage.

Oh, I forgot one more thing; my favorite beverage (alcoholic or nonalcoholic) is chilled and waiting for me as I sit down and relax once I get home.

Ready for another day once I fall asleep on my customized mattress next to my beautiful, very real wife.

Rick Gomez, MD
St. Francis Health Center
Topeka, KS

Describing the ideal pathology practice is like describing the ideal airplane. The specifications are so variable that unless you know what it is used for, you cannot intelligently specify its requirements. As a jet fighter plane differs from a Boeing 747, so does a large multiple hospital or multisystem practice differ from a small, single-community hospital practice or a practice based in an independent reference laboratory. Having completed the required disclaimers lamenting the impossibility of this assignment, let us consider the required elements of any successful practice. Just as every airplane must have an engine, wings, controls, etc., the ideal pathology practice, whatever its size and scope, must have certain basic features.

The ideal pathology practice will have appropriate pathology expertise, either in-house or via relationships with outside consultants, to serve the needs of its customers, for example, patients, physicians, administrators, and other business partners.

It needs a formally defined organizational structure with written agreements defining the relationships between the members. It is not important whether its legal form is a partnership, corporation, or limited liability company (LLC), so long as the structure is well defined and clear.

It needs a mechanism for making major decisions and deciding on strategy. This could be a governing board, a management committee, or in some situations, might be a single individual managing "partner." It should be clear how members can participate or provide suggestions to the governing board. The structure could be a democracy, that is, elected by partners/shareholders or a monarchy, that is, the king/queen rules until he/she dies. In any case, the rules should be clear. It is ideal to have outside expert advice, possibly in the form of an outside board member or via trusted consultant(s) who can provide expertise in different fields deemed important. Over time, this body must develop the ability to make time-sensitive decisions that are not unanimous and act on those decisions. It is common to wait for unanimity on all decisions so as not to offend. This essentially conveys veto power on any issue to the most reluctant adopter and is inimical to rapid, decisive action.

There must be an individual who plays the role of the chief executive officer. This could be a non-pathologist or a managing partner/president who is a pathologist. This individual must have the authority to and be able and willing to make timely day-to-day decisions involving the practice. Perhaps the most important executive function is allocation of resources. There will never be sufficient funds or personnel to accomplish all of the desired goals. The executive must make timely choices as to how to use the available human and financial resources. There must be a clear understanding of the threshold of financial decisions that the executive is able to make independently without board approval.

Revenue sources should be diversified. If a hospital-based practice is the starting point, expanding outpatient/outreach revenue sources is desirable. There is no right number, but 15–25% of total revenue would be a good benchmark to start. This could be accomplished by an internal effort, by a joint venture with a hospital, or by contracting with an independent laboratory. Success in this endeavor requires recognizing the value of sales skills since success in the physicians' office market demands capable representation and a physical presence visiting the physician's offices.

Marketing is a separate discipline from sales, although they are often conflated. While the experience and expertise of both might be combined in one individual, it is valuable to consider them separately. Marketing is the discipline that influences choice among potential "buyers" of services that the pathology group offers. The concept of marketing for pathologists is not necessarily intuitive. Identifying, establishing, improving, and maintaining the pathology group's image can be viewed as a function of marketing, perhaps its most important function. This speaks to the importance of concentrating on the group's image whether at tumor board, conferences or everyday conversation with clinicians. While producing elegantly designed marketing pieces is satisfying and can be an important sales aid, marketing must also analyze the capabilities of, provide advice to, and influence the structure of the practice. Providing information about potential or current customers is also important. Surveys are one method for gathering this information.

It can be advantageous for a practice to have ownership of a business or property that has the potential to appreciate in value. In addition to diversifying the assets of a group, the thought processes involved in dealing with equity versus cash compensation can provide valuable insights into managing a business. One of those educational advantages is a greater appreciation for the disciplines involved in finance along with a greater understanding and appreciation of financial tools.

The ideal practice requires regular, consistently prepared, understandable financial reports. Income statements should be prepared monthly; balance sheets at least quarterly; cash flow statements as often as required to be useful. Accrual-based statements are strongly preferred; particularly if these financial statements are to be used for outside review, financing, or acquisition. These statements should be subjected to annual review by an outside accountant. If a third-party transaction is contemplated in the future, an annual audit is beneficial. Accrual-based statements are also preferred for decision-making based on past history and trends. Budgeting or forecasting future financial performance is also enhanced by accrual-based information.

Other traditional finance functions include paying bills (accounts payable), managing money (treasury), and banking relationships (e.g., establishing credit lines, long-term loans, capital equipment purchases).

Billing should be accurate and complete. Regular audits are recommended, particularly when changes occur, for example, when coding rules or payment rules change. Many practices will use an outside billing service, since billing expertise is difficult to maintain in house, especially in a smaller practice. Billing reports by payor are important. Standard accounts receivable aging reports are also vital. There should be written policies addressing bad debt write-offs, professional courtesy, and collection agency interface.

The practice requires someone to function as a controller, that is, to monitor expenditures.

Human resources functions include payroll and benefits administration, recruiting, orientation, mentoring, and evaluation. Maintenance of insurance products including medical, dental, vision, medical malpractice liability, general liability, and perhaps officers and directors liability is also important.

Al Lui, MD, FCAP
Chief Medical Officer and Chairman of the Board
Pathology, Inc.
Torrance, CA
Co-founder
Affiliated Pathologists Medical Group (APMG)

Generational and Gender Change

In 5 years, the Next Generation of pathologists will have occurred. Most Baby Boomer pathologists will have retired; Generation X pathologists will be managing practices and Millennial pathologists will be a significant percentage of practicing pathologists and a significant force of change. Generation X and Millennial pathologists will demand a balance in work and life. Women, who comprise about 33% of pathologists, will become 50% or more of pathologists. Pathology practices will need to become more flexible in work hours and scheduling. Millennials, as a generation, are less concerned about income and more concerned about socially meaningful careers. They will want a practice that "gives back." As a consequence, Next Generation pathology practices will "adopt" a cause or provide pro bono pathology services, perhaps to a third world country via digital pathology.

Practice Type

Hospitals will continue to consolidate to be competitive and to form ACOs. Pathology groups will be encouraged or forced to merge by the consolidated health-care systems. Revenue for pathology practices will continue to decrease because of declining reimbursement and value-based payment models. Expenses will continue to increase, primarily because of the increasing expense of information technology. Some pathology practices will not be able to adapt to these economics and will be forced to sell or merge their practices. Therefore, solo and small pathology practices will be rare. Within 5 years, these forces will result in four basic pathology practice models.

1. Large academic pathology practices.
2. Large pathology practices that are integrated into large integrated health-care delivery systems.
3. Pathologist employees of commercial/reference laboratories.
4. Large amalgamated practices widely distributed over one or more states, created from the merger of several formerly independent small practices.

Next Generation pathology practices will be large with 100 or more pathologists in one practice being common. Most pathologists will be employees. The large amalgamated and distributed pathology practice will be the last vestige of a practice setting in which a pathologist is an owner.

Practice Governance
Large and distributed practices are going to be difficult to manage and lead. The technical side of practices will need professional managers who will most likely have an MBA and years of health-care experience. These individuals will manage the technical employees, manage budgets, and negotiate contracts. However, the pathologists will need leadership from pathologists who have leadership and management expertise. Not every pathologist has the ability to lead and manage. Practices will need to recruit for pathologists who already have additional training in leadership and management, or practices will need to specifically recruit for pathologists who have the basic leadership skill set and then send them for additional training.

Digital Pathology
The Next Generation pathology practice will interpret digital slides. This will greatly facilitate internal and external consultations. Cross coverage will be facilitated. For example, a neuropathologist can be covered for vacation by another neuropathologist who lives hundreds of miles away. Digital slides will facilitate leveling workload among pathologists on a daily basis. Digital slides will allow for consolidation of histology laboratories, because the time to return the slides by courier will be eliminated. Immunohistochemical and special stains will be available the same day to pathologists who are stationed at hospitals that are many miles from the histology lab. Quality assurance, peer review, concordance studies, and teaching will be easier and faster with digital slides. Pathologists will be able to insource consultations from other countries.

Next-Generation Sequencing (NGS) and Molecular Pathology
The Next Generation pathology practice will be performing NGS. Practices will be doing NGS gene panels on tumors to investigate for actionable mutations. Whole-genome sequencing of tumors will also occur. Allele-specific testing and fluorescence in situ hybridization (FISH) testing will continue to expand, so Next Generation practices will need board-certified molecular pathologists.

Informatics
Medicine is rapidly becoming completely digitalized. The American Board of Medical Specialties has recently approved the subspecialty of clinical informatics. Clinical laboratory results, NGS, and digital pathology will generate enormous amounts of digital information. The Next Generation pathology practice will need pathologists with training and board certification in clinical informatics to help manage and analyze this digital information.

Laboratory Medical Director
The role of the laboratory medical director (LMD) is becoming more complex. The LMD may someday be seen as a subspecialty in and of itself. Successful LMDs will need more training in personnel management, finance, operations, informatics, negotiation, and leadership. LMDs will need specific training in team building and working with other physicians and administrative colleagues. Next generation LMDs will become the LEAN and Six Sigma gurus of the health-care system.

The Next Generation pathology practice will see many changes and have many challenges. Yet, I see the changes as exciting and I believe the Next Generation of pathologists is up to the challenge.

David Hoak, MD
Incyte Diagnostics
Spokane, WA

Another more technical viewpoint sees a future system where diagnostic reporting is assisted by powerful technical tools making work easier and more consistent.

The roles of artificial intelligence in the preparation of pathology reports
Consider the following two scenarios:
A pathologist reviews a two-specimen skin case: He picks up the first slide of the first specimen, scans the barcode on the slide, in a few seconds, the gross description of the case is displayed on the screen. This is a case with specimen 1, a punch biopsy labeled as "Rt FA" and specimen 2, a shave biopsy labeled as "L upper chest." After the pathologist reviews the slides, he dictates into a microphone "Superficial BCC and lichenoid keratosis." In a few seconds, the voice recognition program recognizes the command, and the report will be generated as

1. Skin, right forearm, punch biopsy:
   − Basal cell carcinoma, superficial type
2. Skin, left chest, shave biopsy:
   − Lichenoid keratosis

He can then say "sign out case." In a few seconds, the report will be finalized, without the usual need for key strokes and mouse clicks.

A second scenario: A pathologist has just finished reviewing 18 slides of a 6-part prostate biopsy; every biopsy is benign. He dictates "benign prostatic tissue times 6." In a few seconds, a report with the appropriate headers and intended diagnoses is generated

1. Prostate, left apex, needle biopsy:
   - Benign prostatic tissue
2. Prostate, right mid, needle biopsy:
   - Benign prostate tissue

Then the pathologist can say "Consult Dr. Johnson." A new paragraph, such as "Comment: Dr. Johnson has reviewed this case and concurs." will be added to the end of the above diagnosis and the report will be forwarded electronically to Dr. Johnson for reviewing. Dr. Johnson reviews the case and sends the case electronically back to the primary pathologist. The primary pathologist will then say "sign out case" to finalize the case.

These are two examples of how artificial intelligence, in conjunction with voice recognition and bar-coded slide scanning, can be utilized to assist pathologists in the preparation of the pathology reports.

Pathologists' expertise is in rendering the most accurate and clinically relevant interpretations of the biopsies. Once the interpretation is completed, making that interpretation visible as text is a step that artificial intelligence can play significant roles in facilitating. These roles are more extensive than the above examples demonstrate, and may include, but are not limited to the following:

1. Extracting the information from the preliminary report dictated by pathologist assistants and setting the information in the appropriate place in the final report, such as generating the headers and putting in the appropriate procedure.
2. Standardizing the headers in the final report, such as "Rt" becomes "right" and "punch bx" becomes punch biopsy.
3. Proofreading and correcting certain errors generated by the pathologist assistant in the preliminary report, such as changing "allergic content dermatitis" to "allergic contact dermatitis."
4. Typing the free-text dictation into the appropriate areas in the report without the need for pathologists constantly checking where the dictation is typed—scanning the appropriate slide guides the cursor to the right place in the document.
5. When pathologists give the command "sign out case", the command can use a built-in safety mechanism to keep an unfinished report from being finalized and can do additional proofreading to catch the voice recognition errors such as correcting words with nonsensical meanings, for example, "irrigated seborrheic keratosis."
6. Reminding pathologists by voice to perform certain tasks, such as repeating estrogen receptors/progesterone receptors (ER/PR) if they are negative in the prior biopsy and asking pathologists to check for the number of lymph nodes if it is a colon resection for colorectal carcinoma.

Artificial intelligence in the preparation of pathology reports as described above has already been prototyped and used in routine work. It has resulted in significantly higher efficiency and avoided much of the frustration associated with voice recognition without artificial intelligence. Since the artificial intelligence performs secretarial tasks, it is designated as Secretary-Mimicking Artificial Intelligence (SMILE) [1].

Template building and graphical user interface (GUI) automation have been used in pathology practice; however, artificial intelligence appears to be in its infancy. Its widespread adoption in the future will liberate pathologists from paying attention to the lower-order tasks (lower-order is not a derogatory term here, simply meaning the actual execution of tasks such as where to type the report, repeating content that is already in the report, some proofreading, formatting, reminding, etc.) and enable them to focus on the higher-order tasks that pathologists are specifically trained to do.

Jay J. Ye, MD, PhD
Dahl Chase Pathology Associates
Bangor, ME

Since the Industrial Revolution, tension has existed between the labor force and technology. While technological advances provide increases in efficiency and/or quality, they also bring the threat of marginalization for sectors of the workforce. The health-care industry has resisted the trend toward automation and workforce reduction for the most part. One could argue the ever-expanding IT infrastructure creates additional jobs by adding additional layers of IT staff, administration, coding/billing personnel, etc. that were not in place before. However, with health care spending at unsustainable levels, the industry will be forced to undergo some uncomfortable introspection. What services and roles are vital? Which are overvalued? Which can be automated?

As pathologists, we can choose to view the encroachment of new technologies into our realm as a threat of replacement or an opportunity for enhancement. As whole-slide imaging gains traction some may fear that computer-aided diagnosis is around the corner. However, rather than being threatened by that prospect, I think we should be excited by it and embrace the possibilities. We pathologists add value through expertise and yet relatively little time and effort are devoted to what we are best at. Instead the majority of our time and energy can easily be expended on peripheral tasks that add little value and result in frustration. We often spend more time gathering data and reporting consultations than we do applying our highly honed skills in diagnosis. Can we craft a future where the technology actually facilitates our work rather than hinders it?

I can imagine sitting down to a workstation and logging in for the day. The first screen presents an overview of the day including meetings, outstanding cases to be signed out, a list of new cases, and a filtered list of e-mails identified as "high interest." With a verbal command all new appointments are added to my calendar. An e-mail demanding an immediate response is dispatched with a short dictation. Next, I am prompted to review cases for tumor board since my digital assistant has learned that my preference is to do this at the start of the day. As I scroll down the list, I quickly review a Wikipedia-style page for each patient which contains an updated medical history, summary of care, and an ongoing dialogue about the patient's condition among members of the care team. My digital assistant has highlighted clinicians' questions which appear most relevant to today's meeting. Digital slides are available for review with likely areas of interest already selected. I choose which views to present and draw some annotations on the screen. Next, I review the prognosis and therapeutic options pulled from the most recent literature and copy it to the patient's wiki as well as sending it to my tablet for reference during the conference.

After preparing for tumor boards, I review my outstanding cases. Newly available immunohistochemistry results are automatically graded and imported as well as any other newly available molecular or laboratory data. A provisional description and diagnosis has been entered based on these newly available results. I review the case as well as a summary of the literature data applicable to the case. On a case for which I would like a second opinion, I tell my digital assistant to send the case to a colleague. My colleague instantly receives the request through our secure messaging service and can simply click a link to access all the relevant electronic information. After she reviews the case, the messaging service allows us to talk through the case and review the slides in real time as we reach a consensus.

When reviewing new cases, which have been previewed by my digital assistant, I am presented with provisional findings and diagnoses. Areas identified as significant by the image analysis tools are spotlighted. As I verify the findings, I make a few adjustments which update the differential list in real time. Probabilities for each diagnosis are calculated using demographics, genetic profile, and other relevant information in the patient's chart. When in doubt, I consult a curated image bank to instantly compare entities as well as potential mimics. My assistant has already ordered ancillary tests indicated by prebuilt algorithms. A list of suggested immunohistochemistry stains, molecular tests, and ICD-10 codes is waiting for review.

Later, I compare my cases to the 3D reconstructed images as we try to validate our new tissue scanner. The scanner uses multiple wavelengths and intensities of light to scan entire tissue blocks, much larger than could fit into a cassette. I can view a representation of what the tumor looks like in situ, even nuclear details. However, the advanced imaging techniques capture much more data than I could possibly review and I rely on the analysis software to present only the most pertinent information, including images and fluorescence profiles.

At the end of the day as I am completing the miscellaneous tasks from my to-do list, I pull up the summary for the automated chemistry line. I can quickly scroll through quality control (QC) for the day and identify any QC failures with explanation of how the issue was addressed. Unacknowledged critical values are displayed with a timer that indicates when the online-notification system alerted the patient's physician or other care provider. There is also a list of unexpected laboratory results with recommendations for follow-up testing that can be approved by me or forwarded on to the patient's physician.

There does not seem to be a lot of optimism about the current state of pathology and medicine in general. The current regulatory environment and reimbursement requirements are onerous at best. At least some feel the best days are behind us, but I hope that is not true. While not on the front lines, I believe that we can still add a tremendous amount of value in delivering efficient patient care. Automation of some of our current tasks is likely inevitable, but I believe we can leverage assistive technologies to harness our true potential and be a valuable partner in delivering the highest standard of care to every patient, in every setting.

Chris Williams, M.D.
University of Oklahoma Health Sciences Center
Oklahoma City, OK

Reference

1. Ye JJ. Artificial intelligence for pathologists is not near—It is here. Description of a prototype that can transform how we practice pathology tomorrow. Arch Pathol Lab Med. 2015;139:929–35.

Chapter 24
Bringing It All Together

Michael L. Talbert

Discussion (1st case in Chap. 1): Evaluating an employment opportunity

Using what you have learned in this book, you should now be prepared to evaluate a potential job. This is the hard part that goes into the details, often referred to in business as "due diligence."The first of the broad range of things to consider is fit:

- Establish what you would be expected to do each day and over the long term. Do the duties match what you would like to do?
- Ask how the hiring practice would define success for you at 5 and 10 years. How does that match with your professional 5- and 10-year goals?
- Explore why the position is available. Is there new business, a desire for your subspecialty skills, or are you replacing someone who left (why did they leave?)?

If the fit seems good, consider the structure and finances of the group:

- Is this an independent private practice or a pure employment model? If this is an independent group, is there a partnership track? How are the shares distributed among the partners?
- Is the practice financially successful? Develop a sense of their book of business. Is it dependent on one or two potentially shaky contracts? Are finances improving or deteriorating? Can you get an idea of the payor mix? A well-insured patient population can make a large financial difference.
- How are pathologists paid? You will be offered a starting salary and benefits but should establish expectations over time. How will your salary change in year 2 and beyond? How sure can you be that these expectations will be met? If a partnership track, how many years before you will be considered for partnership, and how is that decision made? How much did the partners make last year? Take time

M. L. Talbert (✉)
Department of Pathology, University of Oklahoma Health Sciences Center,
940 Stanton L. Young Blvd., BMSB 451, Oklahoma City, OK 73104, USA
e-mail: michael-talbert@ouhsc.edu

© Springer International Publishing Switzerland 2016
L. A. Hassell et al. (eds.), *Pathology Practice Management*,
DOI 10.1007/978-3-319-22954-6_24

to understand the benefit package. A lower salary with a great benefit package can be more attractive than a higher salary with limited benefits.

Knowing how the practice is doing now is helpful, but at least as important is how the practice will fare in the future:

- Is the practice growing or shrinking? What are the practice's strengths and weaknesses?
- What does the practice plan to do in the coming 1–3 years? Are they playing offense or defense? Do they have a vision and strategic plan that make sense, and are they executing on those?
- What does the larger market look like? Are there opportunities? Is there a major competitor that seems to be growing? What "tectonic plates" are in motion around the practice—accountable care organizations (ACOs), major health systems, demographic shifts, regional employers?
- If the practice is part of a larger entity, such as a hospital system, the same questions should be asked about the system.

What About the Practice Itself?

- Do you identify with the culture? For example, is there a sense of just getting the work done to pay the bills or is there an overriding sense of mission?
- Do you sense group dysfunction or discord between pathologists?
- Is this the group of people you would like to join to pursue your professional (and personal) goals?
- What level of turnover has the practice experienced? What has happened to any recent hires?

And, of course, the community should be attractive to you and any family members under your roof, but how this is established is a very personal thing.

So, how do you ask and answer the questions above? Many prospective employers would be put off by a candidate who showed up at a first interview with a list of the questions above. The process should be more gradual and speaks to the amount of effort you should put into evaluating a potential position. In some ways, your comfort in discussing answers to the above questions should reflect the comfort you feel with those individuals with whom you would be working. You can learn a lot by asking open-ended questions of various people you meet during the interview process. You may find yourself particularly "connecting" with one or more of the existing pathologists. Save the more sensitive questions until later in the process. If there are two interview visits, a second visit, which would indicate strong interest by the hiring practice, would be an excellent time to seek answers to the more delicate questions.

Do not just confine yourself to asking questions of the hiring pathology practice. If a pathologist has recently left the practice, find out their views and why they left. If you have a connection to a pathologist with another group in the area, he or she may give you a very different view of the practice and its prospects. Talk with physicians served by the group or a hospital administrator if the group is hospital based. While they may be motivated to attract you by "sugar coating" the situation, their lack of true understanding of pathology can often give this away. So, do your homework and really "kick the tires" of any employment opportunities. The costs, both financial and personal, of moving and changing practices are large, and a good initial choice is crucial.

Where We Have Been?

We have now explored the broad field of practice management. We have considered the financial, contractual, people, and market aspects of pathology practice. You should now understand how a practice works financially, how you are paid as a pathologist, and how to evaluate an employment opportunity. We have explored how to assess a practice in a particular market and how to improve a practice. Hopefully you have developed ideas about how to improve your own practice setting.

We have spent a good deal of time talking about people issues. Much of pathology practice management, and management in general, is about people. While people are a practice's most valuable resource, they can also create its most vexing problems. A rift between two senior pathologists can be a greater threat to a practice than changes in Medicare payment rates. This can be compounded by our current environment of rapid change and downward pressure on payments, which engenders stress and may exacerbate underlying people issues within a practice. In our experience, day-to-day people issues can demand more total time than the other aspects of practice management combined. As such, careful recruiting, early identification of problems, a focus on fairness, and a proactive approach to intervention are key. Continually evaluating culture and mood is also essential. With these warnings in mind, though, a high-functioning team of professionals is both fun to be part of and difficult to beat in the market.

Looking Ahead

The practice of medicine and its integral parts are changing at an unprecedented rate. My grandfather was a general practitioner who also worked in public health. Though he died when I was young, I have been told that he would occasionally come home with chickens or eggs as payment for his professional services. Despite his modest income, the work was steady, and my grandfather was a pillar of his community. My father was a pathologist who practiced during the so-called "golden years" of pathology, when income was derived primarily from the clinical laboratory and anatomic pathology was, when compared to today, done for very little. He then practiced through the transition from clinical pathology to anatomic pathology paying the bills. While this was a scary time, pathologists adapted and most practices continued to prosper. Overall, there was a general sense of stability. For my father, hematoxylin and eosin (H&E) microscopy was the central tool supported by histochemical stains, the earliest of immunohistochemical stains, and rarely, electron microscopy. Today, a surgical pathologist does perhaps twice the workload of 25 years ago backed up by the same histochemical stains but with menus of immunohistochemical stains of greater than 100 antibodies. Gene-based studies are now commonplace for diagnosis, prognosis, and to determine therapy. Early automation and fairly advanced process control have come to histology, while an information system assists in constructing evermore detailed reports.

But this feels like the early innings of waves of changes. Whole slide imaging and digital pathology seem almost ready to revolutionize practice. While our efficiency can be greatly increased by the move to digital pathology and digital tools to assist diagnosis, once a slide is digitized, it can be "read" anywhere there is power and signal. Similarly, as sequencing costs fall and bioinformatics improves, possible future scenarios continue to multiply. Will sequencing become ubiquitous or centralized at large centers? Will it be a commodity with the value-added opportunity being in the informatics and interpretation? Or, will proprietary software displace the frontline diagnostic pathologist into a triage role? That sequencing and bioinformatics develop at different rates suggests that a variety of scenarios will be possible. Of course, other technologies such as microRNA expression profiling and proteomic profiling could take a large role in the future and that ignores other promising technologies and approaches yet to be developed.

The continuing impact of Moore's law (now 50 years old), which suggests that information technology (IT) will continue to advance at a dizzying rate, is another game changer. The power of ubiquitous smartphones connected to the Internet with ever-growing computing power and storage (the cloud) will continue to create untold possibilities. Health care has been affected, but really only on the edges. Other industries such as communication, finance, and retail have been upended and remade, with huge winners and losers. IT in health care seems at least a decade behind other industries, but the possibilities are startling to consider, and many developments will be beyond the control of most pathology practices and, indeed, may come from outside of health care.

With these and other changes, the next decade or two promise to be turbulent. A pathologist's specialized knowledge will still be valuable, but the "moat"—the protections and stability of the past—is drying up and being bridged. But all of the above must be tempered by the multi-decade observation that change in health care seems to happen, at best, at one third the rate you think it will. Whether because of the lack of true organization in the health-care system (i.e., it is not a system in the usual sense), the local nature of health-care delivery, or just the sheer size and complexity of health care, the speed of change will be mitigated compared to what seems logical, and change will occur at different rates in different locales.

Hopefully, this book has armed you with a grasp of the present workings of pathology practices and the skill set to evaluate environments and consider the future. Pathology, we believe, has a bright and interesting future, if different. A major College of American Pathologists (CAP) workgroup's effort predicted a growing shortage of pathologists based on current and projected practice patterns [1], although major changes in practice could render that model irrelevant. At any rate, a well-trained pathologist with a good grasp of the concepts explored in this book should have a leg up; hospital-based pathologists have central roles in hospitals and are natural change agents for hospitals and physician practices. So, keep your pathology skills current, be a student of your environment, and engage with your local health-care system. Let us lead the change.

References

1. Robboy SJ, Weintraub S, Horvath AE, et al. Pathologist workforce in the United States: development of a predictive model to examine factors influencing supply. Arch Pathol Lab Med. 2013;137:1723–32.
2. Diamandis PH, Kotler S, editors. Bold. How to go big, create wealth, and impact the world. New York: Simon & Schuster; 2015.

Appendices

Appendix A

Extended Cases

Lewis Hassell, M.D.
    Case 1: Pathologist Workload Management Issues

Introduction

"We're always here at 5 p.m., while you guys are usually on the 9th hole of the golf course at that time!" It was true, reflected Joe, the head of the six-person, two hospital practice serving hospitals about 50 miles apart. Folks usually were long gone over there whenever he called late in the afternoon. And the us versus them mentality that was reinforced by this disparity threatened to destroy the group's esprit de corps. Yet, whenever he looked at case numbers, charges, and other measurables at his disposal, it always seemed the two locations were pretty evenly balanced.

> If you are going to manage, you have to measure.
> Manage things, lead people.

A fundamental question a leader or organizer of a group faces is how to optimize the array of personnel and talent to accomplish the work to be done. With profitability as a bottom line metric of performance, success depends on not devoting more resources (i.e., personnel) and thus incurring cost to an activity that will only generate so much revenue. In an era of diminishing resources when the focus is on providing optimal outcomes, this challenge becomes even greater.

    Additionally, the perceived productivity of an individual within an organization and the rewards they receive for that work influence their sense of self-satisfaction with their work, the environment in which they work, and their interactions with others in the workplace. Thus, the division of workload, the allocation of resources,

© Springer International Publishing Switzerland 2016
L. A. Hassell et al. (eds.), *Pathology Practice Management*,
DOI 10.1007/978-3-319-22954-6

Table A.1 Specimen volumes for a full-time equivalent pathologist under several workload studies. Since each study used somewhat different metrics, the assumptions on which the normalization to the various case types is based are noted in the footnotes

Method	Haber (1995)	RCPath (2006)	CanRCP (2005)	Ku (1998)	FPSC-RVU (2010)
Surgicals	7500	4622[a]	4153[b]	5889[c]	6112[e]
Cyto	6000	10,040[d]	3180	7656	
Autopsy	250	400	264	765	725

RVU relative value units
[a] Assumes average specimen macro/micro score of 4.5 (52 weeks)
[b] Assumes average surgical case = 1.3 L4E
[c] Assumes average KU specimen weight of 1.3
[d] Assumes 1–3 slides/case
[e] Assumes average RVU of 1.3/case

human or otherwise, and the rewards or profits from that work have a major influence on the culture and success of an operation.

An understanding of the history of workload measurement as it pertains to laboratory work is pertinent to see where we are heading, and to appreciate why this task is so fraught with challenges. This perspective will also perhaps illuminate why determining optimal staffing of an organization is so difficult in today's environment. The question, "when do I need to hire an additional pathologist?" was posed and first answered by Seth Haber, pathologist at Kaiser Permanente for several decades. His answer was based on his best estimates of what the components of a pathologist's work were at that time and how much of any component a pathologist who was doing only that could do in a full year. This methodology, essentially a linear, multivariate sum, has been the essence of pathology performance benchmarks ever since, even as other observers and investigators have tweaked the values for the constants and new variables have been added (see Bibliography). Most recently, Cheung et al. have proposed a complexity-based model better suited to the modern anatomic pathology (AP) practice that they believe may be more widely adaptable, though this model also does not account for the full breadth of pathologist activities pertinent to workload equitization. The expectations, however, can vary widely across time (as the complexity of cases changes, medical understanding shifts, treatments evolve, and processes and support systems improve) as well as across systems and international boundaries (e.g., Korea vs. Canada). Table A.1 summarizes the relative projected annual workloads for a full-time pathologist doing just one of the activities (surgicals, cytology, or autopsies) in the AP realm. As can be seen, the time and location context have led to very different conclusions about what constitutes a fully loaded pathologist (Several "best guess" assumptions were required based on the methodology and counting methods used by these studies to allow direct comparison, as listed in the footnotes.).

Attempts to apply meaningful workload metrics to other, nonprofessional aspects of laboratory work have also been attempted. The most notable of these was the comprehensive workload recording methods put forth by the College of American Pathologists (CAP) in the 1960s and periodically updated until the early 1990s [1]. At that time, an expanded comparison set of metrics was offered under the acronym Laboratory Management Index Program (LMIP). It was increasingly recognized that the complexity of methods and clinical settings had made solid comparative efficiency data difficult to derive and rely on. Most laboratories, however, continue to use some form of counting system to measure internal productivity and allow detection of significant shifts in workload.

Another effort to provide useful comparison data such that practices could compare performance and determine potential trigger points for action was put forth by the CAP under the title Path*Focus*™ [2]. This effort was hampered by the need for large amounts of data and limited interest in supplying this data, but it did provide some insight into comparative best practices for some settings, and clearly highlighted the fact that practices are highly variable in performance. No doubt, as the roles of pathologists continue to evolve, the challenge of measuring their activities for comparative purposes will grow in magnitude. Of even more fundamental import will be the question of whether and to what degree these new activities add value to the clinical care of patients, and how that value compares with traditionally counted (and coded) activity.

Aside from hiring brighter people who know how to work hard and fast, efforts to increase productivity in any area of the laboratory can be some of the most significant contributors to improvement, both from a quality of patient care standpoint and from the view of employee satisfaction. Process improvements and upgraded, easier to use tools and support services, if designed with the intent to reduce barriers to accomplishing the work and reduce errors requiring rework or re-handling, not only improve the frequently measured items such as time to report, but also improve the worker's sense of accomplishment and hence job satisfaction and morale.

Environmental structures (such as cultural norms) that reward positive behaviors both from a productivity standpoint and the citizenship standpoint (such as assumption of duties that may not be measured by whatever workload system is in use) can produce dramatic results. In this case, it is important to be cautious about what is measured, since the very act of measuring something tends to affect behaviors. Distribution of work that penalizes good performance, that is, high productivity without commensurate recognition or reward, has been repeatedly shown to normalize production to the mean, rather than raise it.

From an anatomic pathology standpoint, the following are all to some degree "measurable" activities that might enter into a workload assessment equation today.

- Number and complexity of surgicals
- Number and complexity of cytopathology cases
- Number and complexity of Fine needle aspirates (FNAs) and bone marrows (procedures)
- Number and complexity of autopsies
- Extent of supervision and management
- Amount of research and teaching
- Number of medical staff conferences and committees
- Time involved in hospital and lab QA
- Time spent in accreditation and compliance
- Time spent at other sites and travel
- Time spent in continuing medical education (CME) and vacation
- Time spent on-call

In clinical pathology, the range of activities is also broad and becomes more difficult to measure due to this variability and the inherent differences in testing performed and services provided in the context of the organization's mission. At one institution, the following list is generally followed:

- Review/revise procedures (annual)
- Review QC/QA (monthly)
- New test development/improvement
- Staff supervision and morale
- Consultations and interpretations
- Continuing education for staff, clients, etc.
- Publications
- Meeting time and CME

For either an anatomic or clinical pathologist, the following should probably also be entered into the equation:

- Practice management activities
- Business management
- Human resource management
- Physician communications
- Internal consultations
- Organized medicine activities

One consideration when measuring productivity is to actually measure productivity (output or outcome) rather than just activity. As an example, time spent on research is an activity measurement while publications may more effectively measure productivity. Some activities may be time related; for example, a group may be paid on an hourly basis for medical direction or on-call time.

From a more basic standpoint, this issue of comparing productivity is in part the crux of the paradigm shift that occurred following the Omnibus Budget Reconciliation Act of 1989 mandated use of the Harvard Resource-Based Relative Value Scale studies published by William Hsiao in 1988. The entire physician payment system fundamentally changed from "usual and customary" (which some might have interpreted as "whimsical and wishful") to a system that attempted to account for physician time, intensity and liability, adjusted for regional overhead differences (see Chap. 1). As a result, many practices have used the relative value units (RVUs) associated with billing activity as a surrogate for physician productivity, recognizing of course that a sizable number of activities, both clinical and nonclinical, are not measured under this system, and that some activities which hold value may be under-rewarded compared to others. Since these may comprise a disproportionate part of an individual pathologist's time, systems which use RVU's as the "carrot" incentive will potentially penalize certain elements of their practice over others (e.g., gynecologic cytology or clinical consultation.)

Thus, deciding what you measure and how you use productivity data may be one of the most important decisions a leader can make. Behaviors will adapt to what is being rewarded (either directly or indirectly). And "gaming the system" will happen in almost every situation if people know what is being observed and measured, sometimes even if it is not directly influencing the rewards. For example, one observer, on reading the recent publication on the system proposed by the University Health Network in Canada, immediately remarked, "Well I can tell what I'd be doing to look good in that system!" For example, a medium-sized practice hired two new associates around the same time. Both were exceptionally well-trained and pretty hard workers. One was faster than the other in getting their work done, and would often take extra cases from the communal pile as they became available. The other worked more ploddingly and frequently volunteered for tasks that required travel away from the main location. When the slower pathologist became aware that the number of cases being signed out was being monitored by practice leadership, he began coming in a bit earlier and sifting through the pile of cases to claim all of the "gross only" and simple cases, such as fallopian tubes, tonsils, and appendices, to bolster his numbers. Ultimately the group and this slower pathologist decided to part ways as the pathologist's approach to gaming the system became evident.

Case 1: Workload and Productivity

The Hohum Health Care System Hospital (HCSH) and Dienomite Regional Medical Center (DRMC) have recently announced their intentions to merge and have asked you (Dr. Dee "Buzz" Sawh) to lead the merger of the two pathology groups into a single entity. You see this as a great opportunity but one full of great challenges as well. The two hospitals are located 4 miles apart with moderate overlap in their medical staffs, serving a medium-sized city with no other significant regional competitors. Dienomite has a large outreach effort into a variety of nursing homes, clinics, and small health stops both within the city and in smaller communities up to an hour away, including a small critical access hospital. Administration is expecting that you will be able to help them recoup considerable savings in operational costs between the two facilities by consolidating services in various ways to both reflect needs at the two institutions and in the community.

You ponder the organizations and their workforces in anatomic pathology (Table A.2).

Table A.2 data suggest that Hohum pathologists do not have enough work and are spending time screening paps and going to meetings all day while Dienomite pathologists appear more productive. You consider the model of having one pathologist who visits Hohum 1 day a week for part of the day, though it appears that the surgical volume there may increase to balance the load between the sites. You think that the retirement of one of the Dienomite Regional Medical Center (DRMC) pathologists 9 months down the road may not require seeking a replacement based on the current numbers.

Based on the historic variation in vacation taken and cases signed out, you attempt to apply some flexibility in the approach to the matter of time and workload, with some sort of adjustment in pay that takes that into account. At the same time, you are anxious that the group become cohesive, efficient, and begin now to take steps to be more than just a "black-box biopsy reader service."

Table A.2 Data for Hohum HCSH and Dienomite RMC

Parameter	Hohum HCSH		Dienomite RMC	
Operating suites	4	63.4 % usage	12	81 % usage
Primary surgeons	2 Gen'l; 1 Gyn; 2 Uro; 5 Ortho; 2 Plastics	All but one general surgeon and Gyn also work at DRMC	6 Gen'l; 1 ENT; 3 Gyn; 3 Uro; 7 Ortho; 2 Plastics; 2 Neuro; 2 Card-Thor	
Pathologists	2	4 weeks vacation	6 (2 with cyto boards; 1 with transfusion med boards)	2 PA; 8 weeks vacation
Surgical specimens and frozen sections	3550 (23 FS/year)	65 % 88305	16,005 (455 FS/yr)	74 % 88305
Cytology Gyn/Non-Gyn	3K/340	50 Path-perf FNA; no CT	24K/1450	No path FNA; 4 CT
Clinical lab consults	110	Heme; coag; micro; endocrine; transfusion med	266	(Blood smear rev; transfusion med)
Committee Service by Path	Med Exec; Tis/Trans; P&T; Util Rev; Inf Cont	1 prior chief of staff was path	Tis/Trans; Inf Cont; Rad Safety	No leadership history
Autopsy	Two cases	Outsourced to residency program 2 h away at hospital expense	20 cases	Done in house, mostly by PA
Histology output Blk/Slides	5910/7450 (1.26 sl/b)	1 HT, with other duties; all IHC sent out	37,250/81,200 (2.17 sl/b)	7 HT; 2 LA; 90 % of IHC done in house (13,400/year)
Transcription	Path performed	Voice recognition	Digital dictation	3.5 FTE
Tumor boards	One monthly		One weekly	
Molecular tests generated from AP/quarter	10 (mostly Her-2 FISH); 140 HPV		60 Her-2; 25 BRAF; 20 oncoDx; 45 MSI; 40 Kras; 200 HPV; 40 other	Currently only Her-2 FISH done in house

HCSH health care system hospital, *RMC* regional medical center, *IHC* immunohistochemistry, *FISH* fluorescence in-situ hybridization, *FTE* full time equivalent

In histology/cytology, it also appears to make sense to consolidate services. It appears that histology could be moved easily to DRMC with little loss of service and cytology could also be centralized to DRMC. You anticipate that this will result in a savings of about 1 FTE from the staff required at Hohum HCSH and improve utilization of space and personnel at Dienomite.

Discussion Questions:

Based on the numbers presented, and assuming the volume of cases remains stable or grows less than 3 % in the coming year, is the pathology practice adequately staffed?

What patterns do you see that might be cause for concern?

What activities might you want to measure going forward in terms of productivity and why?

What behaviors might be identified as needing encouragement and thus meriting more reward?

Case 1, Part 2

As you get to know the players in your team better, you do a profile based on the individual activity rates for the metrics you have gathered above.

Hohum Pathologists

Dr. Ruff Ryder—General pathology, AP/CP, 22 years in practice, signed out 2100 surgicals in prior year, 1.2 day ave TAT; did 42 FNAs, 3 bone marrow bx, and 250 non-gyn cytologies, half the smear reviews and 15 clinical consults. Past president of medical staff; chairs two committees.

Dr. Joe Giardia—General pathology, AP/CP, 16 years in practice, signed out 1450 surgicals, 1.5 day ave TAT; did 8 FNAs (when Ruff was away), 95 clinical consults, 100 non-gyn and all 3000 gyn cytologies. Likes to evaluate instrumentation in clinical lab; helped design clinical pathways for hospital; introduced reflex testing in hematology for work-up of anemia and in chemistry for evaluation of liver disease.

Dienomite Pathologists

Dr. Silvio Poquet—AP/CP, cyto, 32 years in practice, workhorse who did 500 non-gyn cytologies and 4000 surgicals (1.2 day TAT), in addition to 1/3rd of gyn reviews (8 % review rate means almost 700 cases); also covers CP activities in serology and UA; Only took 3 weeks vacation last year. Does about half of tumor boards.

Dr. Ole Benine—AP/heme, not boarded; 15 years in practice; signed out 250 flow cytometry cases, 100 bone marrows, and reviewed 200 smears from clinical lab. Signed out 800 surgical cases. Took full 8 weeks of vacation; occasionally does tumor board.

Dr. Phil Tracion—CP/Transfusion medicine; lab director and chair of T/T committee, principle interests in coag, 21 years in practice. Serves on national committees

Table A.3 Clinical Lab considerations at Hohum and Dienomite

Clinical Lab tests	123,000		3.5 million	
Clinical Lab FTE	5 MT; 4 MLT; 1 LA		65 MT; 40 MLT; 12 LA; 5 clerical	
Specialty areas	Gen'l Chem; Coag; Heme; BB; Micro; UA and Serology	Virology sent out	Gen'l Chem; Coag; Heme; BB; Micro; Virol; UA; Serology; Flow Cytometry; FISH; TDM	AFB, Molecular oncology and genetics sent out

TDM Therapeutic drug monitoring

and travels 2 weekends, plus 1–3 weekdays per month for these duties; signed out 20 transfusion medicine clinical consults, 60 smear reviews. Took 10 weeks of vacation in addition (although 2 were supposedly for education meetings).

Dr. Cotton Rune—AP/CP, two and a half years out of residency; did 3200 surgicals (1.9d TAT), and 200 non-gyns; oversees microbiology and hence also serves on Infection Control Committee. Rather a plodder, tends to dictate long notes on his reports and order lots of stains. Took 6 weeks of vacation total and was away for one national meeting for a week. Has started to do tumor boards about once a month.

Dr. Tran Xu Dat—AP/CP; 8 years in practice, did 7000 surgicals (1.4 TAT), 250 non-gyns, 10 autopsies (bad luck when he's on call!), clinical lab duties in TDM and FISH testing, and visits the critical access hospital 1 day a month. Attended one national meeting and took 3 other weeks to visit family in SE Asia. Does about one third of tumor boards.

Me, *Dr. Buzz Sawh*—AP/CP, cyto; well qualified from work in another state at Mega-Universe Medical System for 12 years; with current group for only 1 year; did 500 non-gyns, commensurate number of gyns, and small number (278 to be exact) of surgicals (2.1 TAT, but they were complex cases) and three autopsies; sat on the Radiation Safety Committee; helped direct chemistry and evaluated starting up molecular services to complement FISH lab and micro-molecular testing. My golf game has been polished recently by playing regularly with the CEO of DRMC and the chair of the Board of Trustees. No vacation taken aside from doing two lab inspections, and 2 days off for family leave to attend funeral.

What kinds of strategies might be employed to shift behaviors among this diverse group of people towards an "optimal" mix of productive activities?
How might their productivity as individuals be improved?
What kinds of targets or benchmarks might be employed? Which ones should be avoided?

Case 1, Part 3

Enter the Clinical Lab considerations at Hohum and Dienomite—(Table A.3)
Although there are likely to be opportunities to consider consolidation of some clinical pathology services between Hohum HCS Hospital and Dienomite Regional

MC, the respective hospital administrations are not willing to consider consolidations at this time. Your consideration, however, is whether there would be adequate pathologist consultative and medical oversight coverage from the combined group practice, particularly as you consider shifts in pathologist staffing for the future.

What clinical pathology duties and behaviors do you feel are important for the pathologists in the group to have?

What kinds of targets or benchmarks might you consider employing? Which ones would you avoid?

Case 2: Group Leadership Dysfunction

Drake Medical Associates (DMA) is a multispecialty practice that has ten pathologists among its 300 physician employees which also include physicians specializing in family medicine, internal medicine (gastrointestinal (GI) and pulmonary), obstetrics, radiology, and anesthesia. They have a histology lab and a general purpose reference lab to service their owned surgery center and a general diagnostic center with a few niche operations that cater to their high end boutique practice needs in the area of fertility. They also provide reference support for a few of the small hospital labs in their region, though these have been consolidating or folding over the past decade. DMA has locations across Muddle County with one site in a neighboring state.

Dr. Duke, pathologist, is the senior managing partner, and chairs the five physician Executive Committee of DMA. A lot of the legwork for day-to-day operations is handled by their superb practice manager, Marissa, an energetic former CPA and their HR director Hollison. The practice is organized in a matrix fashion, with standing committees for Operations and Facilities, Medical Practice and Quality, Finance and Governance, and Marketing and Customer/Client Services, as well as site-specific Operating Committees. These operate with charters/charges pertinent to the strategic plans and receive reports from sub-teams engaged in specific projects or activities.

The overall operation has been quite successful over the past decade as they have executed on their plan to provide quality, niche services in high value (i.e., well-reimbursed) areas along with some general care for their primary population which tends to be fairly affluent. Muddle County is a suburban area that has had a growing population and a solid economic base of clean industries surrounding the second tier mid-Southern city where they are located. In short, the times have been good to DMA. Physician turnover has been low and productivity fairly high. The practice has had difficulty developing metrics that work well across specialties to equalize work and rewards, a topic always guaranteed to produce differing opinions about who is working hard for someone else's bonus (or even base pay).

But multiple national and regional events have cast some question marks on their ability to continue the double digit growth (and hence hefty bonuses) that the past decade has brought. For example, the significant decline in technical reimbursement for AP lab services appears to have put a crimp in the profit margins for the histology lab. The launch of the new Fertility Center by the downtown academic medical center has diverted public attention away from their offerings in this service line. This was followed by the departure of one of their well-regarded senior OB's—Dr. Jones—to join that center with an attendant loss of his patients. Dr. Duke has not been by the OB and infertility practice site for several months, but Hollison reports that morale was low following news of Dr. Jones' intended relocation.

Marissa reviewed their fertility service line and estimated that Jones' departure would likely result in a 50% decrease in their fertility testing volumes at the lab, potentially impacting the workload of at least two employees, and his surgery center volumes were also high enough to furlough half of an anesthesiologist and a nurse. Given the age distribution of some of these employees, she is fearful that the younger, more recently hired and trained personnel will jump for a new opportunity as they see the writing on the wall with declining volumes, even if only temporary. She was in the surgery center last week for staff meetings, but the issue was not yet public and the supervisor there has not reported any side-bar conversations since. She's been so distracted since hearing of this matter that she has not completed the evaluation of their consideration to acquire an in vivo microscopy-endoscopy capability. And to make matters worse, her college-age son reportedly recently announced that he was leaving school to backpack around South Asia for a year with his girlfriend, rather than finishing his business degree.

Thought questions:

What kind of additional information should the key characters and leaders in this organization gather before their next meeting with the Executive Committee?

How could this information be obtained? What of these informational matters might require action before such a meeting?

What actions or habits on the part of leadership might have alerted Dr. Duke or any of the other practice leaders to the potential defection of Dr. Jones?

What features of a healthy organizational culture do you detect in the description? What might be done to further characterize this culture/organization as healthy or not (e.g., sample questions, and to whom addressed)?

Dr. Duke comes to the next executive committee meeting with his fingers crossed that there is not a general rebellion over the fertility issue and that there are no new regional insurrections over other issues. In his mind, he is figuring that he just needs about three more good years before his retirement fund is sufficiently funded that he can remove himself from this fray in favor of the mountain town where he has built a second home.

Marissa is still stewing inwardly from the harsh words spoken by her husband to their son over his "irresponsible choice" to leave school and head off like a vagabond. She did not want the conversation to go that way, but it got away from all of them in the heat of the interchange. She has most of the data regarding the infertility testing and care lines itemized by provider. They do not look good, but should clearly identify their options—hire new talent and shore up operations in the bridge period or jettison the whole operation as soon as possible to minimize losses.

Holliston has been in contact with a head-hunter for some CVs of known fertility physicians and brings them along. His take on the other at risk employees is not bright. He sees the potential for several key support personnel who live closer to the academic medical center to jump along with Dr. Jones if the salary is right. He's also noted that DMA's salaries for other personnel have dipped below national averages, although still on par with local means. Even though their bonuses have usually put them well over the averages, since those are non-guaranteed and times are getting tough, attitudes and advantage could change quickly.

The other members of the executive committee, physicians from family practice, anesthesia, and two from radiology, enter the meeting a bit tardy, laughing as though they have been drinking at the bar. They had glanced at the circulated agenda prior to the meeting a few days back, but frankly, it had not registered that this might be a meeting of great significance. They have not really heard any mumbling or concerns in their work areas or have been too wrapped up in their own work to worry about the decision of some prima donna colleague who is leaving.

They start their meeting with the usual minutes and old business stuff and the waiter comes by with their drinks, salads and bread. The business gets interrupted and discussion turns to other topics for a bit—an up-coming golf tournament they have been asked to sponsor to the tune of a pretty penny, rumors about one of their client hospitals being acquired by a hospital chain with a different history of service models, and a few personal items. Marissa says nothing during this time, although it is evident she is a bit more than usually frustrated by the dinner-meeting tedium.

Only after the main dinner courses do they move to the "meat" of the meeting— budget projections for the new year given the dynamic of the recently announced resignation. The physicians motion for salaries to increase by a full percentage point with "across the board" salary increases, and Marissa does not put up much of a fight, though she knows that will cut their margin of reserve to virtually nothing. Dr. Duke is not inclined to speak for moderation since he knows his retirement package is based on the average of his last 3 years of earnings. The motion carries and they move on to discuss strategy relative to their non-compete contract clause with Dr. Jones and whether to go after a replacement. The discussion goes long, with lots of commentary, some in jest and other comments obviously not reading a lot of deep significance into the decisions. Marissa again fails to speak up about her projections of dire impacts across several business divisions with the loss of Dr. Jones' business and patients.

As the hour grows late, they realize they have not come up with a strategy per se, but they want to get out of there and quickly develop a stop gap set of instructions to Hollister to start the search for a replacement and to Marissa to institute some cost-saving efforts in the interim to deal with the anticipated changes in workload. The Committee remains split on the legal issues, each perhaps figuring that it could be a precedent they will have to defend to their colleagues who might also at some point turn on them. They opt instead to have Marissa consult their legal firm for an estimate of costs and risks associated with enforcing the non-compete. Further decisions are deferred to next month's meeting.

Thought questions:

Based on this account, what information might have been useful to the participants to make the meeting more productive and effective? Why?

How might the information have changed the course of the meeting? How could you design a way to get those cultural weather events onto the table the next time this group meets?

What are the meeting processes that are unhealthy? What could be done to improve the culture as it pertains to the Executive Committee?

Three months later, the ad hoc recruitment committee is in the process of interviewing the first of three candidates to replace Dr. Jones, who has now been gone for 4 weeks. Two other key employees submitted resignations and are rumored to have taken positions at the downtown mecca. After receiving the opinion from their legal team that the wording in their non-compete clause of the contract was so far-reaching (100 mile limit of any facility with which DMA has a contract!) that it would likely be thrown out as attempting to restrain trade in more than one state, the executive committee opted not to pursue formal action. But the lawyers came away with the work of revising their contractual language to draft a more defensible non-compete clause for the other professional contracts.

Marissa's "worst case" budget projections have been proven to be conservative for the first quarter: Revenues from the pathology lab are down over 30% year over year due to the reimbursement change and the last month's revenues in the fertility lab were as expected, less than half of prior numbers even though the other two fertility specialists stepped up their hours in an attempt to retain Dr. Jones' patients in the practice.

Hollison discovered in his exit interview with Dr. Jones that he had felt slighted by the fact that the incentive bonus structure had a "cap" that essentially curtailed his potential earnings in any given year and that having exceeded that productivity cap for each of the prior 4 years, he was "tired of subsidizing the lackeys" in anesthesia and family practice that he knew were barely bringing in their salaries. He generally harbored no ill-will with DMA, but was looking forward to a less socialistic practice setting in the academic department. In Hollison's recruiting calls to Executive Recruiter, he found a wide range of reported salaries and incentive packages, with DMA offerings in the middle of the range. He plans to recommend to the compensation/and recruiting committee that they reconsider the incentive package and "cap" issue as a result of this information, knowing, however, that it will open the door for "class warfare" within the group over the issue of income disparity between specialties.

Dr. Duke has made some rounding visits with his specialty service chiefs at their various sites and talked with a few of the site directors in the process. When he asked them about issues they needed help with to do their jobs better, he got a wide array of answers—things like streamlining contractual payer relationships so that their patients did not always feel so anxious about getting billed for non-covered services, a number of equipment upgrades, better support for their electronic medical record (EMR) and wider links to incoming data from referral sources. When he asked about any concerns relative to Dr. Jones' departure, most were rather nonplussed and had little idea of the financial impact on the practice. They had yet to see much if any impact on their daily operations. People come and go, life will go on, no big deal. Several brought up new procedural or technical opportunities they would like to see the practice embrace and wondered about getting the funding or support for some of these kinds of new services or ventures. Another family practice (FP) had suggested that the group needed to consider becoming more patient-centered, and possibly look into offering an "off the insurance grid" kind of service or suite of services for patients who wanted to retain them as their health managers for a monthly fee.

As a consequence of his visits, Dr. Duke has his fears relieved and commends them for their forward thinking ideas (which he doubts he will push further in the organization—not wanting to risk his energy or retirement stability with some new costly and unproven venture). Written notes of these rounding visits are never made, so the ideas often seem to vanish into thin air. The older section chiefs have figured this out to the point that they rarely bring up things of that sort.

Thought Questions

Based on what you now know about DMA, rank the overall organization on the following cultural trait axes (1–10, least to most)
Transparency
Integrity
Commitment to do things right
Collaborative
Accountable
Risk-taking
Seeing mistakes as a learning opportunity
Perseverance amid difficulty
In what way would the cultural pulse-taking, or mood-monitoring activities you suggested earlier impact the culture on these parameters?
What other means might you employ to improve the cultural DNA of DMA?

Case 2 Part 2: DMA Revisited

Dr. Duke reviewed what had happened over the last 6 months as he scanned the practice financials. Dr. Li—who had replaced Dr. Jones—was great, but it had taken 4 months to get her on board. During the interim, 70% of Dr. Jones' patients had gone with him, and since Dr. Li was just starting her career, she brought no new patients with her. The other two fertility physicians had nearly burned out from working longer hours. The stress was showing. One of them got divorced. Rumor was that their tempers were starting to be visible even to patients. The lab techs and pathologists had tried to avoid them as much as possible.

Fortunately, that part of the disaster was slowly improving. But that was not the worst of it.

The increased salaries had depleted reserves to the point that with reduced revenues from Dr. Li's new practice, DMA had been unable to pay the attorney bill for the significant revisions to the non-compete clause of the professional agreements. Marissa had been able to stop the blustering attorneys from a lawsuit by getting them to accept a delayed payment, but this required DMA to take out a significant bridge loan to cover that and other operating expenses. And for the first time in the storied history of DMA, when the bonuses came out last Thursday—or stated more accurately—when the bonuses *should have* come out last Thursday, there was nothing. Nada. Zilch.

Dr. Duke picked up the papers and shuffled into the emergency Executive Committee meeting. Four glum physicians sat around the table with their practice manager and human resources specialist. Marissa and Hollister looked pale.

"I've never heard it so bad out there, Walt," said one of the doctors to Dr. Duke. "We have the possibility of a major revolution on our hands."

"How did you let it get so far?" another doctor said to Marissa. "Maybe if you weren't on the phone so much to your hippie son in Nepal…."

"Hold it right there, Bill," Dr. Duke interrupted. "Everyone is entitled to a family life. Marissa has been here more evenings lately than most of the rest of us. And you should blame me, not her. I'm the senior managing partner. I should have seen this coming." He paused. "By the way, I don't think there have been any hippies since you and I were in med school, my friend." The joke eased the tension in the room.

Dr. Duke continued. "I've been doing a lot of soul searching lately and have come to the conclusion that my head hasn't been in the game for several years. I've honestly been more focused on my own retirement than our practice. But now that all of our retirements have been threatened and we probably need to furlough an anesthesiologist and a nurse because of this, I think we've got to make some big changes. We've had a major wake-up call, here, ladies and gentlemen. We need to decide whether we want DMA to thrive or not." He glanced around the room. "What do you think?"

Everybody nodded.

"Well then, we've got a lot of work to do to change things. We've got some comp systems that aren't working, some strategy for the future we need to address, and—he looked at Bill—some things we have to do to change our work culture."

Bill turned to Marissa. "Sorry. I was out of line."

"There's a lot I need to do better, too, doctor." Marissa said. "I'm sorry I didn't share more information with everybody about our financials."

Hollister raised his hand. "Dr. Duke, may I make a suggestion? I know a lot of people who aren't here have ideas that could help. For instance, Dr. Li may be new, but at the employment interviews she said that participating in making decisions that affect her was as important to her as her salary. There are others that feel that way, too. I think it would be a good idea to decide which decisions the Executive Committee needs to make and which ones we could involve more people in."

Thought Questions

What changed Dr. Duke's approach as the senior managing partner? Was it a good
   change or a bad change? Why?
What are the things the Executive Committee needs to work on to improve the practice? Which are most critical? Which are less important? Why?
Which are the issues that need to be resolved by the Executive Committee? Which
   could be delegated to other committees? Which should involve other members
   of the practice? Who should be involved? When? Why?

Case 3: Changing Behavior with Metrics

Utopia University Pathology Department has been trying to improve its financial
situation by ensuring that they are at minimal risk of a Medicare recovery audit
while also maximizing their service-based revenue. Several initiatives have been
employed to improve their processes. One of these involves delegating the final
coding decision-making process to the person most knowledgeable and responsible
for the case sign out. However, their systems are flawed and depend upon individual
inspection of the assigned codes. Joe, the practice manager, begins to track where
the defective codes are coming from and to educate the pathologists on proper coding. Some pathologists consistently perform better on this metric, though none are
perfect. Dr. X appears to be an outlier in terms of performance, but insists he tries
to remember. Positive rewards and recognition for above average performance are
appreciated by some at first, but seem to fade in time. Individual education works
marginally but again seems to decay or be unassociated with a shift in the curves.
   Eventually, Joe realizes that he is going to have to take a different approach to
obtain lasting engagement. He determines to publish the data in the group with
illustration of the means, and outliers on his graphs. The graph includes no normalization data, only gross numbers, so comparison between individuals with differing
roles and total cases is generally meaningless. However, Dr. X clearly appears to
have more cases in his column than the others in the group and everyone else can
see that.

For discussion:

Will Dr. X respond to this "outing" of his lackluster performance with improvement
   in his performance?
What is the role of data transparency in an organization? How does the motive in
   Joe's mind—shame, blame or engagement, influence that reaction, and what can
   he do to most clearly communicate the motive he intends?
What are the roles of benchmarks in improvement? How can their potential to evoke
   complacency be avoided?

The distribution of the data evokes an immediate response, not from the high end
outlier, Dr. X, but from Dr. Y, one of the lowest bars on the graph, who complains

that he is highly offended by such a publication and feels that he has been treated as a school kid, rather than a professional. Joe's reassurances that the sharing of the data was not done to shame or blame, but only to build awareness of the problem, solicit ideas and enlist engagement to solve the problems fails to assuage Dr. Y, who though not likely to resign, remains aloof to appeals to become engaged in new quality ventures.

Case 4: Employee Engagement

Your community has been changing over the years, and your practice is beginning to reflect some of the newer arrivals in your area. The practice of Jones and Bagley that was founded 40 years ago by two staid Caucasian males, graduates of the state school and trained in the regional hospital 150 miles south of you, has grown. They have retired to greener pastures, though Jones still stops in now and then to take afternoon tea or talk. It was only 10 years ago that the group hired its first female on the partnership track and the ruckus that her first request for maternity leave created is still spoken of by the support staff with an odd mixture of humor and amazement. Specialization has impacted the practice as well and today the interchangeability of the principals' skills is rather limited when it comes to making decisions for a client or a case.

The offices are busy, with work moving around the place in all directions. Occasionally, confusion as to who can best handle a case leads to concerns about fairness. The new associates, especially Cirille, are anxious about taking on cases that fall outside their comfort zone, but are sometimes reluctant to speak up given the tenuous nature of their employment as non-partners. XinYin also has some concerns, although you would not know it by looking at her, with regard to the manner of distribution of bonus monies and incentive pay. She also was silent during discussion of a change in the manner of applying for and getting time off. Since she has aging parents on another continent, she is concerned she may find herself in the awkward position of needing to take leave urgently should they fall ill and being put in an uncomfortable stance relative to the other workers. Bob is usually jovial, but has been a bit more sobered of late following the death of his wife from a brain tumor and the recently leaked fact that his single daughter was expecting a child. Antonio, whose father was a long-term representative in Congress, has been testing the waters a bit himself politically and recently broached the subject of going part time so he could fill a seat in the state legislature. Sofique, the newest associate, just completed an overseas adoption and is going out on family medical leave act (FMLA), while at the other end of the pipeline, Patrick O'Donohue, the most senior partner, is believed to have purchased a second home in a warm climate location near his four grandchildren. You cannot tell what his timeline is exactly, but suspect something is imminent. He usually keeps things close to the chest, so you know you may not have much notice.

The practice has discussed taking on a new business line. It is a growing market but one that has been or might be dominated by bigger practices or institutions, but which now seems more feasible for a smaller organization. It will involve significant investment of capital, which the practice can leverage of course and also take a lot of start-up time investment. As this decision is considered, it is evident that several different camps are forming that might be named "Hi-Ho, Let's go!", "No way, Jose! Much too risqué!" and "The Why-ners" (why now, why me, why him, why us, etc.). There also seems to be a significant association between age, gender, national origin, and time in the practice and membership in these three camps.

Questions for discussion:

As the practice manager for this group of culturally handicapped, disparate interests, what course of action would be effective in marshaling the resources to (a) make a decision and craft a plan of action, and (b) create a new culture of engagement?

What individual or cultural "minefields" exist in this scenario that you can foresee? What steps to avoid or confront and defuse these should you take, either openly or in private?

Case 5: Cultural Engagement

You are the leader of an academic department at a medium sized, mid-continent university charged with the triple mission of educating the next generation, expanding the envelope of human knowledge and caring for the patients who come under your purview. You have a long and noble history of these endeavors, but the current generation of faculty and the staff that serve them seem anything but mid-Western. In fact, none of them were born in the state, and even though many of them have lived in the country for most of their lives, your faculty and staff meetings seem more like a model UN than anything else. Two are from Latin countries and are first-generation immigrants. Five are of East Asian descent, though not from the same countries. In fact, the father of one was imprisoned for many years by compatriots of two of the others. Two more are of South Asian origin and are female with young children. Your patriarch pathologist is an Austrian-trained Hungarian who is getting a little hard of hearing. The director of AP has a live-in partner and it is believed they traveled lately to a same-sex marriage state with intent to marry. She seems less interested in organizing the department and getting the mission accomplished than in social activism for more personal interests. The lab manager is a very easy going fellow, notably the only African origined person in the department.

You have five faculty members doing full-time research, two others with partial grant funding, and the remaining (15) are funded out of teaching or clinical revenues. You have a clinical lab operation doing about 5 million tests a year to oversee, and a support staff of six for faculty academic and business matters, including two doing the department's billing.

Your main challenge seems to be getting the group to collaborate on any sort of effort to improve the department's performance on just about any metric, whether it is teaching evaluation scores, resident training survey results or Resident In-Service Exam (RISE) scores, clinical productivity or turnaround time, or even when clinical service meetings should best occur. The most recent dysfunction arose after the AP director put one of the more staunch Latin American Catholics on call 4 weeks in a row, purportedly after overhearing him express an opinion opposing same-sex marriage. Following that action, you have heard that two of the other mid-level faculty have been talking with private practices in the area and two of the young faculty requested leave that you circumstantially discovered was to do a job interview elsewhere.

Questions for discussion:

How would you approach the task of keeping this department from imploding and getting the group to work together cohesively?
Which issues would you approach first?
What kinds of tactics would be useful for the various members of the team, and what kinds of efforts or actions should be avoided?

Case 6: Operations, Strategy, and Budgets

Your highly complex clinical laboratory serves a pediatric specialty practice and inpatient pediatric hospital which receives patients from a large radius. There is tremendous pressure to provide rapid turn-around on even the most mundane tests, since so many patients come from a distance for care. The institution has invested heavily in point-of-care testing capabilities deployed in the clinics and on the floors, but even with these, and their associated higher operational costs, there are some times when certain testing must be sent elsewhere, lengthening turnaround time. The institution has developed a strategic plan to capture the allergy treatment market for children and adolescents and advised you as lab director of this. You have accordingly evaluated means to bring the associated testing into your lab, rather than sending it to a reference lab. After your investment of resources to bring this capability in-house, which involved adding FTE, investing considerable time in test validation, and some capital equipment purchases, things are working fairly well. Unbeknownst to you, a large pharma company has developed a targeted treatment and is touting their superior results to your clinicians, who drop their natural skepticism and embrace the new treatment whole-heartedly. Your clinicians now ask you to send the patient serum for allergen-antibody high sensitivity profiling and targeted treatment development instead of doing the conventional testing you have been doing, thus allowing them to employ the new more effective treatment. Aside from development costs and capital equipment, your operational budget for the old method was US$25,000 per year. The new testing costs US$12,000 per patient, and you have been seeing ten new patients a week.

Questions for discussion:

What is the impact of such a disruption on your budgets?
Which kind of budget bears the hit?
How do you adjust?
What other options do you have?

Case 7: Succession Planning and Group Decision-Making

Bob Founder, President of Founder's Pathology Associates, Inc. (FPA), died unexpectedly last weekend while mountain climbing. He was 59 years old. FPA is the premier provider in the region and now serves 14 hospitals, numerous outpatient clinics and a surgery center. The group has grown to 11 pathologists, two PhDs, two medical technologists, and a practice manager. In addition to servicing the many hospitals, the group provides services to a joint venture laboratory with the largest of its client hospitals, and collaborates in a similar fashion with another hospital where its AP laboratory is located. Total revenues for the operation last year were US$12.5 million in the practice, and an additional US$12.4 million in the joint ventures. Almost all of Bob's time had been spent shepherding the various relationships and business interests of the practice.

The ownership of the practice is equally shared among eight of the other pathologists; the other two pathologists are on partnership tracks, at years one and three of what is usually a 4 year process. Steve, the practice manager, is pretty familiar with the business interests in the practice, but has only been with the organization for 18 months. There are two other senior pathologists, Reuben Jones and Follet McKenzie, who have been with Bob for most of the group's history. Reuben is 62 years old and has recently purchased a farm in Missouri where he likes to spend the weekends. Reub is technically the vice president, primarily for signatory functions—that is, he has signed checks when Bob was away in the past. "FM" as he is called, is the diagnostic whiz in the group, his office piled high with articles, slide folders, and files, the "go to" guy when a hard case comes along. He is 63, healthy and active, with three young grandchildren in another state on the west coast. His wife retired recently from an HR position to spend more time grandmothering.

The rest of the group looks like this:

Missy Marks, 42, surgical path and cyto, with some micro duties, medical director at one small lab; two teenagers and one preschooler at home. Husband does cabinetry in his own business.

Bin Ding Tseitze, 45, clinical chemistry and some surgical path, directs the joint venture lab. Divorced, with kids living with his ex-wife in another state. Bin grew up in Thailand, the son of an American soldier father who died in Vietnam, and a Thai-Chinese mother. His accent is unique.

Rowena ("Row") Gamm, 39, blood banker, but also does heme, directs three small hospital labs and does some surgical path. Married just 3 years ago, has a 2-year old at home and has been sick a bit lately, perhaps due to pregnancy.

Jim Otis, 48, just joined the group about 2 years ago, does general surgical path, clinical path, and anything else he is asked to do. He works slowly on cases and problems when they come to him, though he really prefers to stay in his office. Directs one small hospital lab. Married to a banker; no kids.

Emily Welch, 36, came on board just out of a hemepath fellowship 4 years ago and is now a partner. She directs the immunohematology lab in the joint venture, and visits two small hospitals. Single, she has family on the west coast.

Yung Man Buc, 37, came out of a top AP program in Oklahoma, and did a molecular fellowship there. He is now in his sixth year with the practice, doing almost exclusively AP. He and one of the new hires are working on developing more in-house molecular testing. He has two young sons, ages five and eight. His grandmother from China recently came to live with them.

The political landscape externally is fairly quiet right now for the practice. All the hospital contracts are up to date. The group works with several competing hospitals, but they have been in conversations about collaboration on a few issues. The academic medical center 2 h from FPA's AP lab has recently become more interested in capturing outside referral business, and an adjacent smaller practice was acquired by Ameripath/Quest about 5 years ago and may have been visiting some of your clients with marketing materials.

Internally, things are less calm. Ownership in the group is time-of-service based (one share per year as a partner); ownership in the joint ventures is investment based. Not all have opted into the joint ventures, so although salaries are technically equal, income on the whole is not. There was some dissention about both of the new hires, and allegiances to the practice versus the joint venture versus the "mother ship" largest hospital among the pathologists are occasionally suspected. Working in several different locations, the impression that "no one else is working as hard as I am" is fairly common. The group meets quarterly to go over various reports and vote on a bonus, but a lot of the details of things have not been covered by Bob very thoroughly. Aside from the dissention about the new hires, which centered around whether they were needed or not, as well as which candidate to select, other disagreements have been few, and generally Bob's recommendations have been stamped with approval by the partners.

It is now near the end of the quarter, with the regular group meeting scheduled for 2 weeks hence. Reub and Steve agreed to call a special gathering, even though two partners were out of town, to cover a couple of questions:

Who will be on call for Bob starting on Wednesday?

Who will take over making the schedule (and get the next one out in a week)?

What will be the plan for leadership succession?

Should they immediately place an ad, talk to a locum tenens agency, or hold off?

Oh, and as the group had no corporate life insurance on Bob's life, the buy-out stipulations dictate that you will have to make a payment to his widow for his share of the accounts receivable as of his date of death within 60 days, which will impact whether or not you can declare a bonus this quarter.

Discussion questions:

What aspects of contingency planning did this group miss?
What components of a disaster plan need to be in place to cover unexpected loss of
    key employees or financial duress?
What recruitment practices could have led the group to be facing this crisis better
    equipped to cope?
What resources should be sought or considered outside of the group itself to navi-
    gate through the shift in leadership and governance?

Case 8: The Research Mission (for Academic Practices)

At the request of the College of Medicine Dean, the Vice President of Research
and basic science Chairs were planning a strategic retreat to address the on-campus
research enterprise. Specific questions to be addressed were:
    How large should the research enterprise be?
    How should we focus the research?
    How many graduate students should we have?
    What resources exist?
    What can be eliminated over the next 24 months?
    Over time, the research enterprise does not completely cover its costs and must
be subsidized. While a very successful researcher, with the appropriate amount and
type of grants, may cover much of her salary, the indirects, or grant money for the
research infrastructure, ultimately cannot pay both capital and operational costs for
a university. And, in this progressively more difficult funding environment, no allowance is made to support faculty who either cannot get sufficiently funded or who
are unsuccessful at renewing existing grants. Compounding this is the tendency for
certain non-federal granting bodies such as non-profits to disallow either indirect
costs or even salary dollars. A further challenge faces the growing research programs or if a departing faculty needs replacing; Where would new startup funds
come from when a startup package of seven figures is not unheard of? While some
of the dollars can be assigned through teaching commitments by researchers, this is
generally of limited impact and these dollars as well are under downward pressure
from a funding standpoint. Potentially, money can be transferred from clinical income, philanthropic dollars or endowment dollars can be used to support research,
or contract research can cover some expenses.
    In the case at hand, an organization is taking a step back to ask some funda-
mental questions. Most universities pursue research because it is expected, to build
prestige, to support a graduate program and other teaching programs, to develop
intellectual property and to help create the environment of inquiry that truly defines
a university. Beyond total funding, funding per square foot, and publications, good,
broadly applicable and benchmarkable research metrics are difficult to identify.
Given the realities of today, bigger is not always better (although national rankings

based on total federal funding seem important), but perhaps thought should be given to optimizing outcomes vis à vis the missions as listed above. Questions such as the following could then be asked:

Are we comfortable with the visibility/impact of our research and the resultant prestige?
Is research supporting, complementing or even synergizing with the educational mission?
Are invested research dollars producing a reasonable outcome/return?
How successful are research resources at developing intellectual property? Are we meeting our goals?
Does research support the overall spirit of inquiry at the university?

Appendix B

You and Your Environment: Cases for Group Discussion

Michael L. Talbert, M.D.

You and Your Environment 1—The Value Proposition

Ponder the following and then discuss with members of your practice:

What is your practice's value proposition?
If you are hospital based, why is it your group that is providing the services?

Who might provide the services better?

If you serve the outpatient market, what is your value proposition to that setting?

How would that setting say the value proposition could be improved?

How has your practice's value proposition improved (or eroded) over the past year?
What is the value proposition of the nearest potential competing pathology practice?
What are the value propositions of the regional and national labs that serve your area?
How does your practice's value proposition stack up against your potential competitors' value propositions?
How can you improve your practice's value proposition?

You and Your Environment 2A—Challenges and Opportunities—The Small Private Practice

You are a four person independent pathology practice serving a 200 bed community hospital, Free-standing Community Hospital (FCH), in a metro area of 1.5 million that is otherwise dominated by three healthcare systems that extend across your state. Your practice serves some of the doctors' offices of the physicians who admit to FCH while their clinical laboratory work is performed in the hospital's clinical laboratory and reported using remote printers in the physician offices.

What challenges/risks can you identify?

Some of the largest challenges/risks would include:

- Will FCH remain independent?
- Will FCH remain viable without a combination with one or more systems?
- Would the hospital/medical staff/patients be better served by a larger, more specialized pathology practice?
- Will the physician offices continue to send specimens to you and the lab with the relatively simple reporting system in place; That is, can you hang on to your outside business?
- *What opportunities or potential opportunities can you identify?*
- Can you take an active leadership role in FCH as it evaluates future opportunities?
- As more physicians are employed by hospitals, will the outpatient volume grow and be more tightly attached to you and FCH?
- If FCH joins one of the systems, how might that be advantageous to your practice?

For further discussion:

What would you do if the CEO of FCH told you they were striving to employ as many of the providers serving FCH patients as feasible and launch an accountable care organization (ACO)?

What would you do if you were asked to merge with one of the other pathology groups in the metro area?

How would you respond to the FCH CEO if she told you a national reference lab had pitched a scheme to take over and operate the hospital's clinical laboratory?

What if the CEO also told you that the FCH Board of Directors felt FCH needed to do this for financial reasons in order to continue providing laboratory services?

How would you respond to FCH administration if you were asked to prove the value of your Part A services as part of "a review of all our medical director contracts?"

You and Your Environment 2B—Challenges and Opportunities—The Academic Practice

You are chairman of a mid-sized academic pathology department that is based in a mid-sized tertiary care academic medical center but that also serves two 150-bed community hospitals, each of which is staffed by a single full-time pathologist and a second pathologist who rotates on a weekly basis from the tertiary care hospital. The two smaller hospitals are on separate "old and klutzy" computer systems, while the academic medical center recently installed the "Super Duper" computer system. Your faculty practice plan migrated to a different outpatient system 3 years ago for their outpatient clinics which has been partially interfaced to the "Super Duper" system. Of the community physicians in your system, only the largest practices have an electronic health record but these are not interfaced to either hospital computer system. Your department has an active research program with a moderate level of federal funding but recently, three of your investigators have failed to replace grants that were ending. Educational demands on your faculty are relatively high: you have a well-regarded residency program and three fellowships; your faculty teaches pathology in the medical, nursing, and allied health schools, as well as running a graduate program. State provided educational funding covers less than one third of the required effort while hospital graduate medical education (GME) money just barely reflects the effort involved.

Although your university practice seems to be fairly static, your environment has been changing and the faculty practice plan leaders have been nervous. The multihospital Big Hospital System has been purchasing many of the independent primary care practices and investing heavily in an integrated inpatient and outpatient IT solution that has received national attention. A different not-for-profit regional healthcare system has developed a state-wide network of hospitals, surgery centers, and primary care while advertising incessantly on TV and in print.

What challenges/risks can you identify?

> Information systems
> You are not the largest in your market
> No clear competitive advantage (at least not provided in this scenario)

How do you continue and balance the three missions, education, research, and clinical care?
What potential opportunities can you identify?

> Need to identify competitive advantages
> *What opportunities are there for growth?*
> *What efficiencies can be gained?*
>> Consider upgrading pathology specific IT
>> Can we reconfigure personnel and maintain more at the central location through digital pathology?

For further discussion:
What might you do proactively?

> *At the practice plan level?*
> *For your department?*
> *For your hospitals?*

How would you respond to your practice plan's CEO if he said the system was in talks with a non-aligned 200 bed hospital in the community? What if that hospital was 100 miles away?

Your hospital has informed the practice plan that it is developing bundled pricing, that is, a set price for a particular episode of care, for hip and knee replacements, reduction mammoplasties, and screening colonoscopies. The hospital has asked physicians to standardize their practices around these procedures and develop a single set price for all physician services involved in each procedure. *What would you do for pathology?*

Budgeting for the coming academic year reveals an expected budget shortfall (loss) of 4% of budget for your department. Given the challenging economic times across your college of medicine, the dean will not approve any budget that does not show at least a 3% positive margin. *How might you approach this problem?*

You and Your Environment 2C—Challenges and Opportunities—The Large Private Practice

You are the president of a 15 pathologist regional pathology practice serving two 300–400 bed hospitals, each of which is the major hospital for its respective hospital system (Systems A and B) as well as providing services to the two smaller hospitals in each system which can generally be covered from their central hospitals with scheduled visits for meetings and frozen sections. You and your partner pathologists own a histology and cytology lab with couriers and billing as a separate entity to provide technical component services for anatomic pathology. The lab is located near one of the larger hospitals and all cytology is signed out at the central AP lab. Surgicals are grossed, cut and stained at the central AP lab but slides are "read" and reports generated at each of the two largest hospitals with cases for each system being read at the respective large hospital. The AP lab owns its own reporting system which remote site prints reports as needed at each hospital, surgery center or doctor's office serviced by the group.

There is a third system (System C) in the metro area and region that is about 30% larger than either of the two systems served by your practice which are of similar size to each other.

What challenges/risks can you identify?

> Recent cut in technical component (TC)
> Serving two systems

Challenge of multiple sites
Non-interfaced reporting

What potential opportunities can you identify?

May be dominant player—can continue to develop competitive advantage and grow at the expense of the third system.
Control of means of production, that is, technical component including courier and billing
Size and independence provide some capability to raise capital

For further discussion:

The CEO of System A tells you that "due to competitive pressures, we will only deal with a pathology group that is totally committed to our system and does not provide services to System B." What possible responses would you have?
You are called to a secret meeting by the CEO of System A. After signing a nondisclosure agreement, you are informed that System A and System C are contemplating a merger. What possible scenarios can you envision?
The gastroenterologists of Systems A and B combined to form a large group. With the help of a national consultant, they are contemplating starting a histology lab to handle the outpatient biopsies and hiring their own specialty trained pathologist. They give you 7 days to submit a proposal to provide the histology and/or professional diagnostic services in a manner advantageous to their new megagroup. How would you respond? What range of possibilities can you envision?
System A and System B use a respected national laboratory as the reference laboratory for most testing not done in their laboratories. Over lunch, the regional vice president for business development of a competing national lab approaches you about helping to switch reference laboratories with the promise that it will partner with you and allow you to provide anatomic pathology technical and professional services for the AP specimens it collects in the region. This would represent about 20% additional growth for your practice. What questions would you have? How might you structure a win-win?

References

1. Koss W, Sodeman T. The workload recording method. A laboratory management tool. Clin Lab Med 1992 Jun;12(2):337–50.
2. Martin SA, Styer PE, Assessing performance, productivity, and staffing needs in pathology groups: Observations from the College of American Pathologists Path*Focus* practice activity and staffing program. *Arch Pathol Lab Med* 2006 Sep; 130(9):1263–1268.
3. Suvarna SK and Kay MS. KU activity: a method for calculating histopathologists' workloads. *J Clin Pathol* 1998; 51:530–534.
4. Carr RA, Sanders DSA, Stores OP, Smew FA, Parkes ME, Ross-Gilbertson V, Chachlani N, Simon J. *J Clin Pathol* 2006; 59:835–839.

5. Maung Raymond T, What is the best indicator to determine anatomic pathology workload? Canadian experience. *Am J Clin Pathol* 2005 Jan; 123(1):45–55.
6. Haber, SL Kaiser Permanente: an insider's view of the practice of pathology in an HMO hospital-based multispecialty group. *Arch Pathol Lab Med* 1995, 191:646–9
7. Haber SL, When do you need to hire another pathologist? *CAP Today.* October 1987:40.
8. Cheung CC, Torlakovic EE, Chow H, et al. Modeling complexity in pathologist workload measurement: the Automatable Activity-Based Approach to Complexity Unit Scoring (AA-BACUS). *Mod Pathol* 2015 Mar; 28(3):324–339.
9. Hsiao, W. C., et al. Results and policy implications of the resource-based relative-value study. *New England Journal of Medicine* 1988; 319 (13): 881–888.
10. DHSS. WELCAN Workload measurement for pathology: manual with schedule of unit values. 1988–89 edn. Cardiff: DHSS, Welsh Office
11. Hye Kyoung Yoon, Michele H Diwa, Youn Soo Lee, Gwangil Kim, Sang Yong Song, Kyoung Bun Lee, Han Kyeom Kim, Woon Sup Han and Jeong-Wook Seo. How overworked are pathologists? An assessment of cases for histopathology and cytopathology service. *Basic and Applied Pathology 2009; 2: 111–117*
12. Brimhall B, et al. Critical leadership and management skills for pathology practice. *Arch Pathol Lab Med* 2007;131:1547–1554.

Index

© Springer International Publishing Switzerland 2016
L. A. Hassell et al. (eds.), *Pathology Practice Management*,
DOI 10.1007/978-3-319-22954-6

Printed in the United States
By Bookmasters